A Multimodality Approach to Breast Imaging

A Multimodality Approach to Breast Imaging

Saar Porrath, M.D.
Director
Woman's Breast Center
Santa Monica, California

AN ASPEN PUBLICATION
Aspen Publishers, Inc.
Rockville, Maryland
Royal Tunbridge Wells
1986

Aspen Publishers, Inc.
1600 Research Boulevard
Rockville, Maryland 20850

Library of Congress Cataloging in Publication Data

Porrath, Saar.
A multimodality approach to breast imaging.

"An Aspen publication."
Includes index.
1. Breast—Diseases—Diagnosis. 2. Diagnostic imaging. 3. Breast—Diseases—Treatment. I. Title.
[DNLM: 1. Breast Diseases—diagnosis. WP 815 P838m]
RG493.5.D52P67 1986 618.1'9'0757 86-17465
ISBN 0-87189-356-8

The authors and publisher have made every effort to ensure the accuracy of the information herein, particularly with regard to drug selection and dose. However, appropriate information sources should be consulted, especially for new or unfamiliar drugs or procedures. It is the responsibility of every practitioner to evaluate the appropriateness of a particular opinion in the context of actual clinical situations and with due consideration to new developments. Authors, editors, and the publisher cannot be held responsible for any typographical or other errors found in this book.

Printed in the United States of America
1 2 3 4 5

To the many women that we have saved, and to the many women that we could have saved had their fears not immobilized them

Contents

Introduction

As our knowledge of breast diseases increases, so does our need to be able to differentiate these diseases diagnostically. There is an increasing variety of available tests, bringing with them the increased necessity to integrate our knowledge to aid the referring physician, ourselves, and most importantly the patient.

Our understanding of the influence of hormones on the breast and the way in which they act has been changed during the last few decades. There are now drugs available which influence these hormonal reactions and interactions. Moreover, we have an increased ability to measure their effects on the breast.

The surgical approach to the breast has also undergone remarkable changes. Most breast biopsies are now being done as outpatient procedures. There has been a decrease in the use of the modified radical mastectomy and increased use of lumpectomy and radiation therapy in the treatment of breast cancer. Surgeons are using the more cosmetic periareolar approach to breast biopsies whenever possible. There have been great advances in plastic surgery and its use in breast augmentation, reduction, and reconstruction.

Our understanding of the pathology of breast disease has been aided greatly over the past few decades. Haagensen and others have redefined and regrouped categories, both benign and malignant. The description of the entity "minimal breast cancer" is changing our concept of breast therapy and diagnosis.

Improvements in mammography, in both decreased radiation dosage and improved image, have led to an increased ability to detect smaller legions. New techniques in ultrasound allow us to detect abnormalities we have not previously seen. Diaphanography is undergoing clinical testing to evaluate its usefulness, and thermography is being reevaluated to see what place it might have in the detection and recognition of breast disease. Computed tomography scanning has been tried, found successful, and discarded because of inherent problems. Magnetic resonance imaging is on the horizon, its role undetermined.

With all the new tests and "toys" available to us as imagers, we sometimes ignore the foundation of breast diagnosis: the clinical history and physical examination. It is part of the purpose of this book to integrate the available testing modalities with the history, physical findings, and treatment of breast disease. It is hoped that this unique synthesis of material will aid the physician and nurse practitioner so that he or she can better understand and use these available resources.

Although the detection of breast cancer remains our foremost objective, there are a multitude of benign conditions that must also be recognized and attended to. Patient concerns and complaints must be addressed. With the emergence of the breast specialist there is an increased demand to know more and to use this knowledge. It is no longer sufficient to tell a patient and her doctor that her signs and symptoms are not cancer. Further explanation and perhaps a therapeutic suggestion may be indicated.

It is helpful if the breast imager can understand the problems of the surgeon, and the surgeon should understand both the advantages and shortcomings of the diagnostician. Both must relate to the pathologist to achieve a holistic synthesis of each specific case. The imager must understand what has been done to the breast by the plastic surgeon so that he or she can be of greater assistance in the problem cases. It is this integrated approach that is the base of this book.

The approach here is unlike that in most other books on diagnostic modalities. There is an orientation toward breast disease, not just the identification of cancer.

The diagnostic modalities are discussed in the initial section. In the clinical portion the approach is by pathologic entity, with a discussion of the disease followed by case histories which highlight the diagnostic problems. It is hoped that in this way the reader will obtain a better understanding of the methods that are used by the author at the Woman's Breast Center.

A section on the psychological aspects of breast screening and the role of the breast in feminine identity has been included so that we can better understand and deal with the patients' concerns and fears. We must understand why patient compliance is sometimes poor, and why a referral for a breast examination is just a test to the doctor but a "psychological mastectomy" to the patient.

It is the hope of the author that this integrated approach to breast disease will be useful to all who do "breast work": nurses, nurse practitioners, primary care physicians, radiologists, pathologists, surgeons, and oncologists. It is only by better understanding the diseases that affect the breast and our ability and at times inability to detect and treat these conditions that we can best serve our patients.

Saar Porrath

Acknowledgments

I want to thank the contributing authors for their work and assistance. I wish to thank my office staff for their time and patience. In particular, I want to thank Raj Sandhu, R.T. for excellence of radiographic work and Jean McNeil for assistance in typing and some editing. I thank the invention of the word processor without which this book would not have been possible.

I thank Roman Selicki for his untiring effort to provide perfection in photography for this book.

A special graditude of thanks is given to Flexitherm, Inc. Howard Stern and Phillip Meyers, who graciously underwrote the cost of the color photography so that thermography could be presented in its real form rather than on black and white photos. Their assistance is greatly appreciated.

Most of all, I want to thank my wife, Dr. Toni Bernay, for her assistance, support, and encouragement.

Contributors

Toni Bernay, Ph.D.
Private Practice
Beverly Hills, California;
Assistant Clinical Professor of Psychiatry (Psychology)
Neuropsychiatric Institute
University of California at Los Angeles
Los Angeles, California;
Co-Editor, The Psychology of Today's Woman:
New Psychoanalytic Visions

Ernest Carlson, M.D., Ph.D.
Private Practice
155 W. Hospitality Lane, Suite 100
San Bernardino, California

A. Richard Grossman, M.D., F.A.C.S.
Chief of Staff
Plastic Surgery Division
Southern California Burn Center
Sherman Oaks, California

John R. Milbrath, M.D.
Director, Breast Cancer Detection Center
Associate Clinical Professor of Radiology
The Medical College of Wisconsin
Milwaukee, Wisconsin

Saar Porrath, M.D.
Director
Woman's Breast Center
Santa Monica, California

Otto W. Sartorius, M.D.
Director
Santa Barbara Breast Cancer Institute
Santa Barbara, California

Kathryn White, Ph.D.
Private Practice
Los Angeles, California

Section I

Imaging Modalities, Plastic Surgery, and Psychology

1

Physical Examination

Otto W. Sartorius

Because the breasts are accessible, superficially positioned organs, they should lend themselves to the ready clinical detection of benign and malignant lesions. However, it is just this conclusion that has fostered both high quality clinical examinations on the one hand, and frequent performance of totally inadequate physical examinations on the other. It is the latter that has resulted in low detection rates and abnormally high occult carcinoma detection rates by mammography.

Detection rate disparities are strongly suggested by comparing the Health Insurance Plan (HIP) study with the Breast Cancer Detection Demonstration Project (BCDDP). In the HIP study 45 percent of the breast cancers were found by physical examination alone[1,2] compared with the BCDDP report, which stated that only 7 to 8 percent of the cases were found by physical examination alone. Mammography alone detected 33 percent of the carcinomas in the HIP study in contrast to 43 percent found in the BCDDP.[3,4] Additionally, Mahoney and Csima have reported that of 302 breast cancer patients 29 percent were detected by clinical examination and only 5 percent by mammography.[5]

It is not surprising that these statistical differences should occur. Over the past 10 years significant improvements have been achieved in mammography; yet little has been done to improve the state of the art in clinical examination of the breast. One diagnostic modality has standardized techniques, with interpretation by trained mammographers. On the other hand, diagnosis by palpation is not standardized and is frequently performed by the inexperienced examiner who is often deluded by the breasts' accessibility.

The Examiner in Breast Cancer Detection

Major factors in the success of the clinical examination as a diagnostic modality are the experience, skill, and thoroughness of the examination, and to a lesser extent, the technique employed by the examiner.[6] Experience is acquired through the repetitive palpation of many breasts—those of the young and old, the fat and thin, the firm and soft, those containing lesions and those without. The examiner's experience (thus acquired) matures only through correlation with the underlying pathology. Such correlation enables the examiner to recognize physiologic from pathologic change. It aids in differentiating the fine modularity associated with lobular hyperplasia from multiple small cysts and in noting the difference in the feel of lipomas from that of cysts both hard and soft. It takes experience and pathologic correlation to recognize the differences in palpation between the hard infiltrating scirrhous carcinoma and the circumscribed softer medullary carcinoma. Lastly, experience counts in the ability to appreciate the difficulty of recognizing infiltrating lobular carcinoma in the firm, fibrous breast.

This experiential knowledge of examination, when coupled with the tactile sensitivity developed through repetitive palpations, soon results in the acquisition of a valuable skill. Ironically, the surgical resident put in charge of examinations in breast detection units often lacks the crucial skill. The general surgeon, whose experience also is generally limited to the readily palpable lesion, does not possess the same skill as the internist who examines all types of breasts in his search for abnormalities. If thoroughness is neglected, the examiner's experience and skill are useless.

Every woman coming for a breast examination should be considered to have a minimal, possibly occult, carcinoma. It is the responsibility of the examiner to find that lesion by conducting the most diligent and thorough possible search. Only then can a negative physical examination be considered adequate or, if questionable, the search continued by use of additionally indicated diagnostic modalities such as mammography, fine needle aspiration, ultrasound, and multispectral infrared transillumination. Marchant believed that a good breast examination requires at least 5 minutes, including instruction in breast self-examination.[7,8] However, it has been observed that a house officer never devotes more than 1.5 minutes to inpatient breast examination and not more than 2.0 minutes to the breast clinic examination.

It is the author's opinion that it takes 15 to 25 minutes to perform an adequate examination, depending on the size and consistency of the breasts. Through such diligent search, many minimal carcinomas and the majority of carcinomas between 0.5 and 1.0 cm in size can be detected by palpation.

Technique of Breast Examination

The actual technique of breast examination may differ according to the preferences of the examiner, but it should always be conducted in a methodical, orderly, meticulous manner. Some examiners prefer to inspect the breast initially, followed by palpation with the patient sitting and then supine. The order of this procedure is probably unimportant so long as consistency is maintained. Furthermore, the examiner's demeanor should be calming and reassuring, with alertness to the discomfort and apprehension of the patient. Gentleness in palpating and handling the breast is a necessity.

Most physicians teach that when palpating the breast the examiner should utilize the volar aspect of three or more fingers of one hand in a rotary motion at constant pressure.[9–12] The author employed this technique for many years but found that small lesions, particularly those that were soft or semisoft and deeply placed, escaped detection. Accordingly, this technique is now used only to determine the general texture of the breast tissue and to teach breast self-examination.

It is preferable that the patient first be placed in the supine position with the appropriate arm extended and the breast palpated with the fore and middle fingertips of each hand (Fig. 1-1). A space of approximately 1 cm is encompassed by the fingertips as gentle, varying pressures are applied so as to detect the movement or presence of any underlying lesion. The exploring, slowly "walking" fingers progress systematically back and forth across the breast until the entire organ has been

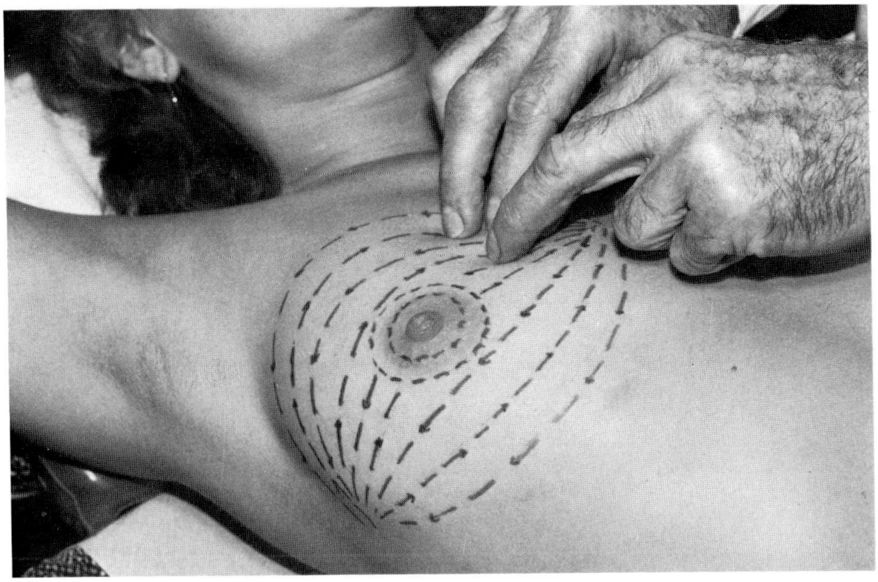

Fig. 1-1 Palpation using four fingertips with the patient in the supine position.

palpated. When palpation detects a discrete lesion, however small, or abnormal tissue thickening, the overlying skin is marked with a felt pen so that this finding can be reevaluated when the patient is in other positions. When the patient has large breasts, the lateral portions of each breast are reexamined with her lying, first on the left side and then on the right side, with the upper arm fully extended. Deep-seated lesions are more easily felt in these positions. Careful attention must be given to the tail of Spence and the subareolar and nipple areas. This author has not found that simultaneous palpation or examination with the examiner at the head of the table as reported by Griboff[13] provides additional information to the methods described.

With the patient in the sitting position, each breast is reexamined. The fingers of one hand extending upward displace the breast forward away from the chest wall, and the fingers of the other hand compress the intervening tissue (Fig. 1-2). Thus the breast is gently compressed between the fingers of both hands and systematically palpated in the manner described above. It often helps to have the patient bend slightly forward while being examined in this position. Attention is also paid to any marked areas noted in the supine position. For more accurate identification or for easier and safer penetration when employing fine needle aspiration, deep lesions occasionally are displaced more superficially by the lower hand.

The patient is then asked to extend her arm over her head, thus tending to compress the breast against the chest wall in a manner similar to that for the supine examination. The examiner now applies gentle traction to one segment of the breast with one hand at the 6 o'clock segment, flatting out to an even greater extent the 12 o'clock segment. The entire examining finger, usually the forefinger or thumb, now irons out the breast tissue. This technique utilizes the chest wall as an ironing board, from the periphery of the breast tissue at the 12 o'clock segment toward and to the nipple (Fig. 1-3). This process is rapidly repeated, segmentally, until the entire breast has been examined. Again, attention is paid to areas that have been previously marked, and new marks are made for areas or lesions requiring further investigation. Small lesions are frequently detected by this maneuver.

The nipples are carefully inspected for asymmetry, retraction, deviation, superficial ulceration, or discharge. The discharge may become apparent through

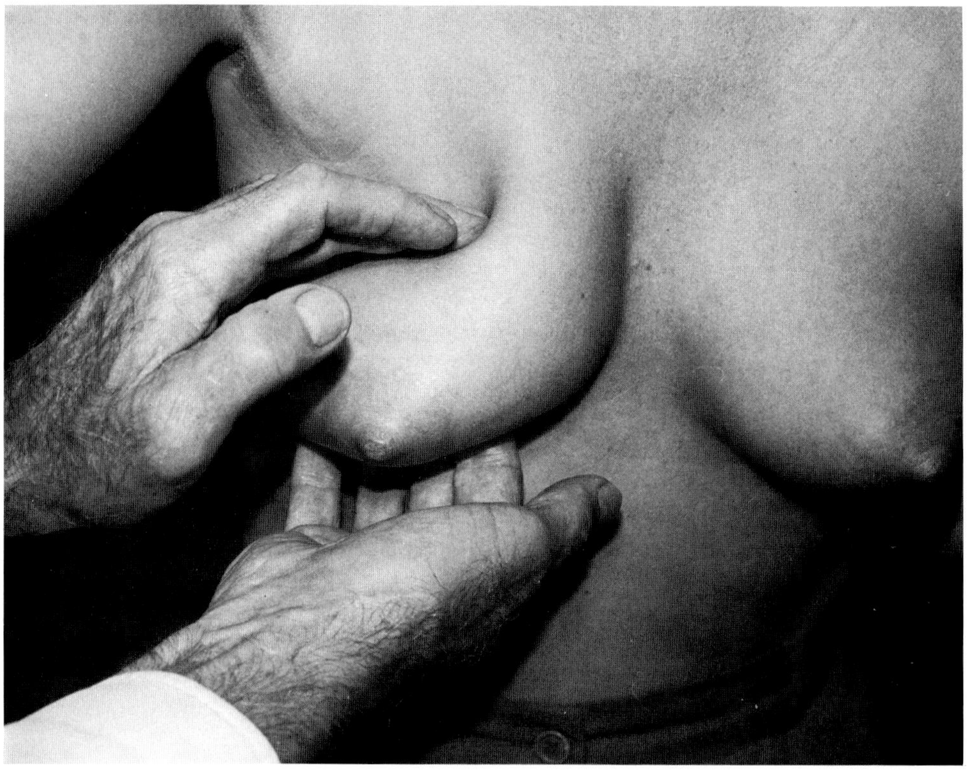

Fig. 1-2 Palpation with two hands using the fingertips. The patient is in the sitting position.

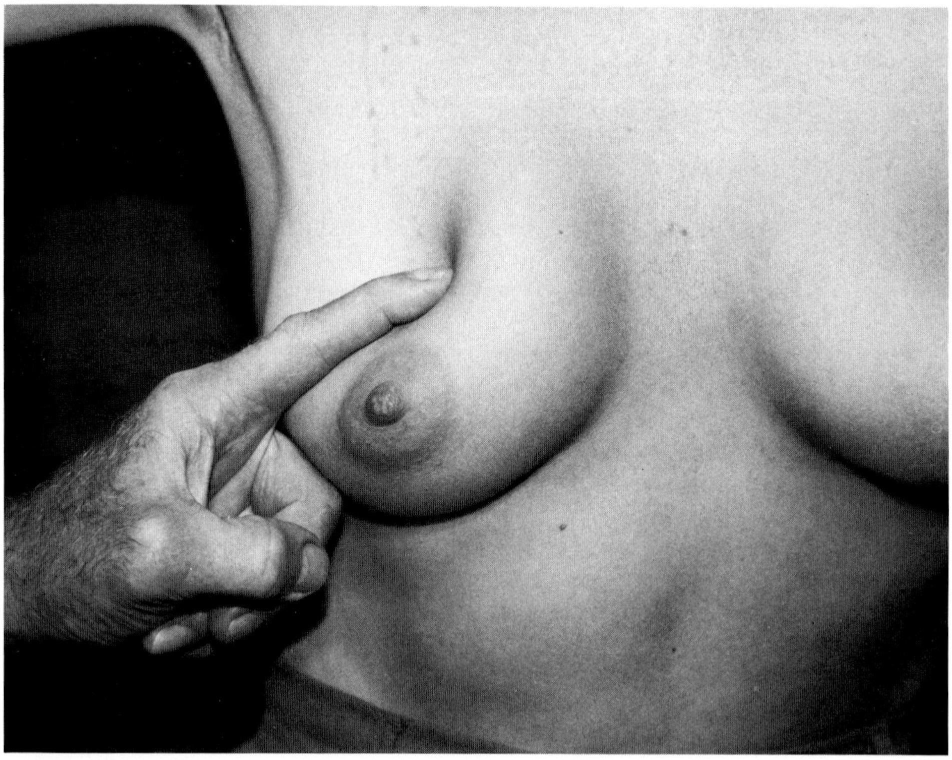

Fig. 1-3 Ironing the breast with the patient's arm extended. Tension with the opposite hand is not shown.

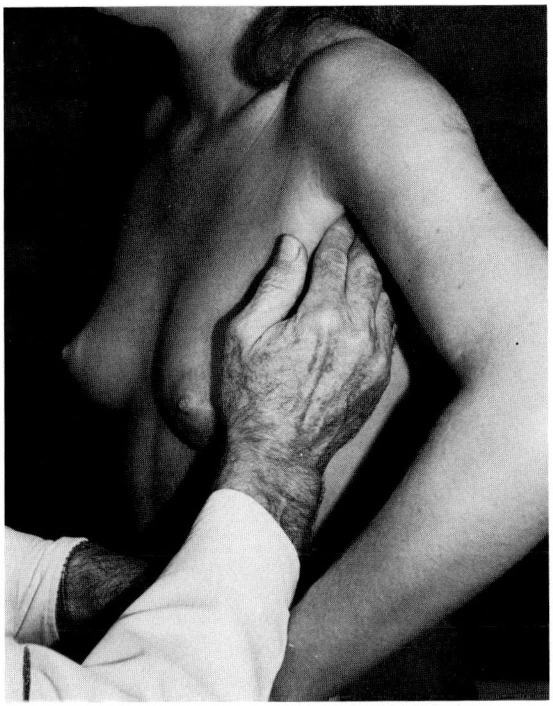

Fig. 1-4 Palpation of the axilla. The arm is supported by the other hand.

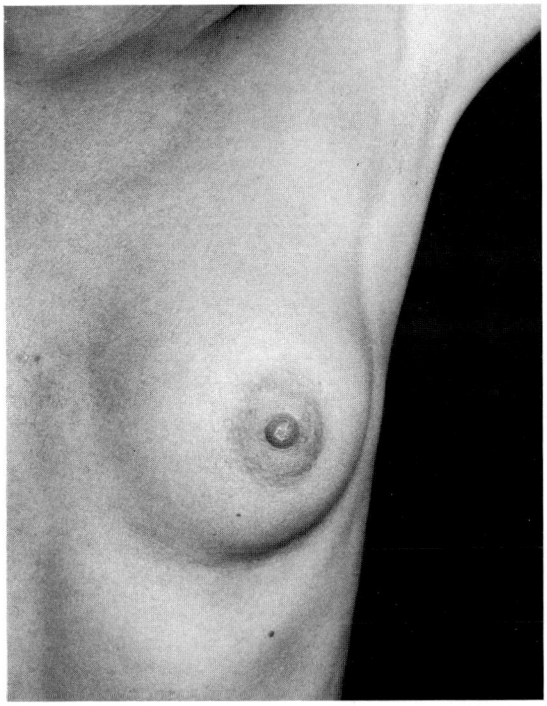

Fig. 1-5 Inspection with the arm fully extended.

these methods: palpation of the areola, expressed by stripping the nipple or using a nipple aspirator. If only a few drops of fluid are obtained, a Hemostix can be used to test for the presence of blood. If more than two large drops of serous or serosanguineous/thin fluid is obtained, further cytologic investigation is indicated.[14]

With the patient in the sitting position, the axillae are carefully palpated, with the patient's arm and forearm being supported and adjusted to the proper height by the examiner's opposite hand (Fig. 1-4). Usually the supra- and infraclavicular areas are not examined except in postmastectomy patients or in those with clinical suspicion of malignancy.

Finally, visual inspection is conducted under good light and with the sitting patient in different positions (Fig. 1-5). The patient's arms are pressed together to contract the pectoral major muscles (Fig. 1-6), and in another position the arms are supported on the examiner's shoulders so the patient may lean forward comfortably (Fig. 1-7). In order to detect slight dimpling or alteration in symmetry, the skin is gently moved over the underlying parenchyma while the breast itselt is slightly elevated. This maneuver allows visualization of even slight contraction of Cooper's ligaments or alteration of Langer's lines. This inspection is carried out in each of the aforementioned positions, again paying special attention to any previously marked areas.

It is essential that the examiner employ an orderly and meticulous technique in the conduct of the physical examination of the breast and graphically document the findings. A sample physical examination check sheet suffices for general observations about breast size, consistency of tissue, and symmetry, and it provides space for detailing multiple lesions according to the nine breast segments (Fig. 1-8). Important details on each detected lesion can be rapidly recorded as to location (on the clock), distance from the nipple, size, shape, consistency, tenderness, and

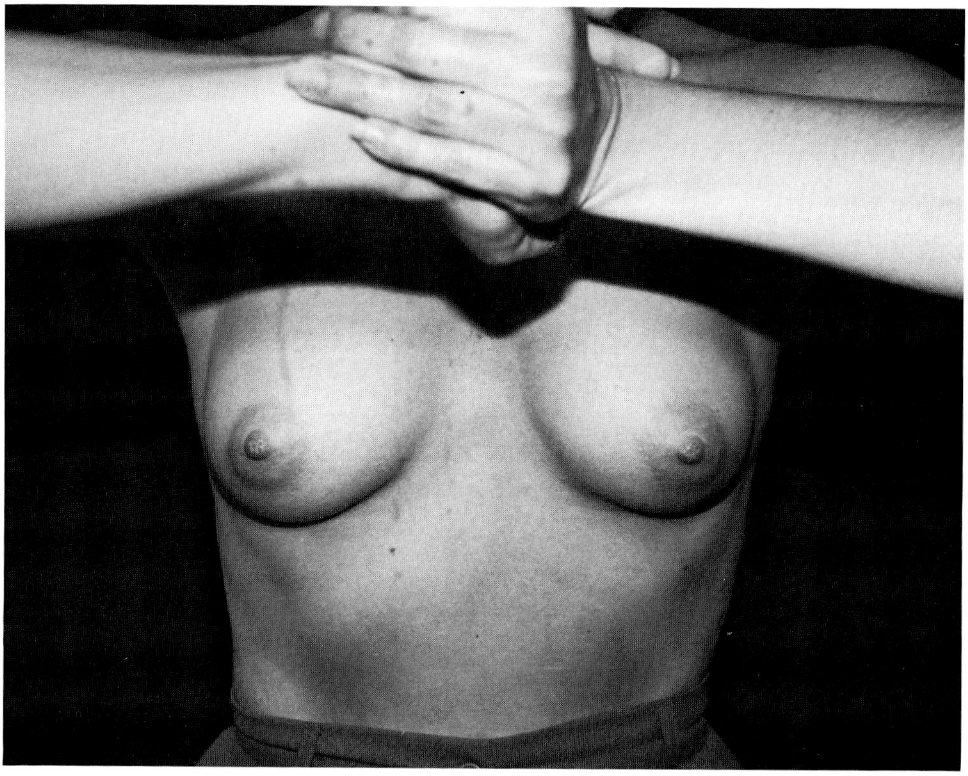

Fig. 1-6 Inspection with the pectoral muscles contracted.

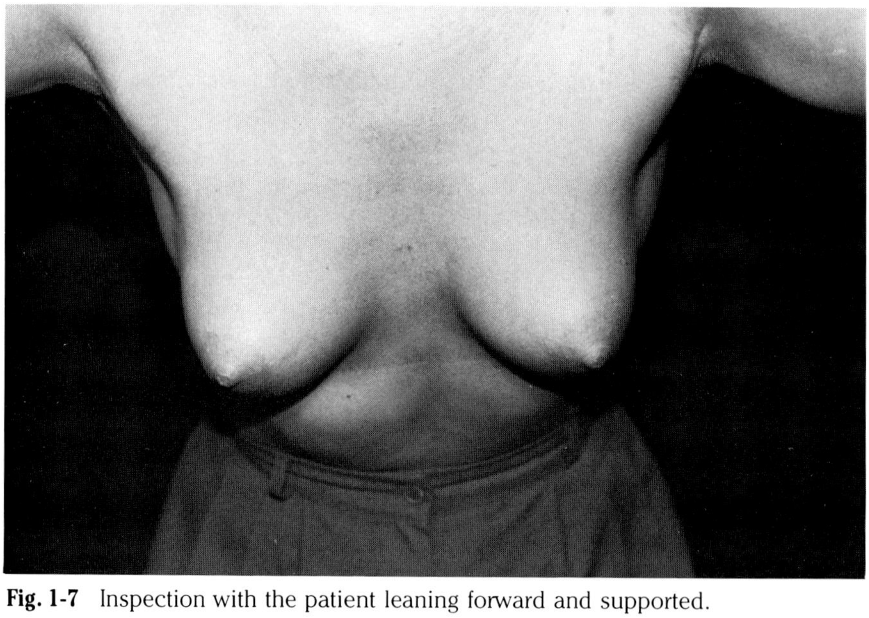

Fig. 1-7 Inspection with the patient leaning forward and supported.

Name ______________________

Exam. No. ______________________

PHYSICAL EXAMINATION: BREASTS

DATE ______________________

Size — Small ☐ Med. ☐ Large ☐ Pendulous ☐ — Consistency — Soft ☐ Nodular ☐ Rt. ☐ Lt. ☐

Symmetrical — Yes ☐ No ☐ — Comment ______________________

Tenderness — Yes ☐ No ☐ — Comment ______________________

Skin: Thickening ☐ Edema ☐ Erythema ☐ Yes ☐ No ☐ Rt. ☐ Lt. ☐ Area <3 cm> ☐ ☐

Prominent Veins — Yes ☐ No ☐ Rt. ☐ Lt. ☐ — Location ______________________

Comment ______________________

Nipple: Size — Small ☐ Med. ☐ Large ☐ — Inverted — Yes ☐ No ☐ Rt. ☐ Lt. ☐ — Normal — Yes ☐ No ☐

Discharge — Yes ☐ No ☐ Rt. ☐ Lt. ☐ — Type __________ Duration __________

Comment ______________________

Axillary Nodes: Palp. — Yes ☐ No ☐ Rt. ☐ Lt. ☐ — Size <1 cm> ☐ ☐ — No. 1 ☐ 2 ☐ 3+ ☐

Consistency — Soft ☐ Hard ☐ — Tenderness — Yes ☐ No ☐ — Moveable — Yes ☐ No ☐

Comment ______________________

LESION: Lesions Present — Yes ☐ No ☐ Single ☐ Mult. ☐ Rt. ☐ Lt. ☐

No. of Breast Segment

1	2	3
4	5	6
7	8	9

	RIGHT SEGMENTS 1	2	3	4	5	6	7	8	9	LEFT SEGMENTS 1	2	3	4	5	6	7	8	9
Location on clock (1-12)																		
Distance from nipple (cm.)																		
Size (cm.)																		
Shape: R-round O-oval I-irregular																		
Consistency: S-soft M-medium H-hard																		
Tenderness: N-none S-slight M-marked																		
Mobility: M-moveable F-fixed																		

DIAGRAM:

RIGHT **LEFT**

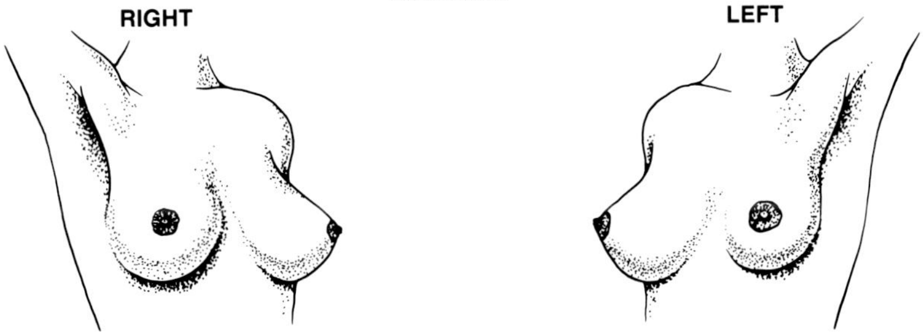

Comment ______________________

Fig. 1-8 Physical examination check sheet.

mobility of the lesion within the breast tissue. The examiner's diagnosis or impression, right or wrong, should always be recorded.

The frequency of physical examinations performed on any given patient varies according to that patient's breast cancer risk factors. When high risk factors are present, examinations at 6-month intervals are required. With moderate risk factors such as hyperplastic disease in a multiparous postmenopausal woman, examinations at 9-month intervals might be appropriate. It is this author's belief that the large majority of women who are at average or low risk should be examined yearly from age 35 notwithstanding the recommendations and guidelines of the American Cancer Society.[15] Regardless of the frequency of physician examination, the patient should be advised to perform monthly breast self-examinations. The merits and problems associated with this form of examination, as currently taught, are beyond the scope of this chapter.

Effectiveness of the Physical Examination

Ultimately the effectiveness of any diagnostic modality depends on the answers to these four questions: How effective is it in identifying an abnormality in the breast (positive finding)? How effective is it in identifying carcinoma or the suspicion of its presence? How effective is it in finding cancer in women under 50 compared to those of 50-plus years? Lastly, how effective is it in detecting small lesions (less than 1.0 cm) compared to larger lesions?

Because mammography has been shown beyond question to have the capability of detecting malignancy in the preclinical state,[4,16] it is the one modality with which the clinical examination can be compared, although the other modalities discussed elsewhere in this book are, diagnostically speaking, synergistic and complementary.

Results

Over a period of 12 years, the author has seen 243 breast cancer patients, all of whom were examined by the technique presented. All had preoperative mammograms reviewed by at least one experienced mammographer. In addition, all patients underwent additional diagnostic procedures such as fine needle aspiration for cytology, contrast ductography with cytology, or needle biopsy or open biopsy performed by the author. All have had definitive surgery with follow-up done by the author, and all pathology specimens including tumor size, cytologic preparations, and permanent sections were personally reviewed.

The term "positive finding" as applied to palpation included any discrete, solid lesion or abnormal tissue thickening that warranted cytologic evaluation by fine needle aspiration, needle biopsy, or open biopsy. Nipple discharge with negative palpation and negative mammographic findings was classified as "negative" for both modalities. When applied to mammography, a positive finding included any density, asymmetry, or presence of calcifications designated by the radiologist, provided the described abnormality was in the same quadrant of the breast as the carcinoma found. Cases listed as "suspicious for carcinoma" by palpation were those in which the recorded impression was suspicious for carcinoma because of the character of the lesion or the presence of indirect signs such as skin dimpling, retraction, or fixation. When applied to mammography, "suspicious for carcinoma" was desig-

Table 1-1 Breast Cancer: 243 Cases, Total Reported as Positive by Palpation and Mammography According to Age Group

		Palpation: Positive		Mammography: Positive	
Age Group	No. of Cases	No.	%	No.	%
<50	66	62	94	49	74
50 +	177	168	95	149	84
Total	243	230	95	198	82

nated when the report included a suggestion as to the probability or possibility of malignancy or included any suggestion as to the advisability of a biopsy.

The effectiveness of the physical examination in detecting a positive finding related to the underlying carcinoma in this series of 243 cases was 95 percent (230 cases) and that of mammography was 82 percent (Table 1-1). It can be seen that mammography was more effective in the older age group (84%) than in those under 50 years of age (74%). When reporting abnormalities as suspicious for carcinoma, mammography did slightly better in both age groups than did the clinical examination, with both methods being more effective in the older age group (Table 1-2).

When comparing effectiveness according to tumor size, the physical examination alone detected more carcinomas than did mammography alone in every size category (Table 1-3). Thus 39 of 243 (16%) were found by clinical examination alone, whereas 7 (3%) were detected by mammography alone. It should be noted that six of the seven carcinomas detected by mammography alone were under 1.0 cm in size. Interestingly, six carcinomas under 1 cm in size (19% of lesions under

Table 1-2 Breast Cancer, 243 Cases: Total Reported as Suspicious for Carcinoma by Palpation and Mammography According to Age Group

		Palpation: Positive		Mammography: Positive	
Age Group	No. of Cases	No.	%	No.	%
< 50	66	38	58	39	59
50+	177	121	68	131	74
Total	243	159	65	170	70

Table 1-3 Breast Cancer, 243 Cases: Total Reported as Positive by Palpation and Mammography According to Tumor Size

		PE+/ Mam−[a]		PE+/ Mam+		PE−/ Mam+		PE−[b]/ Mam−	
Tumor size (cm)	No. of Cases	No.	%	No.	%	No.	%	No.	%
<1.0	32	7	22	13	41	6	19	6	19
1.0–1.9	86	14	16	72	84				
2.0–2.9	70	10	14	59	84	1	1		
3.0–3.0	32	4	13	28	88				
4.0+	23	4	17	19	83				
total	243	39	16	191	79	7	3	6	3

[a]PE, physical examination, Mam, mammography.

[b]Cancers found by cytology and contrast ductography alone.

Table 1-4 Breast Cancer, 243 Cases: Total Reported as Suspicious for Carcinoma by Palpation and Mammography According to Tumor Size

		PE+/ Mam−[a]		PE+/ Mam+		PE−/ Mam+		PE−/ Mam−	
Tumor Size (cm)	No. of Cases	No.	%	No.	%	No.	%	No.	%
<1.0	32	4	13	3	9	13	41	12	38
1.0–1.9	86	11	13	40	47	16	19	19	22
2.0–2.9	70	9	13	51	73	5	7	5	7
3.0–3.9	32	4	13	21	66	3	9	4	13
4.0+	23	1	4	15	65	3	13	4	17
Total	243	29	12	130	53	40	16	44	19

[a]PE, physical examination. Mam, mammography.

1 cm) were detected by cytology and contrast ductography alone, with minimal nipple secretions being the only positive finding.

When cases reported as suspicious for carcinoma were compared according to tumor size, only 4 patients (13%) having lesions less than 1.0 cm in size were so classified by palpation, whereas 13 (41%) were found by mammography (Table 1-4). This percentage differential for mammography expectedly decreased with increasing tumor size, so that the physical examination alone indicated that 29 of 243 (12%) were suspicious for carcinoma, whereas mammography alone indicated 40 of 243 (16%). The ability of mammography to detect minimal lesions is undisputed, but note that of the 13 cases so reported 7 also had a positive physical finding. Note also that the differences in diagnosis for "suspicious for carcinoma" between mammography and palpation were confined to the older age group, and no differences were found between the two diagnostic modalities at any tumor size in the age group under 50.

Conclusions

The need for thoroughness on the part of experienced, skillful examiners who perform breast examinations in a search for breast cancer cannot be overstated. A technique for performing breast examinations has been presented that emphasizes a methodical approach. The detection rates of the physical examination employing the techniques described in 243 cancer subjects have been presented and compared with the rates of mammographic detection.

It is the author's firm belief that a complete, thorough physical examination remains the cornerstone of breast cancer detection. A mammogram complements this clinical examination and should be performed directly as indicated.

References

1. Strax P: The HIP study updated. *Rev Endocr Related Cancer* 10(suppl): 1981; 59.
2. Venet L: The clinical exam in mass screening for breast cancer. *Cancer Detect Prev* 1976; 1(2):365–372.
3. Beahrs OH, Smart CR: The Breast Cancer Detection Demonstration Projects as viewed by the clinician, in Feig SA, McLelland R (eds): *Breast Carcinoma.* New York, Masson, 1983, p 307.

4. Beahrs OH: Comparative merits of mammography and physical examination, in Feig SA, McLelland R (eds): *Breast Carcinoma.* New York, Masson, 1983, p 303.
5. Mahoney L, Csima A: The use and abuse of mammography in the early diagnosis of breast cancer. *Rev Endocr Related Cancer.* 14(suppl): 1984; 175.
6. Moskowitz M: Clinical examination of the breasts by nonphysicians, a viable screening option. *Cancer* 1979; 44:311–314.
7. Marchant DJ: Physical examination and breast self-examination, in Feig SA, McLelland R (eds): *Breast Carcinoma.* New York, Masson, 1983, p 371.
8. Marchant DJ: The breast mass, in Kase NB, Weingold R (eds): *Principles and Practices of Gynecology.* New York, Wiley, 1983.
9. Haagensen CD: *Diseases of the Breast.* Philadelphia, Saunders, 1971.
10. Pilnik S, Leis HP Jr: The clinical diagnosis of breast lesions, in: Gallagher H, Leis HP Jr, Snyderman RK, et al (eds): *The Breast.* St. Louis, Mosby, 1978.
11. Leis HP Jr: The diagnosis of breast cancer. *CA* 1977; 27:209–232.
12. Zimmer TS: Pitfalls and limitations of breast examination. *Hosp Med,* August 1968, pp 13–17.
13. Griboff SJ: Modification of breast examinations by simultaneous palpation. *New York J Med* 1960; 60:3065–3067.
14. Sartorius OW, Smith HS: Contrast ductography for the recognition and localization of benign and malignant breast lesions: An improved technique, in Logan W (ed): *Breast Carcinoma.* New York, Wiley, 1977, pp 281–300.
15. American Cancer Society report on the cancer-related checkup. *Cancer* 1980; 30:194–240.
16. Egan RL, Goldstein GT, McSweeney MM: Conventional mammography, physical examination, thermography and xeroradiography in the detection of breast cancer. *Cancer* 1977; 39:1984–1992.

2

Mammography

John Milbrath

Women living in the United States have an almost 10 percent lifetime chance of developing breast cancer.[1] Breast cancer cannot be prevented, but it can be cured in almost 100 percent of cases if the cancer is found early.[2] Unfortunately, in our society we have taught women to wait until they have a lump in the breast before seeking treatment. Today we have a radiographic test, mammography, that can find cancers 2 to 4 years before a lump can be felt.[3] Most of the cancers found only on mammography are 100 percent curable, and the patients can be effectively treated with less than a total mastectomy.[4] Although mammography is recommended for all women over the age of 35, few women are taking advantage of this life-saving tool.

History

In 1913 the German surgeon Salomon, after radiographically studying approximately 3000 amputated breasts, reported the clinical, radiologic, and pathologic correlates of breast cancers, particularly the invasive characteristics and pattern of spread.[5] Calcifications in cancer were also demonstrated. His work was interrupted by World War I. It was not until 1930 that Stafford Warren, a radiologist, reported on the first in vivo use of mammography.[6] However, because of the unpredictable quality of x-ray mammograms, contemporaries were discouraged and the examination was virtually abandoned. In 1931 Seabold described the radiologic changes occurring during the menstrual cycle and also measured fibroadenomas radiographically.[7,8] In 1932 Lockwood and Stewart radiographically studied the menstrual cycle,[9] and Ries in 1930 showed that it was unsafe to inject iodized poppyseed oil or foreign substances into a duct.[10] In 1953 Leborgne described typical tumor calcifications and emphasized their specificity for certain types of cancer.[11] However, in the United States only Gershon-Cohen persisted in the use of mammography. In 1960 he correlated mammographic images with anatomy and pathology.[12]

A milestone occurred in 1960 when, after extensive experiments with various techniques, Egan reported on a high milliamperage–low kilovoltage technique that resulted in dependable diagnostic images.[13]

During the mid-1960s Gros introduced two innovations in mammographic technique[14]: (1) a molybdenum target that increased the contrast between fat, parenchymal tissue, and calcifications because of the greater photoelectric effect at 26 to 28 kVp; and (2) vigorous compression that eliminated motion artifacts, diminished scattered radiation, and separated structures within the breast. However, the improved image quality was obtained at the expense of an increased surface exposure [8 versus 4 RAD (radiation absorbed dose)]

Xeroradiography, which was developed during the late 1930s but not generally utilized by the medical community until Wolfe's refinements during the late 1960s, represented another important advancement.[15] Xeroradiography employs a photoconductive plate of selenium-coated aluminum as an image receptor. After an x-ray exposure, the resultant electrostatic image is transferred to a piece of plastic-coated paper, resulting in a mirror image. The paper is heated, and the toner particles become embedded in the plastic. The entire developing process takes 90 seconds. Improvements in the technique utilize liquid toner for development and permit a reduction in x-ray exposure.

In 1973 a high definition intensifying screen combined with a single emulsion film was introduced for mammography.[16] Intimate contact between the screen and film was initially obtained by evacuating a sealed, polyethylene bag. The bag has subsequently been replaced with single-screen cassettes that provide intimate film–screen contact. Improvements in the speed of the single-emulsion film have permitted further reduction in the x-ray exposure.

The advent of fine moving grids have greatly reduced the scattered radiation, thereby improving mammographic contrast.[17] Microfocal spot tubes enable magnification techniques that are reported to improve diagnostic accuracy.[18]

Today, both xeroradiography and film–screen mammography are the main mammographic methods utilized. Nonscreen film mammography is used in only a handful of centers. Xeroradiography offers ease of interpretation, convenience because a darkroom is not needed, and increased latitude because of its diminished contrast. Film–screen mammography offers decreased radiation exposure, increased contrast, decreased cost, and less maintenance. Within the past several years there has been a swing from xeroradiography, which was extremely popular during the 1970s especially in high volume centers, to film–screen mammography. Both techniques will continue to be used for the foreseeable future.

Diagnosis Versus Screening

A diagnostic examination is performed whenever a patient has symptoms of a particular disease; the examination groups the population into disease or nondisease categories. A screening examination simply divides a population into two groups, one containing most if not all individuals who are likely to have the disease in question and the other including most if not all individuals who are unlikely to have the disease. When screening for breat cancer, the examination is asked only to identify those women with a high likelihood and those with a low likelihood of having breast cancer.

A low specificity or high false-positive rate is never acceptable for a diagnostic test, but it is acceptable for a screening examination if the sensitivity is high (low false-negative rate).

Screening Studies

From 1963 to 1966 periodic screening with film mammography and physical examination was done to determine its effect on breast cancer mortality rate. This study, under the auspices of the Health Insurance Plan (HIP) of New York, had

62,000 subjects equally divided between study and control groups. Screening consisted of four annual mammograms and physical examinations over a 3-year period. Although one-third of the women never participated in a screening examination, mortality rates were decreased by 30 to 40 percent in the study group starting shortly after the study was begun.[19] Although initial results indicated a lack of mortality reduction for those women in the study group under age 50, more recent analyses indicate a distinct mortality rate reduction of 20 percent, even in this group.[20] A review of the mammograms performed in this study indicates a quality far inferior to that obtainable today.[21] Also, probably as a result of the inferior mammograms, only a handful of minimal cancers were detected in women under age 50.[22]

With impetus from the HIP study, the National Cancer Institute (NCI) and the American Cancer Society (ACS) cosponsored the Breast Cancer Detection Demonstration Projects (BCDDP) at 27 sites throughout the United States. These projects, which began in 1973, were not set up as controlled scientific studies but were designed to demonstrate the application of periodic screening for the detection of early breast cancer to the medical profession and the public.[23]

Of the 4443 cancers found in the BCDDP population, more than 80 percent were detected by the centers.[24] Almost one-third of cancers detected by the centers were either noninfiltrating or small infiltrating cancers less than 1.0 cm in size. More than 80 percent of all cancers showed no evidence of nodal involvement.

The contribution of mammography was substantial. Mammography alone (in the absence of physical findings) found 41.6 percent of the cancer, whereas physical examination alone (in the absence of positive mammographic findings) was positive in 8.7 percent of the cancer patients. The relative contribution of mammography was substantially higher than that shown in the HIP study (Table 2-1). Shortly after

Table 2-1 Breast Cancers Detected During the 5-Year BCDDP Compared with the 4-Year HIP Screening Program

	BCDDP[b]				HIP[c]			
	Ages 40–49 at surgery		Ages 50–59 at surgery		Ages 40–49 at surgery		Ages 50–59 at surgery	
Suspicious modality[a]	No.	%	No.	%	No.	%	No.	%
Mammography only	270	35.4	540	42.1	6	19.4	27	41.5
Mammography + physical examination	381	50.0	638	49.7	6	19.4	12	18.5
Physical examination only	100	13.1	86	6.7	19	61.3	26	40.0
Unknown	11	1.4	19	1.5	0	0.0	0	0.0
Total	762[d]	100.0	1283[e]	100.0	31	100.0	65	100.0

[a]Includes modalities that have findings with one or more features interpreted as suspicious of maligant or benign breast disease.

[b]BCDDP cancers shown here include only those cancers detected following a surgical recommendation made at an annual or early recall screening.

[c]From Shapiro S: Evidence on screening for breast cancer from a randomized trial. *Cancer* 1977; 39 (suppl):2772–2782.

[d]Includes 30 breast cancer cases in which a mammogram was not performed for any reason, such as examination refused, examination not recommended for a woman under 50 years of age, or examination technically not satisfactory. Exclusion of these cases changes the distribution of susupicious modalities to: mammography only, 36.9%; mammography and physical examination 52.0% physical examination only, 9.6%; and unknown, 1.5%.

[e]Includes 17 breast cancer cases in which a mammogram was not performed for any reason, such as examination refused or examination technically not satisfactory. Exclusion of these cases changes the distribution of suspicious modalities to: mammography only, 42.7%; mammography and physical examination 50.4%; physical examination only, 5.5%; and unknown, 1.5%.

Source: Reprinted with permission from *CA* (1982;32). © 1982, American Cancer Society.

the results of the BCDDP were published, the ACS revised its mammographic guidelines to include women down to age 35.[25]

The ability of mammography alone to detect breast cancer and reduce the mortality rate is currently being studied in a population-based, randomized controlled study of 134,867 women living in two Swedish counties. Early results show a 31 percent mortality reduction in the screened group.[26] The only screening method used was a single oblique view mammogram.

Radiation Controversy

During the late 1970s a debate over the relative value of mammography split over from the medical community, causing many women to avoid the most sensitive technique to detect breast cancer.[27] This debate revolved around two points: the lack of a proved benefit of screening women under age 50 and the potential carcinogenic risk of mammography. Women from this era presenting with breast cancers had more advanced cancers than women presenting with cancer prior to the "scare."

Although the results of the HIP study showed a 33 to 40 percent reduction in mortality in the screened population, this benefit was initially restricted to women over age 50. However, later analyses showed a 20 percent mortality reduction in women under 50 beginning around the seventh year, and persisting currently to 14 years, of follow-up. Results of the BCDDP study show a high pickup of minimal cancers especially in women under age 50.[24] Many centers reported a 10 to 12.5 times greater pickup rate of minimal cancers than reported in the HIP study.[28]

The carcinogenic effect of low-level radiation is unknown. However, if there is a risk, it is immeasurably small, especially in women over age 30.[29] Large doses of radiation (1000 times greater than that used in current film–screen techniques) have been shown to cause an increased number of breast cancers, but this increase is confined mainly to women under age 30. Today, although the controversy debate has subsided, the fear of radiation is still cited as one of the chief reasons women do not avail themselves of mammography.

Current State of the Art

Centers currently performing mammography are utilizing either xeroradiography or film–screen mammography. Xeroradiography, which was extremely popular during the 1970s, utilizes a selenium-coated aluminum plate as its recording medium. The resultant image is developed with blue powder and then transferred to a sheet of plastic-coated paper. Xeroradiography does not require a darkroom or dedicated mammographic equipment. Tungsten target tubes give better images than molybdenum target tubes. Ease of interpretation makes this process very popular with high-volume centers. Its readiographic latitude makes visualization of the entire breast including chest wall and axilla very easy. Improved design, utilizing a liquid toner and promising a lower radiation dose, has recently been introduced.

Film–screen mammography is becoming more popular because of its 4 to 10 fold decrease in radiation dose compared to that of xeromammography. Dedicated equipment is essential because vigorous compression and low kilovolt peak are required. Molybdenum targets are preferable to tungsten targets, but units employing magnification occasionally use micro focus tungsten anodes. Photo timing and a reciprocating grid are used in most dedicated systems.

Because of its greater contrast, parenchymal densities are more apparent on film–screen images than with xeroradiography. Calcifications, particularly fine ones, are better visualized on film–screen images.

Results of the BCDDP study showed both processes to be similar in pickup of cancers. Therefore factors other than accuracy should be the major determinants when deciding which method to employ.

As initially espoused by Egan,[13] the accuracy of mammographic interpretation is determined more by the ability of the technologist than it is by the interpretative ability of the radiologist.

Indications

Mammography and physical examinations are the only two methods that are reliably proved to be able to detect breast cancer. Mammography is by far more sensitive than physical examination, although a negative mammogram does not exclude the possibility of cancer, especially in a woman with a palpable mass.

Any patient with a history suggesting breast cancer should have a mammogram. This includes patients with a mass, a thickening, or a nipple discharge. Even patients with cancers that are clinically obvious should have mammograms, primarily to screen the opposite breast.

Because of the proved ability of mammography and physical examination to reduce mortality rates and because of the ability of mammography to detect preclinical cancer that is frequently "minimal," the American Cancer Society recommends mammograms on a periodic basis for all women over age 40 along with a baseline mammogram between the ages of 35 and 40 (Table 2-2).

Future

Both film–screen mammography and xeroradiography, especially after its planned dose-reduction improvements, stand to be the techniques utilized for mammography

Table 2-2 American Cancer Society Guidelines for Mammography and Physical Examination

20 years and older Breast self-examination monthly.

20–40 years of age: A physican breast examination every 3 years and an initial mammogram between the ages of 35 and 40.

40–50 years of age: Periodic mammography every year or two as determined by your own personal history and your doctor's recommendation. Also, an annual physician breast examination.

Over 50 years of age: Annual mammography and an annual physician examination.

If you have a personal or family history of breast cancer, consult with your physician about how often you should be examined and how often you should have mammography before age 40.

Source: Mammography 1982: Statement of the American Cancer Society. © 1982, American Cancer Society.

in the foreseeable future. There is no other technique on the horizon that has the sensitivity of mammography especially for determing minimal cancers. Computed tomography and magnetic resonance imaging are reserved for cases needing special diagnostic information.[30] Thermography appears to have little role.[31,32] Digital mammography, diaphanography, and computed ultrasonography are unproved.[30] B-scan ultrasound is used mainly as an adjunctive study primarily to determine whether a mass is crystic or solid.[33]

A technically suboptimal mammogram is often worse than no mammogram at all. An examination that is so important for the well-being of women requires skilled, interested, and trained radiologists interpreting images obtained by knowledgable, dedicated technologists utilizing dedicated state of the art equipment.

References

1. American Cancer Society: *Cancer Facts & Figures.* New York, American Cancer Society, 1980.
2. Wanebo HJ, Huvos AG, Urban JA: Treatment of minimal breast cancer. *Cancer* 1974; 33:349–357.
3. Fox SH, Moskowitz M, Saenger EL, et al: Benefit/risk analysis of aggressive mammographic screening, *Radiology* 1978; 127:359–365.
4. Montague ED, Spanos WJ Jr, Ames FC, et al: Conservative treatment of noninvasive and small-volume invasive breast cancer, in Feig SA, McLelland R (eds): *Breast Carcinoma—Current Diagnosis and Treatment* New York, Masson, 1983, pp 429–432.
5. Salomon, A: Beitrage zur Pathologie und Klinik des Mammakarzinoms. *Arch Klin Chir* 1913; 101:573–668.
6. Warren SL: A roentgenologic study of the breast. *AJR* 1930; 24:113–124.
7. Seabold PS: Diagnosis of breast diseases by x-ray. *Am Surg* 1931; 93:443–444.
8. Seabold PS: Roentgenographic diagnosis of diseases of the breast. *Surg Gynecol Obstet* 1931; 53:461–468.
9. Lockwood IH, Stewart W: Roentgen study of physiologic and pathologic changes in the mammary gland. *JAMA* 1932; 99:1461–1466.
10. Ries E: Diagnostic lipiodal injection into milk ducts followed by abscess formation. *Am J Obstet Gynecol* 1930; 20:414–416.
11. Leborgne R: Diagnosis of tumors of the breast by simple roentgenography. *AJR* 1951; 65:1–11.
12. Ingleby H, Gershon-Cohen J: *Comparative Anatomy, Pathology and Roentgenology of the Breast.* Philadelphia, University of Pennsylvania Press, 1960.
13. Egan RL: Experience with mammography in a tumor institution. *Radiology* 1960; 75:894–900.
14. Gros CM: Methodologie, symposium sur le sein. *J Radiol Electr* 1967; 48:638–655.
15. Wolfe JN: Xerography of the breast. *Radiology* 1968; 91:231–240.
16. Ostrum BJ, Becker W, Isard HJ: Low-dose mammography. *Radiology* 1973; 109:323–326.
17. McSweeney MB, Sprawls P, Egan RL: Mammographic grids, in Feig SA, McLelland R (eds): *Breast Carcinoma—Current Diagnosis and Treatment.* New York, Masson, 1983, pp 169–176.
18. Sickles EA: Magnification mammography, in Feig SA, McLelland R (eds) *Breast Carcinoma—Current Diagnosis and Treatment* New York, Masson 1983, pp. 177–182.
19. Shapiro S: Evidence on screening for breast cancer from a randomized trial. *Cancer* 1977; 39:2772–2782.
20. Moskowitz M: Minimal cancer redux. *Radiol Clin North Am* 1983; 21:93–113.
21. Gold R: Indications and risk-benefit of mammography. *J Fam Pract* 1979; 8:1135–1140.
22. Thomas LB, Ackerman LV, McDivitt RW, et al: *Report of NCI Ad Hoc Pathology Working Group to review the gross and microscopic findings of breast cancer cases in the HIP study,* in *Final Reports of NCI Ad Hoc Working Groups,* DHEW Publ. No. (NIH) 77–1400, March 1977.
23. *Manual of Procedures and Operations for the National Cancer Institute and the American Cancer Society.* Breast Cancer Detection Demonstration Project, National Cancer Program,

Public Health Service, National Institutes of Health, U.S. Department of Health, Education and Welfare, February 1977.
24. Baker LH: Breast Cancer Detection Demonstration Project: Five-year summary report. *CA* 1982; 32:194–225.
25. American Cancer Society: Mammography 1982: Statement of the American Cancer Society, *CA* 1982; 32:226–230.
26. Tabar L, Gad A, Holmberg LH, et al: Reduction in mortality from breast cancer after mass screening with mammography. *Lancet* 1985; 8433:829–832.
27. Bailar JC: Mammography: A contrary view, *Ann Intern Med* 1976; 84:77–84.
28. Swartz HM, Reichling BA: The risks of mammograms. *JAMA* 1977; 237:965–966.
29. Feig SA: Assessment of the hypothetical risk from mammography and evaluation of the potential benefit. *Radiol Clin North Am* 1983; 21:173–191.
30. Sickles EA: Breast CT scanning, heavy ion mammography, NMR imaging and diaphanograpny, in Feig SA; McLelland R (eds): *Breast Carcinoma—Current Diagnosis and Treatment,* New York, Masson, 1983, pp 233–250.
31. Moskowitz M, Milbrath J, Gartside P, et al: Lack of efficacy of thermography as a screening tool for minimal and stage I breast cancer. *N Engl J Med* 1976; 295:249–252.
32. Schmidt AM, Whitehorn WV, Martin EW: Thermography restriction, *FDA Drug Bull* 1976; 6:32.
33. Sickles EA, Filly RA, Callen PW: Breast ultrasonography, in Feig, SA, McLelland R (eds): *Breast Carcinoma—Current Diagnosis and Treatment,* New York, Masson, 1983, pp 191–205.

3

Ultrasound

Saar Porrath

With the advent of medical ultrasound, the breast, because of its superficial location and its ready accessibility, became an easy organ to study. The relative thinness of the tissue lent itself well to the limited equipment available.[1]

Wild's initial studies during the early 1950s dealt primarily with A-mode delineation of masses.[2] Shortly thereafter, early B-mode detection followed. It is a compliment to the ability of the early investigators that their work was as accurate as it was. Wild and Reid[3] reported a 98 percent ability to delineate a benign state in a series of 77 consecutive breast lesions.[3,4] Howry and his coinvestigators in 1954 reported on the ultrasonic observations of breast carcinoma.[5]

During the 1960 work progressed on an international front with Jellins, Reeve, and Kossoff in Australia, Kelly-Fry in the United States, Wells in England, and Kobayashi and Wagai in Japan.[6–11] These investigators laid down an excellent foundation from which later observers could build.

During this same time automated breast ultrasound was being developed, which allowed investigation of the entire breast with the patient in the prone position. Since the mid-1970s there has been increasing acceptance by the medical community of breast ultrasound and its increased use as a breast imaging modality.

Understanding the Equipment and Its Use

There are advantages and disadvantages to both a hand-held high resolution ultrasound probe, static and real time, and the lower-resolution automated systems. It is perhaps more important to first understand the limitations of breast ultrasound and then to realize the inherent problems with each type of system. Understanding these, the reader will hopefully be able to make his or her own equipment choice.

The ultrasonic beam must reach the lesion in order to adequately visualize it.[13,14] If the transducer strength is not adequate to penetrate the tissue or the (TGC) settings are improper, there will not be enough of the ultrasound beam to "see" the lesion. Ultrasound probes are normally made so that the best resolution is at a set depth. If a wrong-depth probe is used, the lesion may be missed or the resolution so poor as to be nondiagnostic. It is primarily for this reason that many ultrasound probes have a water-path offset which has proved useful for breast delineation.

The anatomy of the breast also plays an important role.[15] Unlike the liver, the breast is a very inhomogeneous structure. Because reflection of the ultrasound beam occurs with a tissue interface, and the breast has many of these, there are many anatomic obstacles to overcome in order to obtain adequate scans: There are fat pockets interspersed within even the densest glandularity, Cooper's ligaments are present throughout the breast, and even in the dense glandular areas the tissue is somewhat inhomogeneous.

With the patient in the supine position, the breast tissue slides easily under the probe and may be difficult to control. A lesion should be stabilized in order to be examined. Because the breast drops against the chest wall, signs such as skin thickening, thickening and pulling of Cooper's ligaments, and retraction are poorly seen. It is also very difficult to examine the entire breast in the supine position with a hand-held probe. However, these disadvantages of the supine position, especially with a hand-held probe, are partially overcome by the reduced tissue volume, giving improved resolution.

The realities are that almost every imaging facility has a hand-held system, the nonautomated systems are less expensive, it is easier on the patient to lie supine, and there is less experience needed to adequately read a limited scan over a lesion.

With the patient in the prone position and using a water-path system, the breast hangs free in the water. This position allows excellent delineation of the skin line. Even the slightest retraction, sometimes not evident clinically, can be visualized. Slight thickening of Cooper's ligaments can be seen. The entire breast can be scanned easily and relatively quickly.

Sometimes the breast hangs too low in the tank or the tissue is too dense to adequately penetrate with the lower-power transducers, in which case the breast must be compressed.[16] Such compression decreases the ability to visualize the skin line and retraction but may increase delineation of the breast lesion and the deeper tissue in the dense breast.

The automated water-path systems are more expensive to buy and maintain than the hand-held units. They also require an expertise to interpret that can be difficult to attain. In the opinion of the author it probably takes at least 300 cases to become even reasonably comfortable with the images.

Economics and comfort in interpretation play an important role in the decision about which type of equipment to use. More important is a question of philosophy. What is the examiner trying to find? Is the breast examination being done solely to detect cancer, to evaluate a particular lesion, or both, or is the breast being examined in toto? If the answer is one of the former, the automated system is not the answer. A single lesion can be well evaluated with the use of a hand-held probe, and in fact the higher-resolution probe can give a better delineation in many circumstances, though not all.

Can the ultrasound detect cancers undetected by mammography and physical examination? The reader is referred to the discussion later in this chapter. Can this detection be done cost-effectively? This value question is difficult to answer—but a deep philosophical question that medicine is being forced to answer. It is the opinion of the author that in a simple screening situation ultrasound is probably not truly cost-effective, although it has been my personal choice to use it in the dense breast where mammography is less accurate.

At the Woman's Breast Center, a significant number of patients are seen for evaluation of breast pain, tenderness, and a variety of other complaints including nipple discharge. In these patients the likelihood of cancer is very small. It is not adequate to simply tell the patient that she does not have cancer. A cause for the symptoms is found if possible and appropriate therapy instituted. In these patients the total examination of the breast by ultrasound can be invaluable. Such examination cannot be adequately done by using a hand-held probe, and the use of the automated system with water-path has been very helpful.

Normal Breast

The ultrasonic picture of the normal breast varies depending on the age of the patient, the hormonal status, and the amount of glandular and fatty tissue.[13–15, 17, 18]

Prepubescent Breast

The early developing breast is a small nubbin of glandular tissue situated behind the nipple. It presents on ultrasound as a dense echogenic area in an otherwise small fatty breast. If it is unilateral, the opposite breast may appear as a small fatty breast.

Adolescent Breast

The developing adolescent breast is densely glandular with little internal fat. The glandular tissue in the smaller breast is cone-shaped. The fat is present posteriorly in front of the pectoralis muscle and surrounding the glandular tissue in the subcutaneous area. The amount of fat is variable depending on the obesity of the patient, which the ultrasonic picture reflects.

Third and Fourth Decades' Breast

The normal female breast during the twenties and thirties is primarily glandular. Unlike the adolescent breast, there is an increase in the amount of fatty tissue present. There is a dense pattern of glandularity (Wolfe DY pattern[19]), with the fat posterior and around the edges. If the breast is less dense, as in Wolfe P2 and P1 patterns, there is an increase in the amount of fat not only posteriorly but interspersed within the glandular portion as well. With an increased number of pregnancies and in women who have nursed, there is a diminution in the amount of glandularity and an increase in the proportion of fat. The fat areas interspersed in the glandular tissue appear ultrasonically as low-level echoes to almost anechoic areas within the dense echoes of the glandularity. Occasionally a fat lobule appears as a well circumscribed low-level area simulating a lesion. Normally there is a break in the well defined contour of the fat lobule if the area of the lobule is examined ultrasonically in all dimensions. It is this break in the contour, often linking the lobule with other areas of fat, that allows the structure to be diagnosed as a fat lobule, not a true lesion.

Premenopausal Breast

As the woman nears menopause there is a generalized decrease in the amount of glandularity and an increase in the amount of fat. The residual glandularity is usually behind the areola and in the upper outer quadrant. The increase in fat occurs in the posterior portion of the breast, the subcutaneous area, and throughout the remaining glandular areas. Although there may be a decrease in the amount of glandularity, there may be residual stromal tissue which shows as bright echogenic areas. The ultrasonic picture must be correlated with the mammogram to properly identify the areas of echogenicity before assuming there is a lesion present.

Postmenopausal Breast

In most patients the postmenopausal breast contains little glandular tissue and is primarily made up of fat. Ultrasonically a fatty breast does not lend itself as well to ultrasound as does a glandular breast. The fat is of low-level echoes, and the ligamentous structures are highly reflective on ultrasound. Because of the diffuse low-level echogenicity and the inhomogenicity of the fatty breast a lesion can be easily missed or not evident on ultrsound.

Benign Lesions

The following discussions on both benign and malignant disease apply to ultrasound in general, with no differentiation being made to the use of the equipment choices discussed above. The discussions here are not meant to be all-inclusive.

Cysts

The detection of cystic structures first by A-mode scan, then B-mode scan, and finally a combination of both has been excellent. The accuracy rate approaches 98 percent, and cysts as small as 2 mm can be seen.

The lesion should be anechoic with increased through transmission. Care must be taken to ensure that the proper TGC curves are used, lest a lesion which has echoes is made to appear echo-free. If the cyst is located far posteriorly, against the chest wall, the ability to detect the increased through transmission may be decreased. Not infrequently, there may be small floating internal echoes visualized within the fluid. These represent small particles within the fluid, conglomerations of the fluid, or small cellular collections. Although in my experience these particles have never represented a malignant lesion, the fluid should be analyzed following cyst aspiration to be sure.

The cyst wall should appear smooth and well defined. Not infrequently there are septations within the cyst which are seen. If irregularities of the wall or internal particles of moderate size (2 mm or greater) are seen, it is best to follow the advice of Tabar et al.[22] and do cyst puncture followed by injection of air into the cyst and a mammogram (called a pneumocystogram). The cyst walls should be smoothly delineated by the air; if they are not, the possibility of an intracystic lesion is raised.

It is very common in the denser glandular breast to find cysts on ultrasound that are not evident on mammography. There may be shadowing evident from the posterior lateral edges of the cyst, which is from the tissue interface or caused by the angle of the ultrasound beam. Care must be taken in these areas to be sure that a lesion is not missed.

Fibroadenomas

Fibroadenomas are usually well defined.[20,21,23,24] The anterior and posterior borders are usually well seen, but the rim is usually not evident. However, there may be increased tissue density due to some compression by the fibroadenoma. Shadowing may be seen from the posterior lateral edges. The tadpole sign described by Kobayashi,[25] with shadowing from the edges and transmission in the center, is not usually seen with any compounding of images.

The echo pattern within the lesion should be fairly homogeneous with low-level echoes. If the TGC settings are improper, the internal echoes can be increased or almost absent. This admonition about proper care when setting up the equipment must be adhered to for all ultrasound examinations.

Not all fibradenomas palpated or seen on mammography are evident on ultrasound. If the density of the lesion is similar to the surrounding tissue, it may not be visualized. The dense calcifications seen within mature adenomas show on ultrasound as very bright echoes with or without shadowing, depending on the beam direction and its intensity.

Although the diagnosis of adenoma can be made with a fair degree of accuracy, it is not accurate enough to obviate the need for biopsy.

Fat Lesions

Fat appears on ultrasound as a low-level echogenic area with bright echoes caused by the surrounding ligaments. As the gain is increased on the ultrasound, the area becomes more echogenic. Lesions within a fatty breast may be difficult to visualize on ultrasound because of a general decreased tissue density.[13–15, 26]

Lipomas appear as low-level or moderate-level echo areas with moderately well defined borders. There may be some increased through transmission. Lesions with fat and tissue such as a fibrolipoma have varying internal density on ultrasound. The amount of internal echoes depends on the amount of tissue other than fat within the lesion. A fibroangiolipoma, for example, is very echogenic.

Duct Dilatation

Ultrasound has the ability to detect even slight duct dilatation with high accuracy. The ducts seen are usually subareolar, although more peripheral ducts can be visualized.[27–29]

In the nonlactating patient the normal duct seldom is more than 1 to 2 mm in width. Often the ducts are seen only as bright linear echos arising from the duct walls, with no clear area, the duct lumen, visualized.

In the lactating breast there is a generalized increased tissue density of high echogenicity with multiple dilated ducts seen radiating from the nipple area that may extend 4 to 5 cm into the breast. Dilated ducts far in the periphery are not usually seen. If ultrasound is done following breast evacuation by either nursing or the use of a breast pump, the size of the duct adjacent to the nipple decreases markedly. This ampulla of the duct, just beneath the nipple, is larger than the more peripheral area. If the duct is filled with inspissated milk, there is echogenicity within the duct lumen. The same is true of grumous material seen in some dilated ducts in the nonlactating patient. Not all the breast and ducts empty equally in the lactating patient, and therefore care must be taken before an area of duct dilatation in these patients is called abnormal.

Intraductal lesions are usually very small and therefore difficult to identify on ultrasound. Unless the duct is dilated or the lesion large, there may be nothing seen. Intraductal papillomas are often accompanied by a distal dilated duct, which can be seen. If the duct dilatation is sufficient to partially surround the lesion, the papilloma may visualize as an intracystic lesion when in reality it is not. The papilloma, if 1 cm in size or greater, may be densely echogenic or almost echo-free: There is no constant pattern.

In the younger, premenopausal patient, there may be some slight duct dilatation seen. It is usually accompanied by a slight bilateral nipple discharge and is related to the patient's hormonal status.

Hemorrhage

The ultrasonic picture of hemorrhage depends on the amount and distribution of the blood within the tissues. It also varies with the duration of time elapsed since the trauma.[17]

When there is a localized hematoma, the borders may be well defined, although if the edges of the fluid collection dissipate into the tissues the ultrasonic picture reflects this as well. Initially the blood presents as fluid and appears anechoic. Within a few days the clots are well organized and present as inhomogeneous dense echoes. About 7 days or more after the initial trauma, the clot begins to liquefy, and the area again appears almost anechoic. During the interval there may be a combination of pictures, with a solid area of echoes floating in the partially liquefied clot.

When the blood is dissipated into the tissues and does not form a well defined fluid area, the ultrasound reflects this by initially showing small fluid areas within the tissue. Later there is increased tissue echogenicity with some shadowing because of the marked density. Ecchymotic areas, if large enough, show skin thickening and an increased density within the normally low-level echoes of the subcutaneous tissues.

Infections

As with hemorrhage, the ultrasonic picture of infection varies with the distribution within the breast and the amount of inflammation present. When there is a localized abscess, the borders are usually well defined. There are some internal echoes within a primarily anechoic area, and through transmission is increased. There may be some increase in density in the surrounding tissues.

Mastitis clinically presents as a diffuse involvement. If the skin is involved there is skin thickening. The glandular tissues appear on ultrasound as increased density and perhaps shadowing. A minimal involvement may appear essentially normal on the scans.

Any infection which involves the skin is reflected on ultrasound as skin thickening and increased echoes within the subcutaneous tissues. Cooper's ligaments may also be thickened owing to some lymphatic involvement that may run along the ligaments.

Duct infections may demonstrate some duct dilatation but the ultrasound is usually normal. Nipple infections may show some enlargement of the nipple and increased shadowing. Montgomery's gland abscesses present as a localized fluid collection with adjacent skin thickening.

Infections such as tuberculosis, if it affects the axillary nodes and causes some lymphatic obstruction, may show an ultrasonic picture similar to inflammatory carcinoma: skin thickening and increased echoes within the subcutaneous tissues. If the infections are localized, as with an abscess, the presentation is similar to that for the abscesses described above.

Fibrocystic Disease

As discussed in the section of fibrocystic disease, this is a wastebasket term and differentiation must be on the basis of the actual tissue present. The ultrasonic presentation is variable, ranging from normal findings to cysts interposed among increased tissue densities. In general there is some increased tissue with shadowing, which varies depending on the severity of the disease. The reader is referred to the section on fibrocystic disease (see Chapter 13) for more specific findings.

Mondor's Disease

There are no ultrasonic findings evident for Mondor's disease.

Male Breast

The male breast under normal circumstances is fatty with a few stromal elements. On ultrasound it appears similar to the atrophic fatty postmenopausal female breast. The fat is low-level to almost anechoic.

Gynecomastia has an appearance similar to that of the prepubescent breast with a nubbin of glandular tissue beneath the nipple. There is usually an increase in the amount of fat as well. The amount of glandular tissue varies from little to a fairly large proportion. There are two types of gynecomastia, one primarily glandular, and the other primarily stromal, or with combination of both. The more stromal elements there are, the brighter is the echo pattern and the more shadowing that is seen. The glandular elements present primarily as solid areas behind the nipple, whereas the stromal elements are more stringy in presentation and tend to flare out more from the nipple area. Other lesions in the male breast present in a manner very similar to those in the female breast.

Scars, Postoperative Breast, Augmented Breast, Postirradiated Breast

Scars as well as the postoperative, augmented, and postirradiated breast are discussed in Chapters 18, 20, and 24, and the reader is referred to these discussions.

Breast Cancer

There have been a large number of studies describing the detection of breast cancers which have been reported since the advent of the use of ultrasound on the breast in 1952. A wide variety of diagnostic signs have been reported. It is beyond the scope of this presentation to review all of these. The reader is referred to the excellent review articles by Kobayashi,[25] Egan and McSweeney,[31,32] and Cole-Beuglet et al.;[33] published elsewhere. The discussion that follows is an overview of basic questions about breast ultrasound.

Can ultrasound detect breast cancer? Is ultrasound a stand-alone procedure, or should it be used in conjunction with other imaging procedures? What are the primary signs an examiner should look for in the detection of breast cancer by ultrasound?

Can ultrasound detect breast cancer? The answer is yes. Egan and McSweeney reported an accuracy of 85 percent in the detection of breast cancer, Cole-Beuglet et al. reported 84 percent,[37] and Barraclough et al. in Australia reported 85 percent.[34] These studies were performed by experienced observers; they reflect the necessity for anyone undertaking ultrasound of the breast not only to do careful examinations but to obtain follow-up results on all cases so that the "misses" can be learned from and explained if possible.

Before further addressing the diagnostic ability of ultrasound, the second issue—if ultrasound can stand alone as a procedure—should be covered. No, it cannot. Ultrasound of the breast is not a screening procedure. It does not have the ability to routinely detect small breast cancers. Although Barraclough et al. reported an ability to correctly diagnose breast cancers of less than 2 cm in 78 percent of patients and Hisa et al. reported a 70 percent accuracy in this same tumor size group, this ability falls off drastically for lesions of less than 1 cm.[35]

Ultrasound should be used in conjunction with physical examination and mammography. Although Kasumi and Tanaka[36] have shown that the microcalcifications of breast cancers can be detected by ultrasound, this experience is not universal.[37] Mammography has the ability to detect minimal breast cancers and cancers smaller than 1 cm with a large degree of accuracy.[38]

Ultrasound and mammography should be viewed as adjunctive procedures, not competitors. Mammography achieves its best results in the fattier, less glandular breast, especially in the older patients, whereas ultrasound is more accurate in the denser glandular breast of the younger patient and less accurate in the fatty breast. Mantalana (personal communication) has noted a 98 percent accuracy when the two procedures are used in conjunction. Harper and Kelly-Fry reported 94.4 percent accuracy rate for ultrasound in 72 proved malignancies. Their results were 100 percent when mammography and ultrasound were combined. Egan and McSweeney[31] showed that 7 percent of their patient's cancers were seen on unltrasound only, not mammography. Half of these had no clinical signs. Although this is a small series, its importance should not be ignored.

There has been an increase in the percentage of cancers that occur in patients under the age of 50,[39] a percentage that has increased more than the overall percentage increase in the general population. In the studies reported by Croll[40] the expected Australian percentage in those under age 50 is 29 percent. Forty percent of the cancers she reported were in women under age 50, reflecting her patient selection. Moskowitz[41] in 1976 as part of the BCDDP program reported that among 8100 screenees, 15 percent of the cancers occurred in those between ages 35 and 44. McSweeney (personal communication) noted that 8 percent of her patients with breast cancer were under age 35.

Primary Signs of Breast Cancer on Ultrasound

Skin Changes

Ultrasound is extremely sensitive to even slight skin thickening. The normal skin line is 2 to 3 mm.[42] Localized skin thickening must be accounted for. Although infection, scars, and dermatologic changes may account for the thickening, care must be taken to search for a possible malignant cause. Generalized skin thickening is seen with inflammatory carcinoma, infection, congestive heart failure, and blockage of the axillary nodes by nonmalignant conditions.

Retraction

Skin retraction is easily detected when the patient lies prone with her breasts extended into the waterbath of an automated system. A slight change in contour or flattening may be seen, or even minimal retraction not evident clinically. Very slight nipple retraction can also be visualized in this position. The pull of the weight of the breast exaggerates any opposite pull by involved ligaments or ducts.

Cooper's Ligaments

Involvement of Cooper's ligaments by cancer often causes an inward pull on these ligaments resulting in the retraction described above. In addition, there may be thickening of the ligaments seen on ultrasound as a dense bright echo extending diagonally toward the skin. This situation can be present even without skin retraction.

Mass Echoes

Most breast cancers present as a mass of diminished echoes to an almost anechoic area. Cole-Beuglet was able to define a mass in 91 percent of infiltrating ductal carcinomas. The greater the tissue reaction anterior to the mass, the less evident is the mass on ultrasound. Medullary carcinomas tend to have more internal echoes than do infiltrating ductal and lobular carcinomas. The smaller the mass, especially those less than 1 cm, the less likely it is that a mass will be evident.

Mass Borders

Most cancers have irregular borders reflecting the invasion into the surrounding tissue. A significant percentage present as a well defined smooth mass. Medullary carcinomas commonly present this way. Cole-Beuglet reported that up to 30 percent of infiltrating ductal and lobular carcinomas also did. It is for this reason that any solid mass must be biopsied, as ultrasound is unable to make an accurate diagnosis.

Posterior Borders

Most cancers have a decreased or absent posterior border. A portion of the entire border may be gone. The diminished echo pattern of the posterior border is different from the posterior shadowing defined below.

Anterior Borders

The tissue reaction anterior to the tumor is caused by tumor spicules with scattering of the ultrasonic echoes. Takehara has termed this reaction the anterior malignant halo.[42] It appears on ultrasound as an irregular area of densely bright echos. It is most pronounced in scirrhous-type cancers. If this echogenicity is intense enough, it may so totally scatter the ultrasound that no pattern can be defined posterior to it.

Shadowing

The total reflection and scattering of the ultrasound beam is termed shadowing. This absence of ultrasonic echoes is reflected on the scans as a black area. The anterior halo and the dense tissue of the cancer may cause marked shadowing. There are two types of shadowing which have been commented on. There is the "dirty" posterior shadowing, which is an area of incomplete shadowing with grayish echoes within the shadow area, and there is the complete, or "clean," shadowing with an almost total absence of echoes within the shadow. The "dirty" shadow is not infrequently seen in dense glandular tissue, whereas the "clean" shadowing is more common with malignancy.

Malignant masses commonly exhibit posterior shadowing. This shadowing may be only a partial posterior shadow of less than the dimension of the mass or posterior shadowing equal to the posterior mass dimension. At times the scattering of the ultrasound is so intense that there is shadowing only present, with no mass discernible.

Conclusion

This overview of breast ultrasound has been presented to acquaint the reader with the varied ultrasonic appearance of many benign and malignant lesions. It is the author's opinion that among the uses of ultrasound are the following:

1. As the primary imaging modality in patients under the age of 30. Mammography is also indicated for any suspicious lesion.
2. For further differentiation of any solitary mass. Ultrasound is done not only for cyst–solid tumor differentiation but for the additional information that ultrasound can provide.
3. For evaluation of the patient with symptoms in order to provide a more definitive answer as to etiology.
4. For evaluation of the pregnant and lactating patient. Although mammography may be extremely important in these patients, in many of them the tissue is too dense to visualize any abnormality except calcifications.
5. As an adjunctive study to physical examination and mammography in patient with dense glandular breasts.
6. As an adjunctive procedure in patients who are at high risk or cancerophobic.
7. For evaluation of the augmented breast and the postirradiated breast.

Even using this list, which may seem overly comprehensive, at the Woman's Breast Center breast ultrasound is used in less than 40 percent of the patients.

References

1. Kossoff G: Quo vadis breast ultrasound, in Jellins J, Kobayashi T (eds): *Ultrasonic Examination of the Breast.* London, Wiley, 1983, pp 9–12.
2. Wild J: The use of ultrasonic pulses for the measurement of biologic tissues. *Surgery* 1950; 27:183-188.
3. Wild J, Reid J: Echographic tissue diagnosis, in Proceedings of the 4th Annual Conference on Ultrasonic Therapy, 1955, pp 47–72.
4. Wild, J: Review of the ultrasonic examination of the breast, in Jellins J, Kobayashi T (eds): *Ultrasonic Examination of the Breast* London, Wiley, 1983, pp 21–30.
5. Howry DH, Stott DA, Bilss WR: The ultrasonic visualization of carcinoma of the breast and other soft-tissue structures. *Cancer* 1954; 7:354.
6. Kelly-Frye E, Harper P: Examination of the female breast by means of mammography, automatic B-mode and rapid real-time ultrasound scanning, in Proceedings of AIUM, p 89.
7. Kobayashi T: Diagnostic ultrasound in breast cancer: Analysis of retrotumorous echo patterns correlated with sonic attenuation by cancerous connective tissue. *J Clin Ultrasound* 1979; 7:471–479.
8. Kobayashi T: *Clinical Ultrasound of the Breast.* New York, Plenum Press, 1978.
9. Kossoff G, Kelley-Frye E, Jellins J: Average velocity of ultrasound in the human female breast. *J Accoust Soc Am* 1973; 53(6):1730–1736.
10. Wagai T, Takahashi S, Ohashi H, et al: A trial for quantitative diagnosis of breast tumor by ultrasono-thermography. *Japan Med Ultrasonics* 1967; 5:39.

11. Wells PNT, et al: Tumor detection by ultrasonic blood flow signals. *Ultrasonics* 1977;15(5)231–232.
12. Wells PNT, Evans KT: An immersion scanner for two-dimensional ultrasonic examination of the human breast. *Ultrasonics* 1968;6:220–228.
13. Cole-Beuglet C, Kurtz AB, Rubin CS, et al: Ultrasound mammography. *Radiol Clin North Am* 1980; 18:133–143.
14. Dempsey PJ Wilson PC: The use of automated sonography in total clinical breast evaluation, in Leopold GR (ed): *Ultrasound in Breast and Endocrine Disease, Clinics in Diagnostic Ultrasound.* New York, Churchill Livingstone, 1984, pp 57–81.
15. Schneck CD, Lehman DA: Sonographic anatomy of the breast. *Semin Ultrasound* 1982; 111(1):13–33.
16. Ezo MG: Tissue compression for the optimization of images in water-path breast scanning. Presented at the AIUM 25th Annual Meeting 1980.
17. Jellins J, Kopssoff G, Reeve TS: Detection and classification of liquid-filled masses in the breast by Gray scale echography. *Radiology* 1977; 125:205–212.
18. Reeve TS, Jellins J, Kossof G, et al: Classification of the sonographic appearance of the normal breast, in Jellins J, Kobayashi T (eds): *Ultrasonic Examination of the Breast* London, Wiley, 1983, pp 149–156.
19. Wolfe, JN: Breast patterns as an index of risk for developing breast cancer. *AJR* Jun 1976;126:1130-1139.
20. Fleisher AC, Muhletaler CA, Reynolds VH, et al: Palpable breast masses: Evaluation by high frequency, hand-held real-time sonography and xeromammography. *Radiology* 1983;148:813–817.
21. Sickles EA, Filly RA, Callen PW: Benign breast lesions: Ultrasound detection and diagnosis. *Radiology* 1984; 151:467–470.
22. Tabar L, Pentek Z, Dean PB: The diagnostic and therapeutic value of breast cyst puncture and pneumocystography. *Radiology* 1981; 141:659–663.
23. Cole-Beuglet C, Soriano RZ, Kurtz AB, et al: Fibroadenoma of the breast: Sonomammography correlated with pathology in 122 patients. *AJR* 1983;140:369–375.
24. Harper AP, Kelly-Fry, E, Noe JS, et al: Ultrasound in the evaluation of solid breast masses. *Radiology* 1983; 146:731–736.
25. Kobayashi T: Current status of interpretative criteria for breast tumor, in Jellins J, Kobayashi T (eds): *Ultrasonic Examination of the Breast*, London, Wiley, 1983, pp 57–64.
26. Behan M, Kazam E: The echographic characteristics of fatty tissues and tumors. *Radiology* 1978;129:143–151.
27. Cole-Beuglet C: Ultrasound, in Basset LW, Gold RH (eds): *Mammography, Thermography, and Ultrasound in Breast Cancer Detection.* Orlando, Grune & Stratton, 1982.
28. Harper P, Kelly-Fry E: Ultrasound visualization of the breast in symptomatic patients. *Radiology* 1980;137:465–469.
29. Matallana R, Orenberg C: Ultrasound diagnosis of mammary duct ectasia, in Jellins J, Kobayashi T (eds): *Ultrasonic Examination of the Breast*, London, Wiley, 1983, pp 319–324.
30. Jellins J, Kossoff G, Reeve TS: The ultrasonic appearance of pathology in the male breast. *Ultrasound Med Biol* 1975;2:43–44.
31. Egan RL, McSweeney MB: Breast sonography—interpretative criteria, in Jellins J, Kobayashi T, (eds): *Ultrasonic Examination of the Breast.* London, Wiley, 1983, pp 307–318.
32. McSweeney MB, Egan RL: Automated breast sonography: Comparison with other imaging modalities, in Jellins J, Kobayashi T (eds) *Ultrasonic Examination of the Breast*, London, Wiley, 1983, pp 325–333.
33. Cole-Beuglet C, Soriano R, Pasto M, et al: Solid breast mass lesions: Can ultrasound differentiate benign and malignant?, in Jellins J, Kobayashi T (eds): *Ultrasonic Examination of the Breast.* London, Wiley, 1983, pp 45–55.
34. Barraclough BH, Jellins J, Barraclough BM, et al: Breast ultrasound, the Australian perspective, in Jellins J, Kobayashi T (eds): *Ultrasonic Examination of the Breast*, London, Wiley, 1983, pp 177–186.
35. Hisa N, Kaneda S. Enomoto K, et al: Diagnosis of small breast cancers by linear-array realtime scanner, in Jellins J, Kobayashi T (eds): *Ultrasonic Examination of the Breast*, London, Wiley, 1983, p 133.

36. Kasumi F, Tanaka H: Detection of microcalcifications in breast carcinoma by ultrasound, in Jellins J, Kobayashi T (eds): *Ultrasonic Examination of the Breast*. London, Wiley, 1983, pp 89–97.
37. Lambi RW, Hodgden D, Herman EM: Sonomammographic manifestations of mammographically detectable breast microcalcifications. *J Ultrasound* 1983; 2:509–514.
38. Sickles EA: Magnification mammography, in Feig SA, McLelland R (eds): *Breast Carcinoma; Current Diagnosis and Treatment*, New York, Masson, 1983.
39. Kelly-Fry E: Breast cancer screening for younger United States women, in Jellins J, Kobayashi T (eds): *Ultrasonic Examination of the Breast*, London, Wiley, 1983, pp 265–273.
40. Croll J: Ultrasound as the decision maker in young patients with breast cancer, in Jellins J, Kobayashi T (eds): *Ultrasonic Examination of the Breast*, London, Wiley, 1983, pp 257–264.
41. Moskowitz M: Significance of minimal breast cancers detected on screening, in Feig SA, McLelland R (eds): *Breast Carcinoma: Current Diagnosis and Treatment,* New York, Masson, 1983, pp 327–332.
42. Kopans DB, Meyer JE, Proppe KH: The double line of skin thickening on sonograms of the breast. *Radiology* 1981;141:485–487.
43. Takehara Y, Hisada Y, Yamada K: Ultrasonic diagnosis of early breast carcinoma—advantages of high-frequency transducer, in Jellins J, Kobayashi T (eds); *Ultrasonic Examination of the Breast*, London, Wiley, 1983; pp 83-88.

4

Transillumination Light Scanning (Diaphanography)

Ernest N. Carlsen

Transillumination light scanning is a noninvasive procedure for examining the breast. It is based on the principles of light scanning and light absorption. The process is an adjuvant procedure to ultrasound, mammography, and physical examination.

Transillumination has been used in medicine for more than 150 years. Its earliest use was for observing babies for hydrocephalus. More recently transillumination has been used to "see through" testicular hydroceles.[1] The transillumination process for breasts was first discussed by Ewing in 1928.[2]

Clinical use of light transmission through the breast was first reported by Cutler in 1929.[3] His group found that by using a high-intensity light in a darkened room breast abnormalities could be visualized by the dark-adapted naked eye. Unfortunately, the process required large amounts of light, thereby producing large amounts of heat. When evaluating the technique Cutler found that the technique had limited ability for distinguishing cystic and solid lesions.

Improvements in the techniques were reported by Gros et al.[4] They developed a water-cooled high-intensity light source that decreased the heat and improved the brightness of the transmission. They also added the capability of obtaining a permanent record, which was best accomplished by using a black and white infrared film. Problems persisted, however: The apparatus was bulky, and the examination required long exposure times. Gros named the process diaphanography.

Ohlsson and his group designed a smaller, hand-held unit, the diaphanoscope.[5] The unit contained a variable light source, fiberoptics, and an air-cooled fan. The images were recorded by a single reflex 35-mm camera system on infrared film using a photoscopic flash unit built into the hand-held unit.

Clinical evaluations from this unit was first reported by Ohlsson et al.[6] and Isard[7] in 1980. It was recognized by these observers that there was a differential in the absorption of visible and infrared light by various lesions. However, most authors subsequently thought that the diaphanograph (infrared film image) did not add any significant data but did improve the discrimination in the younger, dense breast.

In 1980 Carlsen[8] introduced the use of infrared detection equipment linked to television monitors. This innovation provided a better standardization of the technique by providing a live image that could be viewed during the examination and filming. Better coverage of the breast can be ensured. Because of the video nature

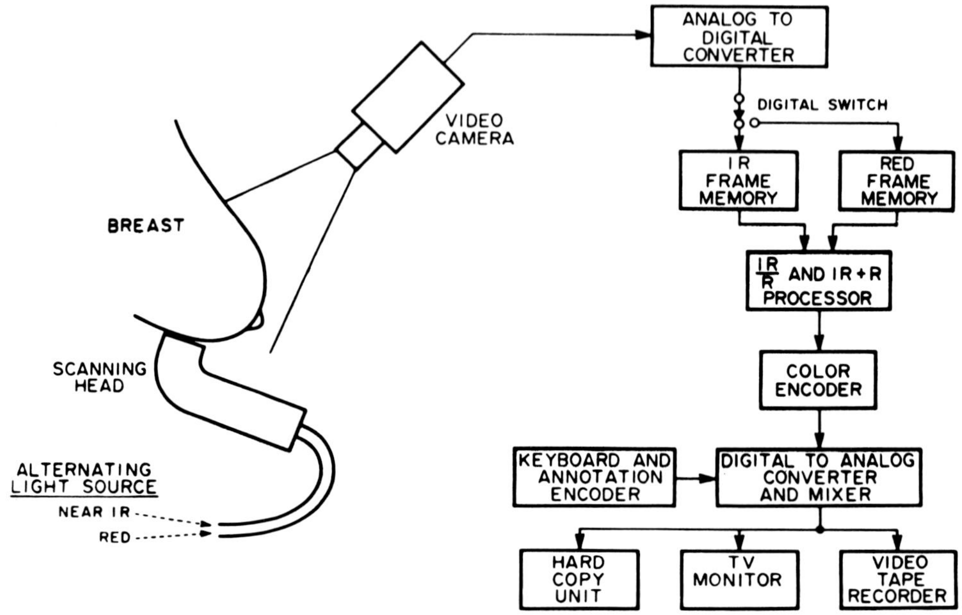

Fig. 4-1 Multispectral light scan system of spectrascan.
Source: Reprinted with permission from *Radiographics* (1984;4:989). © 1984, Radiological Society of North America, Inc.

of the image, Polaroid prints, 35-mm images, or video tape can be obtained. MacDonald's group[9] in 1980 and Mallard[10] in 1981 reported on high-sensitivity television camera techniques. Morton and Miller also reported on the design of a unit which combined film and video diaphanography.[11]

Digitization of the image provides further enhancement techniques.[12] The process of transmission spectroscopy became possible. The process uses selected electromagnetic wavelength bands in the visible and near-infrared range to provide information on the particulate arrangements, the molecular bounding, and the vascularity of the tissue. The technique is a mirage of spectroscope and transillumination.

Figure 4-1 describes a commercial system (Spectrascan, Inc.) that digitizes the signal and processes the information into a final image.[13] Sequential transmission of two wavelength bands are digitized and stored separately. The final image is created from the two digitized images. Two types of processing are performed and displayed in a single image. The intensity (transmission) information is summed (1R + R) and presented as an image relating intensity to brightness on the screen pixel by pixel. The stored data are also used to generate a transmission ratio of 1R to red wavelengths (1R/R). The image display is in real time and is displayed on a color monitor. The ratio data are displayed in color. A variety of process functions are available for postprocessing. Transillumination provides information that is qualitatively different from that obtained by radiographic mammography or ultrasound.

Physics Review of Transillumination

Light is described as both a wave and a particle. Both descriptions are necessary to explain the interaction of light with tissue. In the electromagnetic radiation range, visible light represents only a small portion of the wavelengths (between 400 and 700 nm).

Interaction of Light with Tissue

When light shines on matter, the light can be reflected from the surface, transmitted through the substance, absorbed, or scattered by the molecules of the matter.

Transmission

Transmission is the light that passes through, without interacting with the molecules. This is much like light passing through glass or a vacuum. The incident photons retain their original energies and directions. Usually there is also some degree of reflection, absorption, and scattering.

Reflection

Reflection occurs at surfaces such as the skin and at internal interfaces. Reflection can occur as spectular (related to smooth surfaces), diffuse, or a combination of the two.

Absorption

Absorption is a phenomenon by which a photon of light contacts a molecule and is absorbed, losing its energy to the absorbing molecule. The field of spectroscopy deals with this phenomenon. If a given photon collides with a specific molecule at a proper angle, the photon is absorbed and the molecule is excited from its ground state to a higher energy level. The energy is deposited into vibratory or rotational molecular bond interactions. The excited molecule reverts back to its ground state by giving up this "extra" energy as heat or by reemission of a photon. Both fluorescence and phosphorescence are included in this phenomenon.

Scattering

Scattering occurs when a photon of light either retains its energy or a portion of its energy after collision with molecules. Rayleigh scattering is caused when the photon interacts with molecules or particles that are smaller than the photon's wavelength. The amount of scattering is inversely proportional to the fourth power of the wavelengths. Thus short wavelengths (e.g., light yellow light) scatter more severely than long wavelengths (e.g., infrared light). The scattering is caused by particles larger than the wavelengths (up to 10 wavelengths). The larger scattering particles scatter light at a lower range of exponentials. All of the above phenomena are involved and contribute to developing the image for diagnostic purposes.

Instrumentation Principles

Transillumination systems have two basic components: a light source and a detection system. The amount of transilluminated light (N) can be expressed as $N = No \exp(-\mu L)$ where No is the amount light incident on the tissue and μ is the attenuation coefficient along the light path (L).

Light sources can be described by their spectral output. Several light sources have been used in the range from 400 to 1000 nm. The location of spectral peaks influence the type of image, which is dependent on the particular absorption characteristics of the tissue and the spectral properties of light source. Transmitted light is defined as that light received by the detector. The detector efficiency must be characterized. The detection unit must be sensitive to wavelengths from 400 to 1200 nm. The light transmission appears to be related to tissue type and wavelength.

Mechanisms

Several investigators have attempted to explain the mechanisms involved in the tissue–light interactions. The dominant absorbing substance in the breast is the hemoglobin present. The greater the quantity of blood, the greater is the decrease in transmission. Watmough demonstrated that this situation could happen because of neovascularity.[14] The carbon- and nitrogen-containing radicals appear to the involved in the quantum absorption phenomena.[15,16] These absorptions involve rotational and vibratory motion of the atomic bonds in the molecules.

Fatty tissue transmits well in the 600 to 1200 nm range.[17] No glandular tissue tends to absorb more than fatty tissue. Most of this differential aborption is in the visible region and probably represents the difference in hemoglobin content. Overall attenuation of the light, however, is more likely due to scattering differences between fatty tissue and fibroglandular tissue.[12]

Spatial Resolution

The spatial resolutions of the object to be seen in the breast are dependent on the size of the object and its proximity to the surface of the breast on the detector side. The loss in resolution for deep breast lesions can be explained by light diffusion, interference of scattered wavelengths, and a smaller beam width. The spatial resolution problem can be reduced by a good examination technique.

Examination Technique

The examination is performed in a darkened room with the patient seated facing the examiner. The patient leans slightly forward to allow the breasts to freely fall from the chest wall. Routine views include the craniocaudad, nipple, lateral, medial, and inferior view of each breast. The light source must be placed correctly to permit even illumination of the breast surface that is being viewed by the detector. Chest margins must be clearly visualized. The image size should be adequate to fill the monitor screen but should not cut off the breast image at the edges. The image is best achieved by firm compression. Routine views using the two-wavelength technique requires a balancing of the input light to allow an appropriate dynamic range for the ratio information.

Diagnostic Criteria

The interpretation of breast transillumination is dependent on the detection system. Basically, absorption and vascularity are common to all systems. If available, additional information may be obtained from the ratio information (R value). The absorption of all wavelength groups is evidenced by a dark area. The terms mild, moderate, and marked are usually used to describe the relative levels of absorption. Absorption can be focal, regional, or include the entire breast.

Vascularity can be variously described as clusters of blood vessels (hypervascularity), an abrupt increase in vessel diameter (caliber change), fine branching of major vessels, and small vessels that appear to start and stop. Vascular differences between each breast are evaluated. These differences are not generally used as a criterion for carcinoma, although they may raise suspicions and may be important when compared to the previous studies of the same breast.

The "R-value shift" can be focal or regional and is evidenced by "out of place" color. An R-value shift is a sensitive means of evaluating changes in the internal tissue structures.

The image is analyzed for absorption, asymmetry, vascularity, R-value shift distortions in architecture, nipple retraction, and uneven light transmission.

Clinical Studies

Clinical studies of more modern breast transillumination had its beginning in 1976 with published results by DiMaggio et al.[18] (Table 4-1). These studies used multiple modalities and showed a synergistic effect between the modalities. The series had an overall accuracy rate of 86 percent for 37 cancers. The transillumination equipment was a light transmission system utilizing visual inspection in a darkened room.

In 1979 Ohlsson's group, with a series of 1250 patients, reported that 8 of 9 cancers were correctly identified. This series was later expanded to include 1575 self-selected women among whom 11 of 12 cancers were detected.[5] Four of five occult cancers were detected by transillumination. In an early series by Wallberg

Table 4-1 Breast Transillumination Studies Between 1976 and 1984

Major investigator	No. of patients	No. of biopsied	No. of cancers	Sensitivity (%) Mammography	Sensitivity (%) Light	Ref.
DiMaggio			37	91	86	18
Ohlsson	1575		12	60	92	5
Wallberg	520	275	31	90	90	19
Hussey	51		12	92	92	20
Carlsen	143	148	25	84	92	8
Angquist	259		26	73	77	21
Holliday	176	30	24		83	22
Brown	250	39	15	93	93	23
Carlsen	3293	78	78	82	92	8
Isard	200	200	104		77	7
Marshal	1000	91	34	85	76	24
McIntosh	450	84	14		93	25
Girolamo	523	94	21		75	26
Sickles	1239		83	96	53	27
Bartrum	1200		37	89	80	a
Brown	725	118	47	92	88	a
Merritt	1775	324	64	76	77	13
Benson-Cooper	266	94	46	98	89	28

[a]Personal Communication.

and Alveryd, a sensitivity of 0.90 was achieved for both mammography and transillumination (diaphanography).[19] The series included 520 patients referred for mastodynia, nipple discharge, or a palpable mass. These results were encouraging, although only a few of the lesions were minimal carcinomas. In 1981 Anquist et al. reported on 26 cancers in 259 patients[21]: mammography's sensitivity was 73 percent and that of diaphanography was 77 percent.

Isard, using the equipment designed by Ohlsson, reported on 57 cancers with an accuracy for transillumination of 72 percent.[7] Holliday and Blamey performed double-blind transillumination on 176 patients with an 81 percent accuracy for cancer detection.[22]

Carlsen in 1980 described the use of specially designed transillumination equipment with encouraging early results: a sensitivity of 92 percent based on a selected series of patients being referred for biopsy. There were 25 cancers in the 145 patients. Mammographic sensitivity was 84 percent.[8]

Brown and Shipper[23] had a double-blind study on 250 patients that has now been expanded to 725 patients with 118 biopsies and 47 cancers. The mammographic sensitivity was 92 percent. The light sensitivity was 88 percent. These studies used a commercially available Spectrascan (Brown, personal communication). Carlsen subsequently reported on 3292 patient examinations: 78 cancers were detected with a sensitivity of 92 percent; mammography had a sensitivity of 82 percent; 17 of the carcinomas were nonpalpable.[12]

McIntosh studied 450 patients[25]: There were 84 biopsies performed with 14 cancers found. The light sensitivity was 93 percent with a specificity of approximately 90 percent. Merritt et al. reported a double-blind series of 1,775 patients.[13] There were 323 biopsies reported in the study, with 63 cancers found. Mammographic and light scanning sensitivities were similar at 76 and 77 percent, respectively. Because of the selection criteria many of the patients in the study had dense breasts on mammography. The average tumor size was less than 2 cm; 28 percent of the cancers were less than 1 cm in diameter. The complementary nature of the two examination techniques is illustrated by the fact that the combined sensitivity was 90 percent in the series.

Marshal et al.[24] performed double-blind transillumination and mammography on 1000 patients referred for mammography. Of the 34 cancers biopsied because of palpable or mammographic findings, 26 carcinomas were identified by diagnosticians with less than 4 months' experience. The same transillumination examinations were later shown to experienced interpreters, who detected 32 of the 34 carcinomas. Mammography diagnosed 29 cancers, for a sensitivity of 85 percent. The blinded transillumination sensitivity was 76 percent.

Bartrum and Crow studied 1200 patients in a double-blind study. In the original study 34 carcinomas were found by palpation and mammography.[29] Patients with only a light scan positive were not biopsied. The sensitivities for mammography and light scan are 89 and 80 percent, respectively (personal communication). At subsequent follow-up, since the publishing of the series, four additional carcinomas have been identified, all originally positive only on light scan.

Benson-Cooper and Castor of the Cross Cancer Clinic in Canada examined 266 patients in a double-blind series.[28] Ninety-four biopsies were performed with 46 cancers noted. Mammography sensitivity was 98 percent and that of Spectrascan transillumination 89 percent.

Sickles studied 1239 patients using diaphanography equipment that was assembled from a conglomerate of parts from several technologies. No special care for fine tuning of the technique or equipment was described. Eighty-three cancers were observed. In this nonscreening population mammography showed a sensitivity of 96 percent and diaphanography 53 percent.[27]

Conclusions

Even though transillumination light scanning is still in its infancy compared to techniques such as mammography and ultrasound, it has shown promise as a detector of breast cancer, separate and independent from palpation, mammography, or ultrasound.

Ohlsson, Wallberg, Carlsen, Bartrum, Merritt, and Benson-Cooper all found carcinomas by transillumination not found by mammography. In fact, Merritt et al. found a true synergy between x-ray mammography and transillumination. They were able to increase their sensitivity from approximately 78 percent to 90 percent.

Nonpalpable carcinomas were found by most of the studies. The sensitivity differs not only with the experience of the interpreter but also with the type of equipment used. Even though the sensitivity at this stage of development is less than that of mammography for occult cancers, transillumination can be used in those patients who would not be having a mammogram, under American Cancer Society guidelines, because transillumination can find cancers that are not palpable.

Mammography with its proved reliability is the single test of choice for finding occult carcinoma. On the other hand, if more sensitivity is sought, the nonionizing imaging techniques such as transillumination and ultrasound should be added for a multimodality approach. Continued investigation of these techniques will further define their exact roles.

The reader is referred to later chapters for the usefulness and description of transillumination for specific entities.

References

1. Curling TB: *Hydrocele: A Practical Treatise on the Disease of the Testes, and of the Spermatic Cord and Scrotum.* Philadelphia, Corey & Hart, 1843, p 145.
2. Ewing J: *Neoplastic Diseases*. Philadelphia, Saunders, 1928.
3. Cutler M: Transillumination as an aid in the diagnosis of breast lesions. *Surg Gynecol Obstet* 1929;48:721.
4. Gros CM, Quenneville Y, Hummel Y: Diaphanologic mammaire. *J Radiol Electr* 1972;53:297.
5. Gundersen J, Nilsson D, Ohlsson B: Diaphanography for assessment of mammary changes. *Lakartidningen* 1979;76:1425.
6. Ohlsson B, Gundersen J, Nilsson D: Diaphanography: A method for evaluation of the female breast. *World J Surg* 1980;4:701.
7. Isard HJ: Diaphanography: Transillumination of the breast revisited. Presented to the 4th Annual Meeting, Society for the Study of Breast Disease, Philadelphia, 1980.
8. Carlsen EN: Transillumination light scanning. *Diagn Imaging* 1982;3:28.
9. Hussey G, MacDonald AF, Nichols D, et al: Diaphanography—a comparison with mammography and thermography. *Br J Radiol* 1980;54:163.
10. Mallard J: The noes have it! Do they? Silvanus Thompson memorial lecture. *Br J Radiol* 1981;54:831.
11. Morton R, Miller, SS: Infrared transilluminations using photography and television (videoscopy). *J Audiov Media Med* 1981;4:86.
12. Carlsen EN: Transmission spectroscopy: An improvement in light scanning. *RNM Images* 1983;13:22.
13. Merritt C, Sullivan M, Segaloff A, et al: Real time transillumination light scanning of the breast. *Radiographics* 1984;4:989.
14. Watmough DJ: Diaphanography, mechanisms responsible for the images. *Acta Radiol Oncol* 21:1982.
15. Hardy JD, Muschenheim C: The radiation of heat from the human body. IV. The emission, reflection and transmission of infra-red radiation by the human skin. *J Clin Invest* 1934; 13:817.

16. Coblentz WW: *Investigation of Infra-red Spectra. I. Infra-red Absorption Spectra,* Publication No. 35. Carnegie Institute of Washington, 1905.
17. Cartwright C: Infrared transillumination of the flesh. *J Opt Soc Am* 20, 1930.
18. DiMaggio C, Muzzio PC, et al: Transillumination of the breast. *Radiol Med* 62:401, 1976.
19. Wallberg H, Alveryd A: Investigation with diaphanography, mammography and cytological examination in diagnosis of breast cancer. Report of Huddinge Hospital, Sweden, 1978.
20. Hussey G, MacDonald AF, Nichols D, et al: Diaphanography—a comparison with mammography and thermography. *Br J Radiol* 1980; 54:163.
21. Anquist K, Homlund D, Liliequist B, et al: Diaphanoscopy and diaphanography for breast cancer in clinical practice. *Acta Chir Scand* 1981;147:231.
22. Holliday HW, Blamey RW: Breast transillumination using the sinus diaphanograph. *Br Med J* 1981;283:411.
23. Brown R, Schipper H: Electronic diaphanography as an adjunct to the early diagnosis of breast cancer. Presented at 13th International Cancer Congress, Seattle, 1982.
24. Marshall V, Williams D, Smith K: Light scanning: evaluation of a new modality to screen for breast cancer. Presented at Radiological Society of North America, 1982.
25. McIntosh D: Breast light scanning, a real time breast imaging modality. *J Can Assoc Radiol* 1983;34:288.
26. Girolamo RF, Leis HP Jr: Diaphanography: a fourth dimension in the diagnosis of breast disease? *Breast* 1982;8:16.
27. Sickles EA: Breast cancer detection with transillumination and mammography. *AJR* 1984;142:841.
28. Benson-Cooper D, Castor W: Computer enhanced "lite" scanning of the breast. Presented at the Canadian Radiologic Society Meeting, 1985.
29. Bartrum R Jr, Crow H: Transillumination light scanning to diagnose breast cancer: A feasibility study. *AJR* 1984;142.

5

Thermography

Saar Porrath

The use of body heat to aid in the diagnosis of disease dates to ancient civilizations. Hippocrates used a layer of moist mud on the abdomen to determine the site of infections. The mud overlying the abnormality would tend to dry out the soonest, signaling an underlying "hot" area. The medical imaging of heat has now advanced to where the newer heat detection cameras can differentiate the heat from individual sweat glands.

Breast thermography was started by the observation of Lawson[1] that the temperature of the blood exiting a tumor was higher than the blood entering it. The initial work utilized thermocouples embedded into the tissue. As military equipment for heat detection became declassified following World War II, the ability to detect the heat emitted from the breast by external means was available.

Thermography has evolved into three detection methods: infrared, contact, and microwave. The body emits infrared rays which are electromagnetic waves of a defined wavelength. Because they are invisible to the human eye they must be detected by specialized equipment. This is usually done by focusing the infrared rays using a mirror optical system onto a supercooled detector made of mercury–cadmium–telluride or indium antimonide. The cooling is done with liquid nitrogen. The infrared energy is converted to an electrical signal that is then displayed on a cathode ray tube. Photography of this output provides a permanent image. This system is called telethermography. A version of telethermography termed computed thermography uses similar detectors arranged in rows that are then linked to a computer. The telethermography images, originally displayed in black and white, are now also available in colors graded to the shades of gray, black, and white.[2]

Contact thermography utilizes cholesteric crystals, which have the ability to react to heat by changing their internal pitch. Pitch, simplistically, is the height of the crystal. As this pitch changes it reflects a different color when viewed with white light.[3] Originally the cholesteric crystals were painted onto the body using a black base, an effective but extremely time-consuming and messy procedure. More recently the crystals have been embedded in a rubberized sheet, initially stiff, but later flexible, allowing direct contact of the crystals with the skin to reflect skin temperature. This image is recorded on photographic film.

Microwave thermography is the newest of the techniques. It detects microwaves emitted by the body at lower wavelengths than infrared. The microwaves are detected by the use of an antenna positioned close to the body. These signals are then directed to a special tuner, where they are converted to a readable image.[4–7]

All of the above systems have resolutions of 0.1 to 0.2° C. This degree of temperature resolution has not been found to be necessary in breast thermography, which normally uses temperature ranges of 0.5° C or greater.[6,8]

Breast thermography, although accepted throughout Europe, has become very controversial in the United States. A review of the controversy is outlined here, although based on personal experience this author is somewhat biased in favor of thermography.

Clinical Studies

There are two French studies involving large numbers of patients. The first is the work of the Marseilles Cancer Institute,[4,9] which reported on 4716 consecutive cases of proved breast cancer seen between June 1970 and December 1982. There were a multitude of tests used on many of the patients, although all patients did not undergo all of the tests. Their results showed that physical examination was positive in 4121 of 4716 cases (88%), mammography in 4147 of 4424 cases (94%), thermography in 4138 of 4716 cases (88%), ultrasound in 616 of 646 cases (95%), and needle aspiration cytology in 2111 of 2204 cases (96%).

Of particular interest is the subgroup that was singled out, the patients with early breast cancer. This group, with 680 patients, included only those with a tumor less than 2 cm in diameter. Mammography was positive in 75 percent of the cases, physical examination in 60 percent, and infrared thermography in 72 percent. They found that if mammography and physical examination only were used there was a false-negative rate of 20 percent, which decreased to 3 percent with the addition of thermography. (This approach needs to be explained further. The addition of thermography often led to needle aspiration or further testing of an area, but surgery was not done on the basis of a positive thermogram alone.) Of the 165 T0 breast cancers, cancers that were nonpalpable and under 2 cm, physical examination was obviously negative in all. Mammography was 46 percent positive. Thermography was 85 percent accurate. More importantly, 53 percent of these cases were originally detected by thermography only, which necessitated close follow-up so that the cancers were later seen by another method.

The second of the French studies to be mentioned is that of Gautherie, Gros, and co-workers. These examiners, utilizing a classification of thermography, examined 58,000 women over a 12-year period. The patients were classified by a scale of I to V. Approximately 90 percent of the patients in class Th IV and Th V were shown to have cancer. It is the Th III group that is of particular interest. A class Th III thermogram is an equivocal or borderline thermogram in the Gautherie-Gros classification. There were 1563 women in this group, 2.5 percent of the total. Follow-up was possible in 1527 of these patients. On initial examination 282 (18%) were found to have cancer. The others were followed for as long as 12 years. On the basis of testing (mammography, ultrasound, needle biopsy) 784 (51%) were called normal, and 461 (30%) were diagnosed as benign disease. Of the normal group, negative on all examinations but with an equivocal thermogram, 177 were found to have cancer within 2 years and an additional 121 within another 2 years. The final figure was 198 of 784, giving a cancer rate in this total group of 38 percent. Of the group of 461 who were diagnosed on mammography, ultrasound, needle biopsy, or a combination of these procedures as having benign disease, 44 percent were found to have cancer. Other European studies (especially noteworthy are those of Stark in England) have also shown that in their hands a positive thermogram had a high risk for the detection of cancer.[13–15]

Isard[16,17] in the United States has been one of the leaders of breast diagnosis and the multimodality approach. Although his classification of thermograms differs from that of the French, he found thermography to be positive in 72 percent of 270 breast cancers; and if the equivocal group was included, 85 percent of all cancers were within the thermographically significant group. Hobbins has found a positive thermogram to be 10 times the risk of a positive family history.[18]

If these and other studies are positive, what then are the negative studies. There are three that are of note: those of Threatt, Moskowitz, and the experience of the Breast Cancer Detection Demonstration Project (BCDDP).[19]

Threatt et al.[20] organized a group of 576 thermograms (515 patients), which were divided into three categories. The first group was comprised of normal women who had no breast cancer over a 5-year follow-up. The second was an "incident cancer" group discovered to have cancer after a normal screening. The third group had normal screening visits and interval cancers. The thermograms were read blindly by 10 expert thermographers. There was no significant difference in the readings of the three groups. The strength of this study is in the relatively localized nature of the cancers and its screening aspect.

There are two studies by Moskowitz et al. that are of note.[21,22] The first was a blind reading of thermograms of both normal and cancer patients. There was no difference between the ability of experts and untrained readers in detecting the thermograms of the patients who had early breast cancers or stage I cancer. In addition, neither group was able to detect with any significant accuracy the cancer patients. The second study by Moskowitz et al. was on a group of prebiopsy patients who were later differentiated into biopsy-proved proliferative disorders, benign non-proliferative disease, and normal patients. The thermograms were read by an expert thermographer who could not find any difference between the groups.

The third negative experience of note was that of the BCDDP. There were 27 centers selected as part of this important study. Thermography was included by all the centers participating. When the interval results were reported at 3 years, the overall results of thermography were about 50 percent. Thermography was discontinued at most of the centers.[23]

Discussion

How can these opposite results, as well as the ability of some observors and the inability of others to find thermography useful be reconciled? It has been this author's observation that many physicians have undertaken breast thermography with little understanding of the need to, or how to, obtain excellent thermographic images. In addition, most readers of thermography look for hot or cold areas using no other system of classification.

From a technical aspect thermography must be obtained under standardized conditions. The room must be cooled and draft-free. The patient must be unclothed in the areas to be examined and allowed sufficient time for the skin overlying the breast to equilibrate to room temperature.[24] Approximately 50 percent of the patients referred to the Woman's Breast Center because of a positive thermogram done at a primary care physician's office are actually normal when the thermogram is obtained under more stringent conditions.

There are a number of thermographic reading or classification systems: those of Tricore, Gautherie, Isard, Hobbins, and others. Each of these systems in the hands of its proponent has produced excellent results. The imager who undertakes breast thermography should understand the differences of these systems and adopt one system to be used so that the readings are standardized.

The experience of the BCDDP is perhaps a prime example of the need for standardization. Of the 27 centers, most of the reviewers had no prior experience with thermography and were given a training course before starting. Their results reflect their inexperience, with less than 50 percent accuracy. There were three centers run by experienced thermographers—Isard, Haberman, and Abernathy—that reported excellent results. For example, Abernathy (personal communication) reported that 44 percent of the patients who developed cancer after a normal first screening with physical examination and mammography had a positive thermogram prior to detection of the cancer by other means.

One of the reasons for the difference in acceptance of thermography in Europe, and the dissatisfaction in the United States, is the difference in the role of thermography. Too much was expected of breast thermography in the United States. It was advertised by clinicians and commercial companies as a stand alone test to discover breast cancer. In the European experience thermography was never meant to be used by itself, but was used as an integral part of an overall approach to breast cancer diagnosis. A positive thermogram does not necessarily mean that the patient has a breast cancer. Thermography is used by the French to identify patients who are at higher risk. These patients are then followed closely. It also prompts a more careful scrutiny of the tests to be sure they are normal.

There has been frustration because, unlike a positive physical examination or a positive mammogram, a positive thermogram does not direct the surgeon to the site of the cancer. For those readers who have not performed thermography, this is an important point to understand. Thermographic findings are nonspecific. A deep cancer may appear as a hot nipple or a central cancer as increased vascularity inferiorly. The site of the cancer is not delineated on thermography in many cases.

There are numerous causes of a positive thermogram. Among them are anatomic variants with prominent superficial veins on one breast, blockage of a main venous channel such as the superior vena cava with collateral circulation, benign lesions, hormonal changes to the breast, improper technique of obtaining the thermogram, and infections.

Surgery in the form of biopsy should not change the thermographic pattern of the breast.[25] Breast augmentation does not usually affect the thermographic pattern. The use of a silicone gel implant may, however, affect the heat distribution, as the silicone implant absorbs more of the heat from the underlying tissues and decreases the overall temperature of the breast. This is not true of silicone injections in the breast.

Huber et al. reported on the use of thermography of the breast for the detection of hormonal changes of the breast, specifically progesterone shortage.[26] Porrath reported on an entity called hormone mastitis.[27] The patients were primarily in their thirties and forties. They presented with moderate to severe breast pain of 3 to 8 weeks' duration, with little change of the pain during the menstrual cycle. The pain was usually unilateral. Physical examination, mammography, and ultrasound were normal, whereas the thermogram was equivocal (Gautherie class III) in almost all of these patients. The pain was unresponsive to cessation of caffeine or dietary changes. These patients, as in Huber's study, were treated with topical progesterone cream. The pain resolved in almost all of the patients, and the thermogram became normal within a short time. It can be argued that application of progesterone for the relief of the pain may have been no more effective than the application of any cream to the breast if it were not for the resolution of the thermographic abnormalities.

Thermography is very sensitive to any infection or inflammation within the breast. It has proved excellent in the follow-up of infections; if the thermogram remains positive, further antibiotics are needed. It has proved especially useful in the evaluation of the augmented breast with pain, quickly ruling in or out infectious processes or rejection phenomena. A normal thermogram virtually assures the observer that there is no infection or rejection process.

When evaluating breast pain, a normal thermogram rules out infection or hormonal mastitis. When evaluating other benign conditions, thermography may play a moderate role. The role is further discussed in Section II, later in this book.

The basis for using thermography in the follow-up of patients with lumpectomy and radiation therapy has been well documented by Gautherie.[28] He showed that when the breast temperature does not return to normal following irradiation there is a greater chance of a recurrence.

There have been numerous reports in the literature[9,16,27] demonstrating that patients with cancer who have a more positive thermogram (Th IV or Th V) have a worse prognosis than those who have either a normal or "cold cancer" and an equivocal thermogram. This finding may be simply a function of the size of the tumor and the amount of its infiltration rather than being related to the inherent aggresiveness of the cancer. The use of thermography in treatment has been advocated in inflammatory breast cancer. Advocates recommend treating the inflammatory breast cancer with chemotherapy until the thermogram becomes normal, then proceed with mastectomy.

Summary

The use of thermography in the detection of breast cancer has been sumarized. The reader is referred to the original articles for further evaluation. Thermography is advocated as an adjunctive procedure and should not be used as a stand-alone evaluator for the presence of breast cancer. A positive thermogram must be explained, however, as should any positive test. A thermogram should not be called a false-positive test until the etiology of the abnormality is explained or the patient followed for a sufficient time interval to be sure that the thermogram has not signaled an undetected breast cancer. A positive thermogram often causes the imager to evaluate the other tests more closely, sometimes finding something that may have been overlooked initially. It can be said that all examinations should be carefully looked at; although this statement is true, in reality a second look can be useful.

Thermography has a place in the diagnosis of benign disease, especially with infections. It is the only objective test for the evaluation of hormonal problems in the breast and their treatment.

References

1. Lawson R: Implications of surface temperatures in the diagnosis of breast cancer. *Can Med Assoc J* 1956;75:309–310.
2. Milbrath JR: Thermography, in Baset LW, Gold RH (eds): *Mammography, Thermography, & Ultrasound in Breast Cancer Detection.* Orlando, Grune & Stratton, 1982, pp 143–149.
3. Katz S: Evaluation of design requirements for a liquid crystal thermographic system, in Gautherie M, Albert E, Keith L (eds): *Thermal Assessment of Breast Health*. Boston, MTP Press, 1984, pp 11–17.
4. Amalric R, Giraud D, Altschuler C, et al: The contribution of the infrared thermography to the integrated diagnosis of early breast cancer, in Gautherie M, Albert E, Keith L (eds): *Thermal Assessment of Breast Health.* Boston, MTP Press, 1984, pp 11–17.
5. André J, Barthelemy R, Lefeuvre S, et al: Heating blood in extracorporal circulation with a high-frequency electromagnetic field: Effect of microwaves on blood, in Gautherie M, Albert E (eds): *Biomedical Thermology,* New York, Alan R. Liss, 1982, pp 257–268.
6. Ring EFJ: Technical advances in thermal imaging, in Gautherie M, Albert E, Keith L (eds): *Thermal Assessment of Breast Health.* Boston, MTP Press, 1984, pp 3–10.

7. Szmigielski S: Immunological response of mammals to microwaves, in Gautherie M, Albert E, (eds): *Biomedical Thermology.* New York, Alan R. Liss, 1982, pp 227–246.
8. Schaeffer J, El-Mahdi AM, Carr KL: Thermographic detection of human cancers by microwave radiometry, in Gautherie, M, Albert E (eds): *Biomedical Thermology.* New York, Alan R. Liss, 1982, pp 227–246.
9. Amalric R, Giraud D, Altschuler C, et al: Does infrared thermography truly have a role in present-day breast management? in Gautherie M, Albert E (eds): *Biomedical Thermology.* New York, Alan R. Liss, 1982, pp 269–278.
10. Gautherie M, Gros G: Breast thermography and cancer risk prediction. *Cancer* 1980;45:51.
11. Gautherie M, Haehnel P, Walter JP, et al: Improved survival rate of breast cancer patients with an early diagnosis based on initial thermal assessment and subsequent follow-up, in Gautherie M, Albert E, Keith L (eds): *Thermal Assessment of Breast Health.* Boston, MTP Press, 1984, pp 11–17.
12. Gautherie M, Haehnel P, Walter JP, et al: Long-term assessment of breast cancer risk by liquid crystal thermal imaging, in Gautherie M, Albert E (eds): *Biomedical Thermology.* New York, Alan R. Liss, 1982, pp 227–246.
13. Stark AM, Way S: The significance of an abnormal breast thermogram. *Acta Thermogr.* 1976;1:33–37.
14. Stark AM: The value of risk factors in screening for breast cancer. *Eur J Surg Oncol* 1985;11:147–150.
15. Stark AM, Way S: The screening of well women for the early detection of breast cancer using clinical examination with thermography and mammography. *Cancer* 1974;33:1671–1679.
16. Isard HJ: Breast disease and correlation of images: Mammography-thermography-diaphanography, in Gautherie M, Albert E (eds): *Biomedical Thermology.* New York, Alan R. Liss, 1982, pp 321–328.
17. Isard HJ: The many faces of breast images, in Gautherie M, Albert E, Keith L (eds): *Thermal Assessment of Breast Health.* Boston, MTP Press, 1984, pp 221–227.
18. Hobbins WB: Thermography, highest risk marker in breast cancer. *Proceedings of the Gynecological Society for the Study of Breast Disease,* 1977, pp 267–282.
19. Porrath S, Bernay T: The role of thermography in the multimodality approach to breast cancer diagnosis, in Gautherie M, Albert E, Keith L (eds): *Thermal Assessment of Breast Health.* Boston, MTP Press, 1984, pp 156–166.
20. Threatt B, Norbeck JM, Ullman NS, et al: Thermography and breast cancer: An analysis of a blind reading. *Ann NY Acad Sci* 1980;355:501–519.
21. Moskowitz M, Fox SH, Brun del Re R, et al: The potential value of liquid crystal thermography in detecting significant mastopathy. *Radiology* 1981;140:659–662.
22. Moskowitz M, Milbrath J, Gartside P, et al: Lack of efficacy of thermography as a screening tool for minimal and stage I breast cancer. *N Engl J Med* 1976;295:249–252.
23. Baker L: Breast cancer detection demonstration project: Five-year summary report. *CA* 1982;32:194–225.
24. Ring EFJ: Standardization of thermal imaging in medicine: Physical and environmental factors, in Gautherie M, Albert E, Keith L (eds): *Thermal Assessment of Breast Health.* Boston, MTP Press, 1984, pp 29–36.
25. Porrath S, Sandhu R, McNeil J: Thermography in the post surgery and post plastic surgery breast, in *Proceedings of the American Academy of Thermography,* Los Angeles, 1984. In press.
26. Huber CJ, Pons JY, Patrau A: Breast fibrocystic disease and thermography. *Acta Thermogr.* 1980;5:48–50.
27. Porrath S: Hormone mastitis. Presented at a meeting of the Society for the Study of Breast Disease, San Francisco, 1984.
28. Gautherie M: Temperature and blood flow patterns in breast cancer during natural evolution and following radiotherapy, in Gautherie M, Albert E (eds): *Biomedical Thermology.* New York, Alan R. Liss, 1982, pp 21–64.

6

Contrast Ductography and Duct Fluid Cytology

Otto W. Sartorius

Contrast ductography, combined with duct fluid exfoliative cytology, can be a powerful tool for the diagnosis and localization of benign and malignant intraductal lesions of the breast. Historically, contrast ductography is not a new diagnostic modality. There are numerous reports in the literature attesting to its value in the location of occult intraductal lesions that produce spontaneous nipple discharge. During the late 1930s Hicken et al.[1,2] reported on 625 contrast ductograms obtained by injection through a 27-gauge needle of stabilized thorium dioxide solution or carbon dioxide. Such neoplasms as lipomas, fibromas, papillomas, cysts, galactoceles, and carcinomas were reported as having been visualized and diagnosed by this method. Only three breast abscesses developed. Later, Reis and Mesirow[3] and Romano and McFetridge[4] cautioned against the use of this procedure after finding severe tissue reaction, with occasional abscess formation, secondary to the radiation effects of colloidal thorium dioxide. The subsequent availability of water-soluble contrast media served to rekindle interest in mammary ductography. This interest resulted in excellent studies by Góes,[5] Björn-Hanson,[6] Funderburk et al,[7,8] Quimet-Oliva and Herbert,[9] and Threatt and Appelman.[10] These studies were performed almost exclusively on spontaneously discharging ducts, using blunt 27- or 30-gauge needles.

One of the major problems with the technique of contrast ductography has been the difficulty of entering a duct with the needles or cannulas available. There have been instances of not being able to enter a spontaneously discharging duct. Furthermore, the rigid needle may result in penetration of the duct wall, causing extravasation of contrast material and discomfort to the patient. Another limitation of the technique is that it cannot be applied to a nondischarging duct. The surface orifice of a nondischarging duct either cannot be visualized or is too small to permit entry of the blunt needle or cannula. In 1972 an improved technique for visualization of the mammary duct system was developed for the detection and localization of cytologically positive, but otherwise occult, lesions.[11,12] The development of ultra-thin nylon catheters (0.008 inch outside diameter) together with enhanced visibility of the duct orifices provided by a dissecting microscope with 20× to 80× magnification, has made contrast ductography a relatively simple, rapidly performed, painless procedure (Fig. 6-1).

Mammary ducts yielding spontaneous discharge or abnormal aspirated fluids can be readily cannulated, thereby providing a reliable method for the detection and localization of intraductal lesions or disease states. Contrast ductograms aid in the

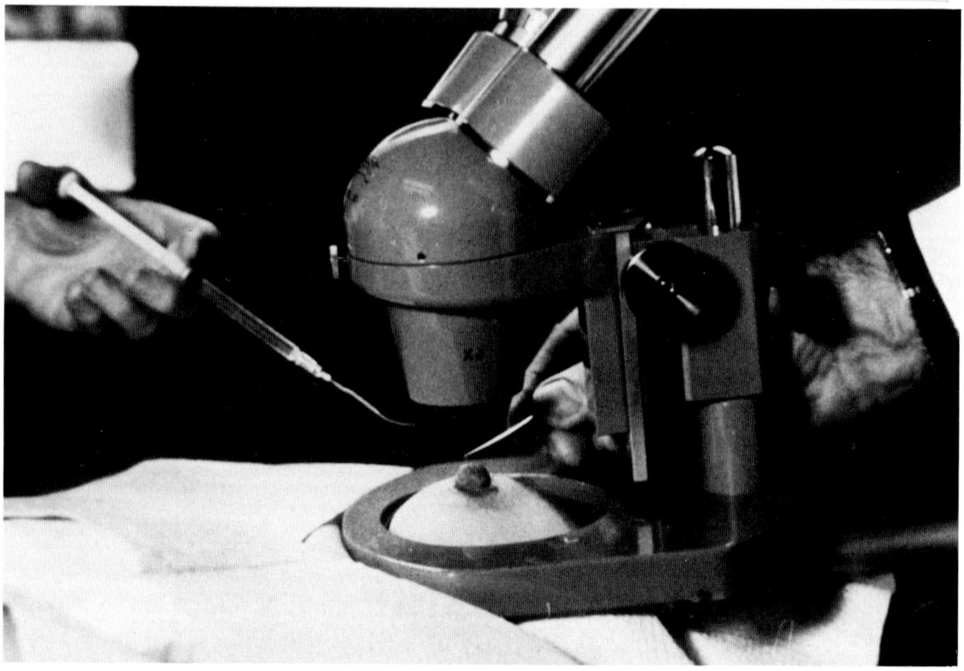

Fig. 6-1 Dissecting scope mounted on an adjustable arm and stand for correct positioning over the breast.

visualization and diagnosis of dilated ducts as well as lesions in direct communication with the ductal system, e.g., fibroadenoms, communicating cysts, and intracystic papillomas. Clustered calcifications, including those occasionally seen in degenerated papillomas or fibroadenomas, and the extravasation associated with infiltrating carcinomas can be identified with more accuracy.

Details of the technique and the interpretation of the resultant radiographs have been presented elsewhere.[1,2] After obtaining satisfactory lateral and cephalocauded x-ray views of the ductograms, 0.5 ml of sterile isotonic solution is injected into the duct via the catheter for reaspiration, collection, and cytologic evaluation. This aspirate provides an abundant number of duct-lining epithelial cells and may contribute significantly to the cytologic interpretation obtained from the initially aspirated duct fluid. Methods of aspirating fluid from the nipples are described in detail elsewhere.[13,14] Briefly, the aspiration device (Diagnostic, Inc., St. Paul, MN) is used to apply negative pressure to the nipple (Fig. 6-2), and the obtained fluid is collected with a 21-gauge needle and a 3 cc disposable plastic syringe that contains a small amount of isotonic solution. The fluid thus obtained is immediately mixed with 3 cc of Polyonic R148 (Cutter Laboratories, Berkely, CA) containing 20% alcohol, tested with a Hemostix for the presence of blood and sent for cytologic evaluation.

The classification for breast duct cells is described elsewhere.[13,14] Briefly, cells are classified as normal or hyperplastic; papillary groups; atypical hyperplastic cells; and "consistent with carcinoma" (Fig. 6-3). For an adequate diagnosis, approximately 50 to 100 well preserved duct epithelial cells must be present either as single cells, small groups, or as organized groups for the specimen to be considered satisfactory. When cells fit more than one category, the specimen is graded into the most abnormal cytologic category observed.

The greatest usefulness of contrast ductography combined with duct exfoliative cytology is apparent in patients having spontaneous nipple discharge and to a lesser,

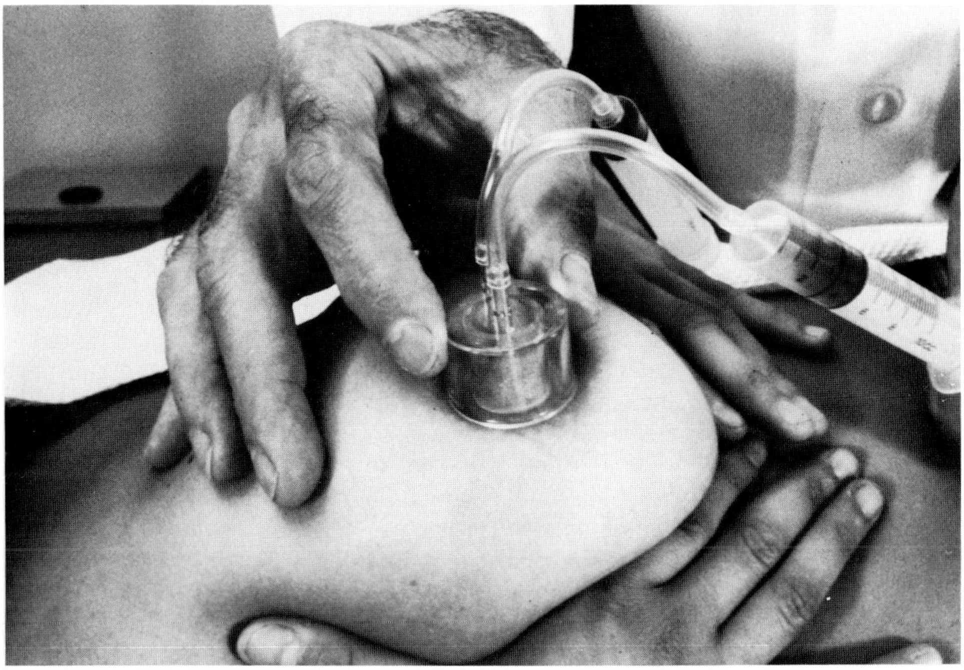

Fig. 6-2 Aspiration device is placed over the patient's nipple while the patient compresses the base of her breast with both hands.

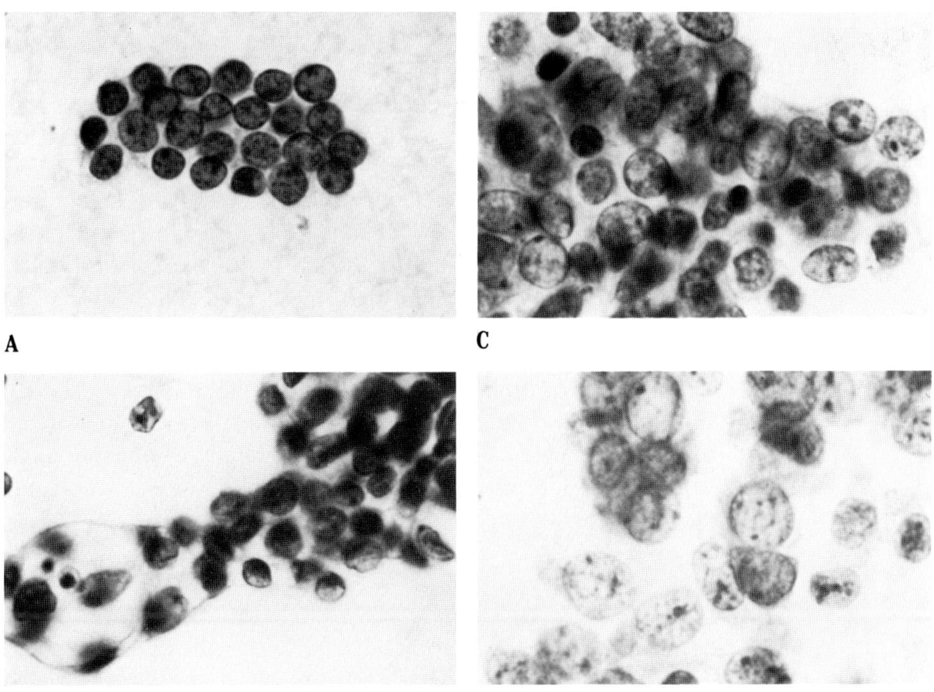

A C

B D

Fig. 6-3 Duct epithelial cell classification: **(a)** Normal ductal cells, uniform in size and shape. **(b)** Hyperplastic cells having a semblance of structure and suggesting papilloma. **(c)** Atypical hyperplastic cells showing nuclear alterations. **(d)** "Consistent with carcinoma." There are multiple enlarged abnormal nuclei, and cells lack cohesiveness. (×1250) but significant extent with aspirated duct fluids. The management of patients with spontaneous or abnormal secretions from the nonlactating nipple has been controversial. When spontaneous secretion or the finding of abnormal nipple fluids is associated with a palpable mass or positive mammographic findings, the problem has been less controversial and surgical biopsy is the indicated procedure.[5] However, most women with abnormal nipple fluids do not present with other positive findings, leaving the diagnosis in doubt.[15,16] In these cases of otherwise spontaneous nipple discharge, surgical procedures such as complete excision of all of the central primary ducts,[17] complete excision of a major duct system,[18,19] or total mastectomy[20] have been performed for spontaneous bloody discharge. In some cases such surgical procedures have been performed without benefit of a preoperative diagnosis, without knowledge of the extent or localization of the causative condition, and without knowing if surgical intervention could have been avoided.

Ironically, however, fluid expressed from the nipple or withdrawn by aspiration is largely ignored and attributed to physiologic secretion.[17] It is not generally appreciated that the nonlactating breast is a functioning organ that secretes and reabsorbs fluid continuously. Proteolytic enzymes within this fluid degrade the exfoliated ductal and lobular epithelial cells, thereby permitting reabsorption via the ductal venous plexus. Sphincters located a few millimeters beneath the duct orifices on the nipple surface serve to prevent the escape of this ductal fluid under normal conditions. By applying mild suction to the nipple, this fluid can be aspirated from a large proportion of nonlactating women.[14]

Spontaneous discharge of breast fluid occurs when various disease processes have disturbed the balance between secretion and reabsorption of the fluid to the point where intraductal pressure exceeds the restrictive action of the sphincter.[14] At lesser pressures or at an earlier stage in the development of the disease process, similar fluid may be aspirated. Spontaneous secretion may appear suddenly owing to intraductal bleeding. In other instances it may be detected only indirectly as tiny spots on undergarments. This author holds untenable the oft quoted statement that duct fluids obtained through suction are physiologic and have no pathologic significance.[17,18,21] Certainly, many fluids so obtained do not signify a disease state, for as pointed out above there exists physiologically constant secretion and reabsorption of intraductal fluid in the normal breast. However, intraductal pathologic lesions do develop and can be diagnosed by their exfoliated cells.[22,23]

That the epithelial cells of the primary ducts are capable of secreting fluid can be justifiably assumed by the observation that the duct between an occluding papilloma or other hyperplastic lesion and the terminal sphincter is always dilated with fluid. When emptied, the duct rapidly fills with increased pressure, the spontaneous secretion recurring only when the pressure again increases. It has been observed that this reaccumulated fluid is similar chemically to physiologically obtained duct fluid and differs only in its content of exfoliated cells, which reflects the disease process.

Results

A total of 471 breast disorders, including 24 carcinomas, were evaluated by the combined use of duct fluid cytology and contrast ductography. Of these cases, 140 patients presented with spontaneous discharge, and 331 were investigated because of abnormal nipple aspirates. The latter group was comprised of (1) those patients having either grossly bloody fluid on nipple aspiration or a copious amount of thin yellow or other pigmented fluid from a single duct orifice, and (2) those patients

Table 6-1 Spontaneous Discharge Diagnosed by Contrast Ductography and Cytology

	Patients		Surgery	
Type of lesion	No.	%	No.	%
Intraductal papilloma	61	43.5	61	100
Papillomatosis, duct hyperplasia	46	33	7	15
Duct ectasia, duct dilation, and cysts	19	135	0	0
Adenosis or sclerosing adenosis	6	4	1	17
Carcinoma	8	6	8	100
Total	140	100	77	55

whose aspirated fluids were either Hematest-positive or were reported on cytology to contain papillomatous cell clumps, atypical cells, or cells suspicious for malignancy.

Spontaneous Fluid

Of the 140 patients examined because of spontaneous discharge (Table 6-1), 61 (43.5%) were found to have intraductal papillomas, 49 of which (80%) were occult to other diagnostic modalities. Four were multiple, three were intracystic, and three were classified as multiradicular (growing into side ducts). The duct fluid was usually yellow, thin in consistency, and abundant. Bloody or Hemastix-positive fluids were found in 52 (85%). On contrast ductography, the projection of the lesion into the lumen produced a smoothly marginated negative concave image, similar to the image illustrated in Fig. 6-4. This type of image has not been observed with any other intraductal lesion or disease process. All of the papillomas were associated with evidence of ductal dilatation, presumably the result of increased fluid secretion. When the lesions produced complete obstruction of the duct, the resultant ductal dilatation was observed to occur between the lesion and the nipple; with incomplete blockage, dilation could be seen beyond the lesion. In two cases the increased fluid secretion produced localized ductal dilatation, resulting in cyst formation containing an intracystic papilloma (Fig. 6-5).

Spontaneous secretion is frequently found in association with generalized disease entities subcategorized under the misleading label "fibrocystic disease." In this series 71 (51%) of the cases fell into this general category. Of these, there were 46 (33%) cases of papillomatosis or ductal hyperplasia (7 of which exhibited sufficient duct cell atypia to warrant biopsy), 19 cases of duct ectasia or duct dilatation with or without cyst formation (Fig. 6-6), and 6 cases of adenosis or sclerosing adenosis, one of which had cell atypia and required biopsy. As a rule, these disease states are not improved by surgical intervention. Yet this group comprises a large percentage of all patients undergoing surgery for abnormal nipple secretion. For example, duct hyperplasia or papillomatosis, in the absence of significant cell atypia, is commonly seen in women between the ages of 30 and 50, and is one of the more common components of the "fibrocystic complex." Recognition of this benign condition is important as the increased cellularity and resultant hypersecretion may be associated with duct dilatation and spontaneous discharge. This condition accounts for approximately one-third of the cases, which if unrecognized may cause the patient to have unnecessary surgery. Recognition of papillomatosis is readily and simply accomplished by cytologic study that reveals (1) many foam or degenerating epithelial cells and (2) single or small clumps of cohesive duct cells that are uniform

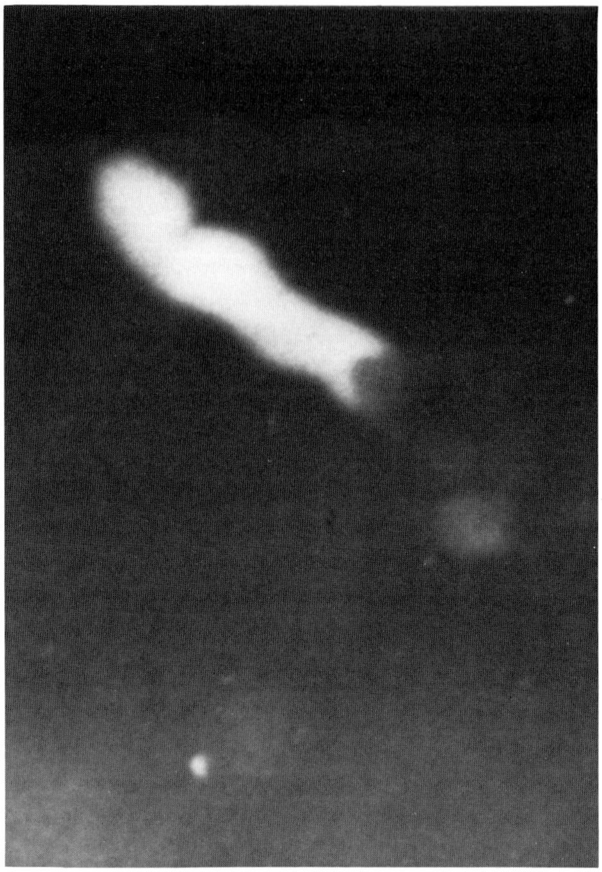

Fig. 6-4 Solitary papilloma in a 71-year-old woman with spontaneous discharge of yellow fluid. Cells were positive for papilloma. Note the convexity into the contrast column.

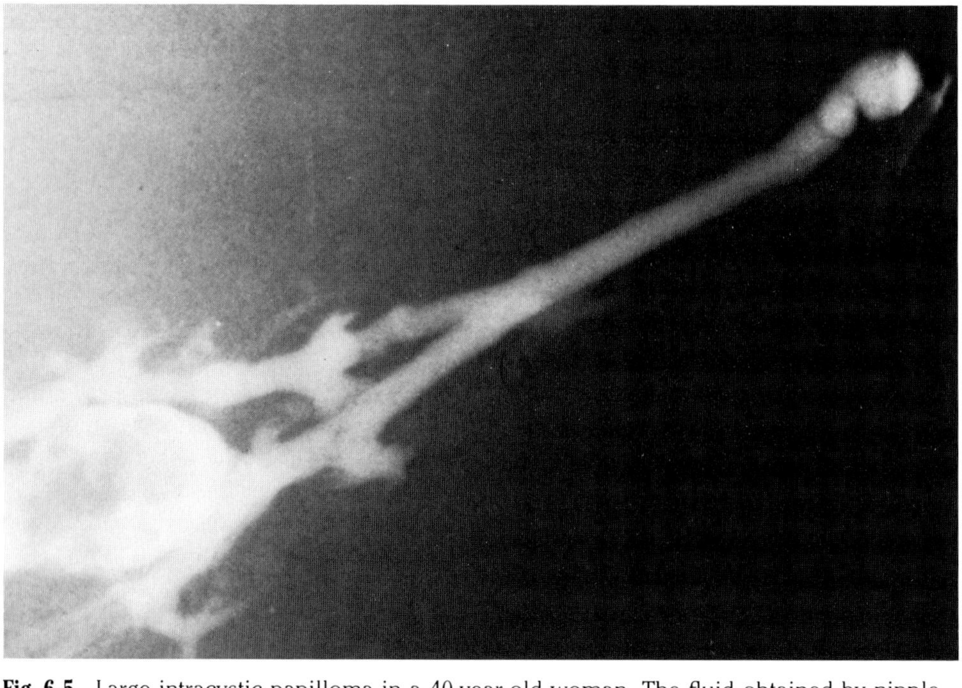

Fig. 6-5 Large intracystic papilloma in a 40-year-old woman. The fluid obtained by nipple aspiration was Hematest-positive.

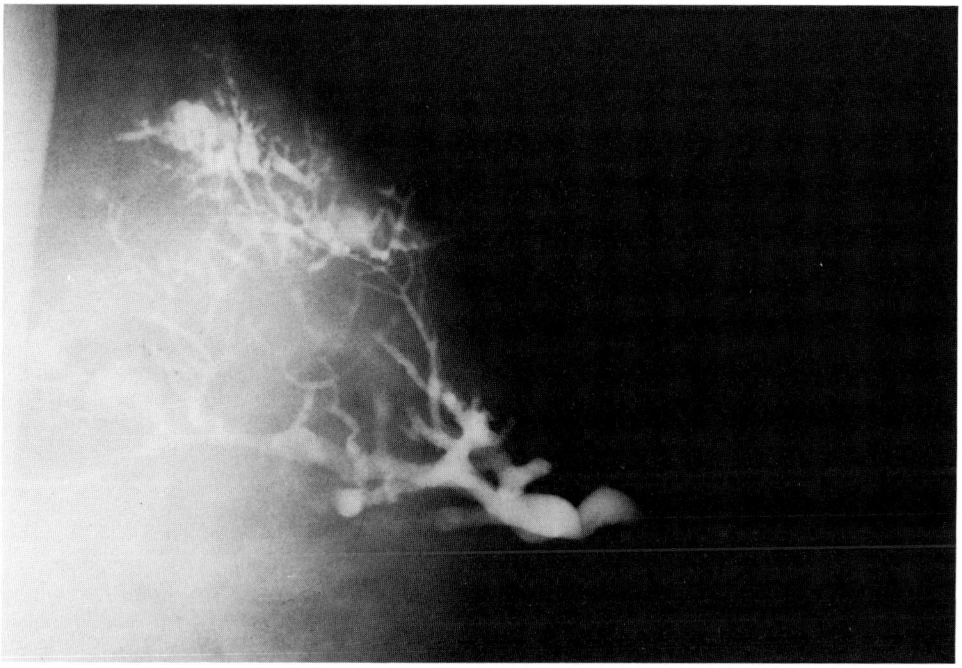

Fig. 6-6 Dilated ducts with papillomatosis and cyst formation in a 46-year-old woman.

in size and exhibit normal or slightly atypical nuclear morphology. Contrast ductography confirms the diagnosis, with areas of irregularity of the duct wall produced by the piling up of cells. There is also duct dilatation, frequent "accordian-like" pleating of the duct wall, and blockage of many small duct branches.

Contrast images of duct ectasia and duct dilatation are self-explanatory. The duct fluids from duct ectasias are usually green and of a thick consistency; they can be very abundant. Clear, watery fluid has been reported to be associated with carcinoma.[17] In my experience, only 1 of the 143 cases of carcinoma reviewed had spontaneous discharge of clear duct fluid. However, it is not uncommon to find clear fluid in the aspirates from young women on birth control pills, in cases of adenosis, or in occasional cases of papillomatosis. It is my impression that the closer a hyperplastic intraductal lesion is located to the nipple, the earlier is the appearance of spontaneous discharge. A small number of cases were found with purulent discharge from one nipple or spontaneous physiologic fluid discharge from both sides. These conditions are not relevant to this discussion.

Eight patients with carcinoma presented with spontaneous discharge, five of which were either grossly bloody or were Hemostix-positive. The detection of breast carcinoma by duct fluid cytology and contrast ductography was particularly effective for tumors 1 cm in size or smaller. Three (37%) of these patients had no palpable mass and negative mammograms (Fig. 6-7). Positive cytologic findings diminished as the lesions approached the 2 cm size and were negative for all those more than 4 cm in greatest diameter. Evidence presented previously[12] and confirmed by subsequent studies[14] has clearly demonstrated that large infiltrating lesions disrupt the duct wall, resulting in extravasation of fluid into the interstitial spaces (Fig. 6-8). When the integrity of the duct wall is disrupted, fluid is not readily aspirated from the ductal system, and these carcinomas can rarely be detected by fluid cytology. However, in cases of intraductal carcinoma, contrast ductography can be very help-

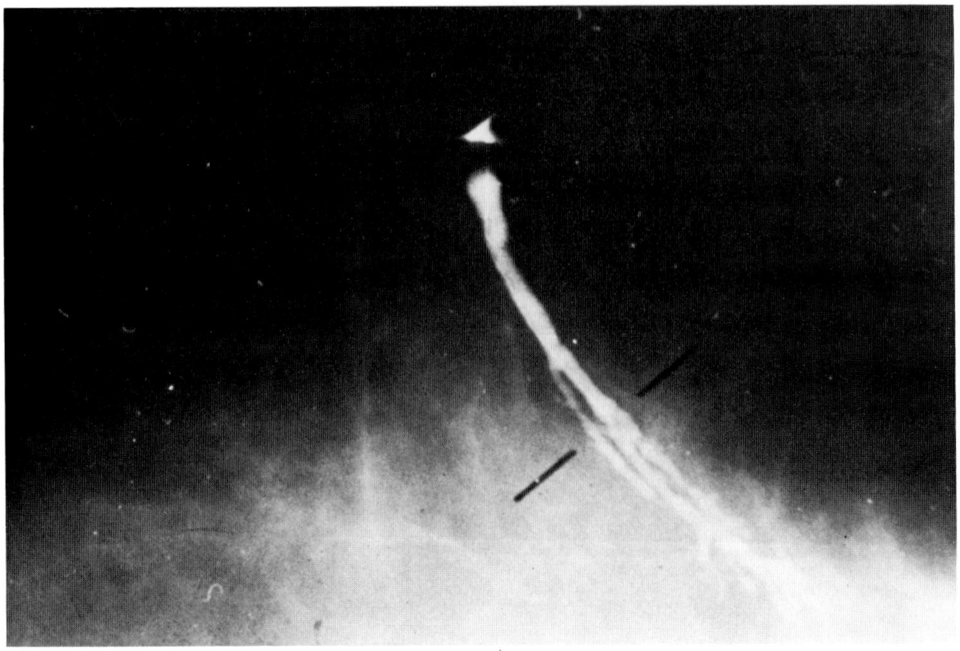

Fig. 6-7 Intraductal occult carcinoma with cells consistent for carcinoma by nipple aspiration and contrast ductography.

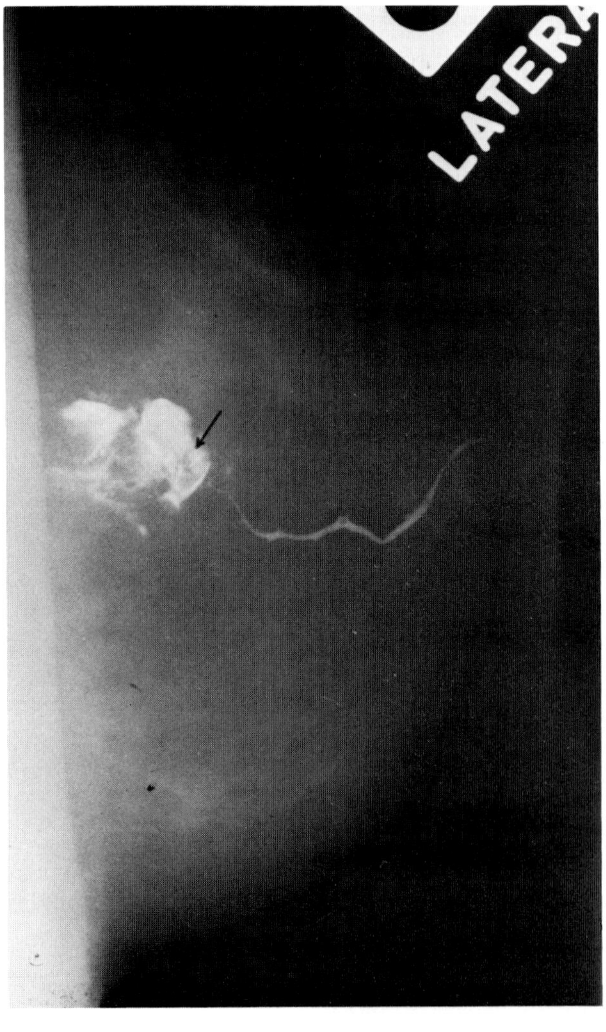

Fig. 6-8 Contrast ductogram of a 40-year-old woman with an 0.8 cm infiltrating duct carcinoma revealing extravasation of contrast material at the carcinoma site (arrow).

ful in detecting a point of infiltration and thus be of assistance to the pathologist and surgeon alike. The type of the detected malignancies included intraductal, infiltrating ductal, and infiltrating lobular carcinoma.

The intraductal lesion localized by contrast ductography is amenable to a simplified surgical approach. Prior to the surgical procedure, a sterile 4-0 monofilament nylon suture is cut to reflect the distance from the nipple surface to the lesion as visualized on the ductogram (Fig. 6-9). The marker or suture, having a knot at its top, is then introduced and inserted to its full length into the proper duct. A drop of collodion is placed on the knot of the marker, serving to hold its position, and a small Telfa or other covering prevents inadvertent displacement of the marker.

At surgery, through an appropriately placed incision near the the base of the nipple (Fig. 6-10), the duct containing the clearly visible suture marker (Fig. 6-11) is identified, isolated from the adjacent ducts, and carefully dissected free until the distal end of the suture can be seen. Then the lesion, together with the attached duct, is more widely excised, examined (Fig. 6-12), and sent to the pathology department for permanent section. This technique ensures that the lesion is found and correctly identified and that the integrity of the adjacent ductal systems is maintained. The approach is simple, nonmutilating, and efficient; moreover, it is done at minimal discomfort and cost to the patient.

Nonspontaneous Aspirated Fluids

Among the group of 331 women in whom either abnormal fluids or atypical cells were found on nipple aspiration, 55 subsequently underwent surgery: 27 had papillomas, 8 atypical hyperplasia, 3 florid adenosis with cell atypia, and 17 carcinoma

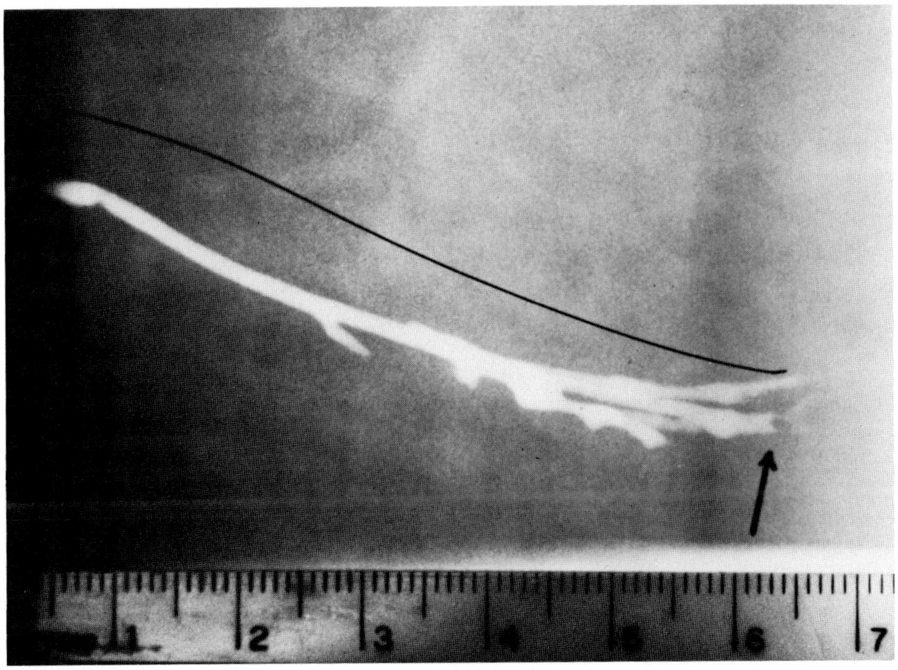

Fig. 6-9 A 54-year-old woman with bloody fluid containing papillomatous clumps on nipple aspiration. The 6.5 cm 4-0 monofilament nylon marker is cut to length preoperatively.

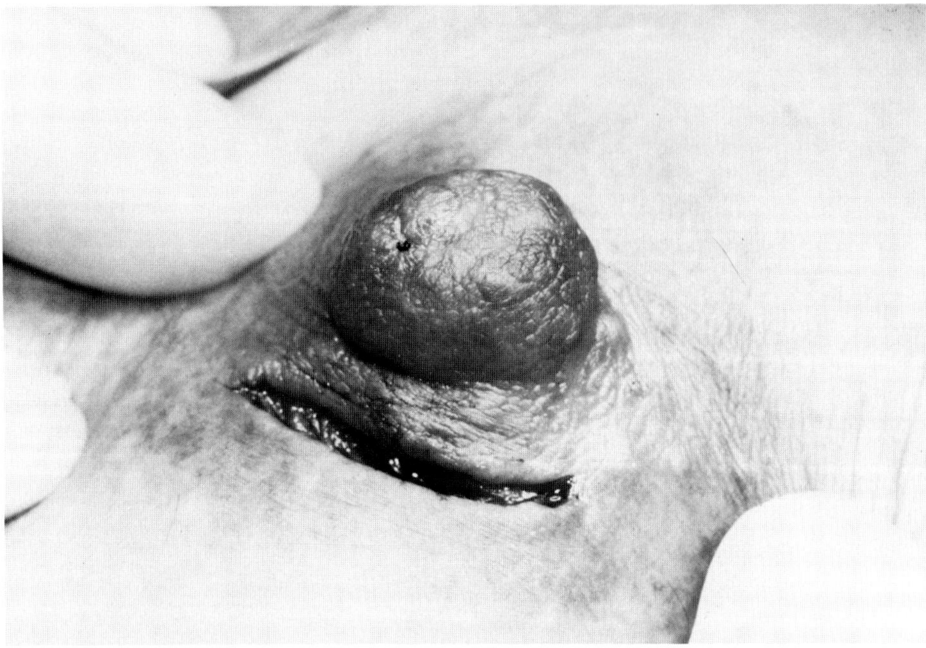

Fig. 6-10 A 2 cm incision near the base of the nipple. Note the knot of the nylon marker at the surface of the nipple.

(Table 6-2). Some of the papillomas were slightly smaller in size, the ducts less dilated, and the lesions located slightly farther from the nipple than those which presented with spontaneous discharge. Of the 17 carcinomas visualized by contrast ductography, diagnosed by cytology, and confirmed by biopsy, 3 were minimal lesions, occult to both palpation and mammography.

Table 6-2 summarizes the distribution of diseases detected by these techniques. All cellular aberrancies found in the spontaneous discharge were likewise

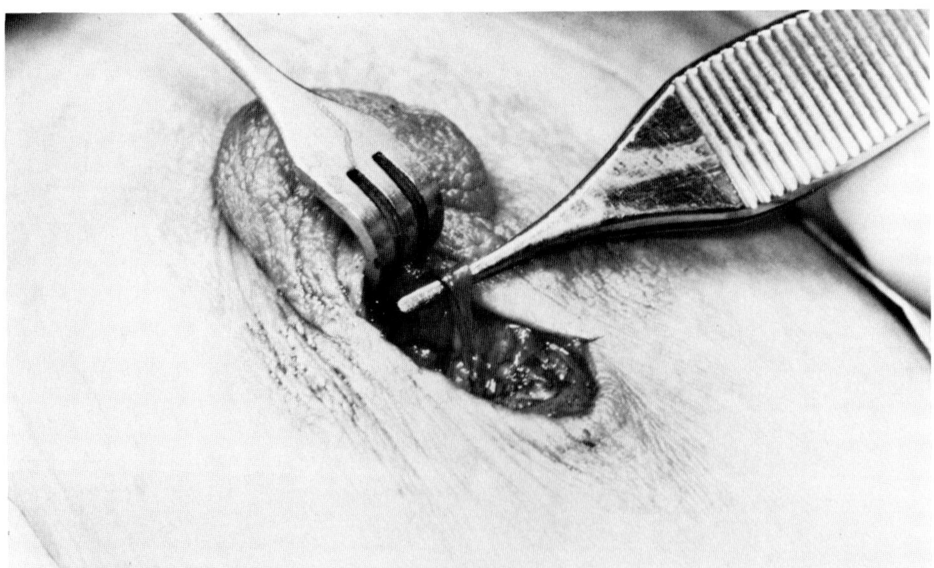

Fig. 6-11 The central duct containing the previously inserted suture has been isolated at surgery, and the contained suture is clearly visible.

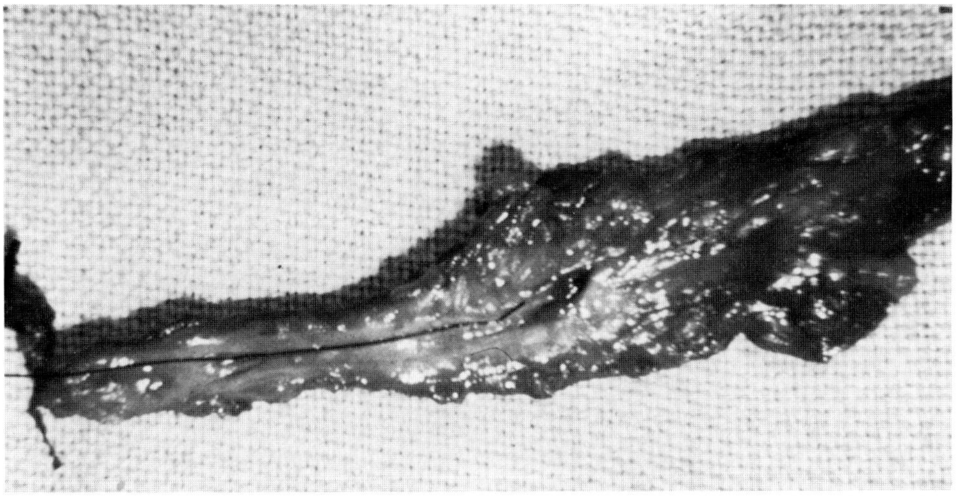

Fig. 6-12 Specimen shows the dissected duct, which has been opened, disclosing the inserted suture leading directly to the lesion.

found in aspirated duct fluids. As documented in previous publications,[12,14] the various types of disorder could be distinguished by the duct pattern or filling defect as imaged on the contrast ductograms. For example, a generalized disease such as papillomatosis, with or without cysts, can be readily distinguished from a localized intraductal papilloma.

Conclusion

Employing the combined techniques of duct fluid cytology and contrast ductography, a high level of confidence has been gained in the differential diagnosis and localization of surgical and nonsurgical conditions.[12,14]

Some authors have regarded contrast ductography as being too difficult, having a significant failure rate, and being time-consuming. Such criticisms have had a fair degree of validity if the ducts giving rise to spontaneous discharge must be cannulated with blunt lymphangiographic needles. The ducts yielding abnormal fluids or cells on nipple aspiration cannot be successfully cannulatd with this method.

Table 6-2 Nonspontaneous Duct Fluid Aspiration Diagnosed by Contrast Ductography and Cytology

	Patients		Surgery	
Type of lesion	No.	%	No.	%
Intraductal papilloma	27	8	27	100
Papillomatosis, duct hyperplasia	96	29	8	8
Duct ectasia, duct dilation, and cysts	130	39	0	0
Adenosis or sclerosing adenosis	61	19	3	5
Carcinoma	17	5	17	100
Total	331[a]	100	55	17

[a]Includes nipple aspirates containing blood, an abnormal volume of fluid from one duct, or cytologic reports of papillomatous clumps, atypical cells, or cells classified as suspicious for malignancy.

However, development of the technique of using ultrathin catheters and a dissecting scope with a 20× to 80× magnification has negated these criticisms. With a little practice, it takes less time to insert a catheter into a duct orifice, from which fluid can be obtained, than it does to take a lateral and cephalocaudad x-ray film for contrast imaging. Patient discomfort has been negligible, and no complications have been observed in more than 2600 contrast ductograms performed over a 15 year period.

The simplified surgical procedure employing insertion of a preoperative marker has been used in all cases in which detection of the lesion was considered to be a problem. It was employed to locate all small lesions sited more than 2 cm from the nipple and all occult intraductal carcinomas, and it was used in all cases of suspicious clustered calcifications as shown on mammography. This surgical technique leaves all other primary ducts intact, a point we consider important in the event of the development of a subsequent lesion in another lobe. Scarring is minimal, discomfort practically nil (postoperative Tylenol or acetylsalicylates suffice), and the cost low, as the procedure can be done in either the office or outpatient department, depending on facilities and the location of the lesion.

Lastly, it is recommended that interested radiologists, physicians specializing in breast disease, and all breast diagnostic centers include the technique of contrast ductography in their breast diagnostic armamentarium. With the cooperative efforts of interested cytopathologists using this technique, carcinomas will then be detected at an earlier state, benign conditions will be differentiated from premalignant or malignant lesions, and unnecessary surgery will be avoided. Ultimately, the problem of managing patients with spontaneous discharge and those with abnormal aspirated mammary duct fluids will be minimized.

References

1. Hicken NF: Mammography: The roentgenographic diagnosis of breast tumors by means of contrast media. *Surg Gynecol Obstet* 1937;64:593.
2. Hicken NF, Best RR, Hunt HB: The roentgen visualization and diagnosis of breast lesions by means of contrast media. *AJR* 1938;39:321.
3. Reis RA, Mesirow SD: Studies in the evaluation of mammography. *JAMA* 1938;110:1900.
4. Romano SA, McFetridge EM: Limitations and dangers of mammography by contrast mediums. *JAMA* 1938;110:1905.
5. Góes JS Jr: 1965. *Contribuicao Para o Estudo Semiologico da Mama Pela Mastografia Intraductal,* thesis. University of São Paulo, São Paulo, Brazil.
6. Björn-Hansen R: Contrast mammography. *Br J Radiol* 1965;38:947.
7. Funderburk WW, Syphax B, Smith CW: Contrast mammography in breast discharge. *Surg Gynecol Obstet* 1964;119:276.
8. Funderburk WW, Syphax B: Evaluation of nipple discharge in benign and malignant diseases. *Cancer* 1969;24:1290.
9. Quimet-Oliva D, Herbert G: Galactography: A method of detection of unsuspected cancer. AJR 1974;120:55.
10. Threatt B, Appelman HD: Mammary duct injection. *Radiology* 1973;108:71.
11. Silverstein MJ, Sartorius O, Zarem HA: Pathology of the breast for the plastic and reconstructive surgeon, in Goldyn RM (ed): *Plastic and Reconstructive Surgery of the Breast.* Little, Brown, Boston, p 59.
12. Sartorius OW, Smith HS: Contrast ductography for the recognition and localization of benign and malignant breast lesions: An improved technique, in Logan W (ed): *Breast Carcinoma.* New York, Wiley, 1977, pp 281–300.
13. Sartorius OW, Smith HS, Morris PL, et al: Cytologic evaluation of breast fluid in the detection of breast disease. *J Natl Cancer Inst* 1977;59:1073–1080.

14. Sartorius OW: *Fluid Cytology and Contrast Ductography: Breast Surgery, University of Minnesota Medical School*. Miami, Symposia Press, vol VIII, book I, 1981, pp 79–92.
15. Atkins H, Wolff B: Discharges from the nipple. *Br J Surg* 1964;51:602–606.
16. Copeland M, Higgins T: Significance of discharge from the nipple in nonpuerperal mammary conditions. *Ann Surg* 1960;151:638–647.
17. Leis HP, et al.: Nipple discharge: Significance and treatment. *New York J Med* 1967;67:3105–3110.
18. Urban J, Egeli R: Non-lactational discharge. *Cancer* 1978;28:130–140.
19. Urban JA: Excision of the major duct system of the breast. *Cancer* 1963;16:516–520.
20. Madalin HE, Clagett OT, McDonald JR: Lesions of the breast associated with discharge from the nipple. *Ann Surg* 1957;146:751–763.
21. Leis HP Jr: The diagnosis of breast cancer. *CA* 1977;27:209–232.
22. Ringrose CA: The role of cytology in the early detection of breast disease. *Acta Cytol (Baltimore)* 1966;10:273–275.
23. Saphir O: Cytologic examination of breast secretions. *Am J Clin Pathol* 1950;20:1001–1010.

7

Plastic Surgery

Richard Grossman
Saar Porrath

The varieties of plastic surgery on the breast are presented so the reader will have a better understanding of what the plastic surgeon has done and can appreciate why the breast feels or appears as it does. The theoretical purpose of plastic surgery of the breast is the attainment of what the patient idealizes as the "perfect" breast for her. For the small-breasted woman the original use of silicone injections and the later use of implants allowed her to become "bustier" and in her mind sexier. For the very large-breasted woman reduction surgery made her more "normal." Uplifts changed the contours and made the breasts look younger. Breast reconstruction after mastectomy rebuilt what was lost. Psychology and surgical constraints dictated what was done to the breast.

The surgical procedures, exclusive of reconstruction, are based on the concepts of Stromberg, McKissock, and Pitangy. Reductions, uplifts, and enlargements, exclusive of simple implant insertion, are all variations of the marking and excision of the breast tissue with preservation and, if necessary, movement of the nipple areolar complex. In essence, each procedure attempts to reconstruct the normally shaped breast with the nipples pointing in a perpendicular line from the body.

In all of these surgical procedures, multiple scarification occurs. This scarification may take the form of either hypertrophied, widened scars or keloids. These are usually in the horizontal lines in the inframammary fold, around the areola, or in the axilla. In addition to the external signs, internal scarification takes place as well.

Reduction Mammoplasty

Bilateral reduction mammoplasty, whether for gross gynecomastia or cosmetic improvement, usually follows the same surgical lines. The idea is to reduce the large, pendulous breast with the nipple pointing toward the ground and to return the nipple–areolar complex to a more perpendicular position.

Usually the tissue in the inferior aspect of the breast and the upper pole are removed. A "keyhole" is created in the supraareolar area encompassing the nipple and areola to accommodate the elevation and to reposition the nipple–areolar complex. This change forms a vascular bridge to the nipple–areolar area, often sacrificing the continuity of the ductal system. The portions of breast tissue are then apposed in as near a conical fashion as possible.

With extremes of size it may not be possible to do this, and the inferior portion of the breast may have to be amputated and the nipples placed in a more natural position with a full-thickness graft. In these instances the areolar complex can survive, but the height of the nipple cannot, as it must be defatted to maintain the blood supply. The nipple is usually replaced at the apex of the cone of reconstruction.

When the right and left sides of the breast are coapted after removal of the center core, scarification usually occurs internally along this suture line. In addition, because the normal ductal configuration in the tissues and egress to the nipple have been interrupted, there is the increased potential for ductal problems, e.g., cysts, plugged ducts, and dilatation. It may be difficult or impossible for the woman to nurse following reduction surgery. If there is a significant weight gain after reduction surgery, with fat accumulation within the breast, the scarification may cause the breasts to be asymmetrical.

These changes in the internal configuration of the breast and the scarring may be visualized with the imaging procedures described elsewhere in this book. The scarred areas may be seen on mammography as increased density or a distortion of tissue. On ultrasound there is increased shadowing from the scarred areas. Small cysts or dilated ducts may be seen. On light scanning there is increased absorption of light around the areolar area much in the shape of the "keyhole" used at surgery. The scars can be visualized on physical examination. There are also ridges of tissue formed by the surgical apposition of the remaining tissues.

Augmentation Procedures

Silicone Injections

Fortunately, the injection of free liquid silicone into the breast for purposes of enlargement has been banned by the Federal Drug Administration (FDA) the United States. Popular for about 15 years, the procedure was imported from Asia during the 1960s. The silicone was an oily suspension of silicone particles injected directly into the breast by needle. The free silicone became encapsulated by fibrous tissue in the breast, and a tissue reaction ensued. Over a long time interval, the silicone coalesced into nodules. In addition, the silicone was noted to migrate along soft tissue planes. Silicone particles have been reported in the arms, back, abdominal wall, and even in the lower extremities. It is impossible to determine on physical examination that a nodule is silicone alone or a tumor. As the silicone migrated under the skin, there was reddening of the skin and even ulceration of the silicone through the epidermis. The silicone nodules were often painful, and surgical removal occasionally resulted in a draining tract.

Partial removal of the breast or subcutaneous mastectomy has been done to relieve these problems, but a bilateral mastectomy with reconstruction is the procedure of choice. This is drastic surgery for a benign condition, however, and the symptoms must be severe to warrant it.

The diffuse nature of the silicone, its nodularity, the change in configuration of the breast, and the marked hardness of the breast that silicone causes lead to problems during physical examination. It is virtually impossible to detect small or, at times, even large masses or cancers within the breast.

Thermography may show increased vascularity and heat from the skin reactions but is usually normal otherwise. On light scanning there is an inability to adequately penetrate the breast because of the extreme tissue reaction. Occasionally silicone nodules, if well defined and superficial, show an increase in light transmission. On mammography the diffuse silicone particles can be seen. However, the density and conglomeration of these particles can hide glandular tissue or lesions, and mammographic accuracy is markedly reduced owing to the silicone. There is diffuse shadowing and increased density on ultrasound. The solitary nodule may show up as an area of decreased echoes, almost simulating a cyst.

Implantation

There are three basic types of implants: the saline implant, the silicone gel implant, and silicone gel surrounded by a saline bag. The implant is placed in one of two positions, the submammary or the subpectoral site. In the submammary position the implant is placed behind the breast tissue and in front of the pectoralis muscle. A pocket is formed in the tissue in which the implant is placed. In the subpectoral position the edge of the pectoralis muscle is elevated into an avascular plane and the implant inserted into the pocket that is formed. The edge of the muscle is either reattached or not, depending on the preference of the surgeon.

The implant occasionally changes position. It slides within the pocket that has been formed by the surgery. Such sliding is more common when the implant is in the submammary position but can occur even when it is located behind the pectoralis muscle. The usual movement is laterally and superiorly toward the axilla, dictated by the surgical mode of making the pocket, with the inferior and medial aspects a tighter seal.

The most common complication is firmness of the implant, caused by a capsular contraction. The capsule is the fibrous area that forms around the implant, and as it thickens there may be some compression of the implant. This hardening has occurred with all types of implant, although the incidence of hardening appears to be decreasing with the newer implants. The plastic surgeon may attempt a "closed capsulotomy" to break the fibrous band. This technique is done by the plastic surgeon interlocking his or her fingers and manually squeezing the breast in the hope of disrupting the underlying tissue and forcing the implant through a tear in the fibrous capsule. It is a very painful procedure which may be temporarily successful. Unfortunately, the fibrous capsule not infrequently reseals and the hardening recurs. Many patients go through a series of "closed capsulotomies," each successive one proving less successful.

The hardening of the capsule and the results of the closed capsulotomy are not evident on the imaging procedures. What may be seen mammographically or on ultrasound is a slight buckling or wrinkling of the underlying implant, which causes indentations or a double-edged effect of the implant, easier to demonstrate with a silicone gel implant. With the saline-bag or double-bag procedure there may be wrinkling of the implant caused by the pressure.

There are occasions when the force of the capsulotomy ruptures an older implant, with leakage of the material (saline, silicone, or both) into the tissues. The saline is not seen as it is absorbed, but the partially deflated implant is visualized. The silicone that has been extruded may form "bubbles" or may migrate along tissue planes.

Occasionally there is spontaneous delayed leakage from a saline implant. The saline bag or outer bag of a double-bag implant may be pricked by a needle during closure. A clot or fibrin material may temporarily seal the leak, only to be later disrupted by slight trauma or by the pressure of a chronic capsule contraction. The partially or completely deflated implant is apparent on physical examination as well as on mammography and ultrasound. Removal and replacement of the ruptured implant should be done as soon as it is recognized, for the capsule will continue to contract, resulting in a smaller pocket for the newer implant.

Saline implants have a valve that is used to inflate the implant. Not infrequently there is a dense fibrotic reaction around this valve that may cause a nodule which can be mistaken for a mass or carcinoma. This reaction can be recognized by the use of mammography correlated with physical examination, and its recognition may prevent unnecessary surgery.

Cysts can form adjacent to implants, or the implant may form a pocket or bulge. Mammography and ultrasound can demonstrate both of these circumstances. It is imperative that the implant not be needled inadvertently lest leakage occur.

Subcutaneous Mastectomy

The purpose of subcutaneous mastectomy is to remove as much breast tissue as possible and replace the tissue with an implant. This procedure is initially done through a submammary incision. Flaps of skin and subcutaneous tissue are created, and the breast tissue is dissected away from the overlying skin and nipple. Care is taken not to disrupt the blood supply to the nipple–areolar complex. The dissection is carried out posteriorly, and the breast tissue (the glandular element) is lifted intact from the pectoralis fascia. The dissection must be carried into the tail of Spence area to remove this glandularity as well. Following this dissection an implant is placed either directly beneath the created flaps, or the pectoralis muscle is sectioned and the implant placed behind the muscle.

This operation, which came into vogue during the late 1960s, was done to decrease the patients' risk of breast cancer. It was not designed as cancer surgery but, rather, as a preventive procedure. Women with a strong family history of breast cancer and breast disease were candidates, and prime candidates were women who had had multiple biopsies that demonstrated fibrocystic disease. Women who were cancerophobic were also considered for this surgery. Unfortunately, the indications were "stretched" by many surgeons, and less than ideal candidates were operated on. Currently the procedure is less common, and stricter guidelines are usually adhered to.

The complications of the procedure have done much to diminish its frequency of use. If the skin flaps are cut too thin, the blood supply is endangered and the implant can erode through or the skin necrose. The neurovascular supply to the nipple and areola can be compromised if this area is shaved too thinly, which can result in either permanent loss of sensation to the nipple or even necrosis. In order to decrease this risk surgeons did a two-stage procedure. The dissection was done initially. The skin flap was then allowed to adhere to the pectoralis fascia in the hope that revascularization would occur. An implant was inserted during the second stage and worked moderately well in the small-breasted woman. In the large-breasted woman or in women whose nipples were initially present below the inframammary line, the skin wrinkled and crinkled when it adhered to the pectoralis fascia. These wrinkles remained even after the implant was inserted, causing an unsatisfactory cosmetic result.

It has been estimated that 85 to 95 percent of the glandular tissue can be removed, thereby decreasing the risk of later breast cancer markedly. Although they are unusual, cancers have occurred in patients after subcutaneous mastectomy.

The patient who was initially at high risk should still be followed closely. Because of the procedure, physical examination may detect a large percentage of lesions that develop. On mammography and ultrasound, the small amount of glandular tissue, usually behind the nipple or in the axillary tail, can be well delineated. The position of the implant, in front of or behind the muscle, is easily seen. Diaphanography can demonstrate an increase in light transmission through the implant, and a lesion is often evident with diminished light transmission.

Mastopexy

Mastopexy is a term used by plastic surgeons to imply a reshaping of the breast. Either because of the normal attrition of age combined with gravity or postpartum changes, the breasts "hang." Mastopexies are in reality skin–brassiere reductions with elevation of the nipple to a more attractive position. There are multiple surgical approaches, the most common being the creation of a keyhole position above the nipple. The skin of this keyhole is removed and the dermis and breast tissue coapted. The skin margin at the superior aspect of the areola and the skin at the upper edge of the keyhole are then brought together. This maneuver elevates the nipple–areolar complex. The skin beneath this area is excised and pursestring sutures applied as necessary.

There is scarring along the surgical margins, especially in the inferior aspect of the breast. In addition, the breast tissue of the inferior portion of the breast may be folded over, causing an increased density on mammography and ridges on physical examination. The scarred area demonstrates shadowing on ultrasound.

Occasionally a small implant is used posteriorly to help support the breast and aid in the rebuilding process. The implant helps to "fill out" the upper breast.

Breast Reconstruction After Mastectomy

Reconstruction of the postmastectomy breast has seen great improvements, with a great variance in techniques. The basic approach is creation of a pocket and insertion of an implant into this new pocket. The extremes of reconstruction use an abdominal skin and muscle flap with blood supply intact or rotation of a latissimus dorsi muscle and skin flap from the back. These flaps are positioned over the breast area to create the pocket.

With the simpler methods, an implant is placed through the lateral portion of the mastectomy site, with undermining of the skin. The implant may be placed beneath the skin but is usually put behind the pectoralis muscle. A small gel implant is placed in the created pocket, and the patient is urged to massage the area to create a larger pocket. After the second surgery and insertion of a larger implant, the reconstructed area optimally has attained a reasonable size. Occasionally a number of surgeries with implant insertions of progressively larger size are necessary. The opposite breast may be reduced to bring it more in line, in terms of size, with the new breast.

Another technique allows insertion of an inflatable saline implant behind the muscle. The size of this implant is slowly increased by injection of saline, over weeks to months, through a specialized valve in the axillary line. When the appropriate size has been attained, either the implant is left in place or another implant is used.

The nipple and areola are created using either a portion of the opposite areola or full-thickness skin grafts from the upper inner thigh, which gives a close to normal color match. The elevation of the nipple complex is made by taking composite grafts from the ear or subcutaneous tissue from beneath the great toe, or by using foreign substances such as collagen.

The skin recurrences of breast cancer can be easily seen after reconstruction, but deep recurrences along the pectoralis muscle may be difficult to see.

There is an increasing tendency for immediate reconstruction at the time of mastectomy. Psychologically it is of value to many women to have this option.

Male Breast

Gynecomastia is the most common reason a man consults with the plastic surgeon for breast problems. Although most cases of gynecomastia regress during the late teens or early twenties, occasionally the enlarged breast causes psychological problems or concerns. Such concerns may lead to removal of the tissue.

This surgery is done through an elliptical incision in the inferior margin of the areola. The breast tissue is dissected out, an approach similar to that used for subcutaneous mastectomy. A portion of fat is usually left over the pectoralis muscle to prevent a stepladder deformity. The skin in the man usually contracts down against the fat tissue, giving a good cosmetic result. The nipple buds are usually left in place so as to give a good prominence to the nipple.

Breast cancer in men is almost always treated with a modified radical mastectomy. Reconstruction in men is a rare surgical procedure.

Bibliography

Birnbaum LM, Hopp DD, Mertens BE: The role of iodine-releasing silicone implants in prevention of spherical contractures in minc. *Plast Reconstr Surg* 1982;69:956.

Clegg HW, Foster MT, Sanders WE Jr, et al: Infection due to organisms of the *Mycobacterium fortuitum* complex after augmentation mammoplasty: Clinical and epidermiologic features. *J Infect Dis* 1983;147.

Cole-Beuglet C, Schwartz G, Kurtz A, et al: Ultrasound mammography for the augmented breast. *Radiology* 1983;146:737–742.

Corso PF: Plastic surgery for the unilateral hypoplastic breasts. *Plast Reconstr Surg* 1971;50(2).

Cronin TD, Gerow FJ: Augmentation mammoplasty: A new "natural feel" prothesis. Excerpta Medical International Congress Series 66. Proceedings, Third International Congress of Plastic Surgeons, Washington, DC, 1963, pp 41–49.

Courtiss EH, Goldwyn RM, Anastasia GW: The fate of breast implants with infections around them. *Plast Reconstr Surg* 1979;63:812.

DeCholnoky T: Augmentation mammoplasty, survey of complications in 10,941 patients by 265 surgeons. *Plast Reconstr Surg* 1970;45:513–527, 573–577.

Devitt J: Fibrocystic disease of the breast is not premalignant. *Surg Gynecol Obstet* 1972;134.

Freeman BS: Techniques of subcutaneous mastectomy with replacement, immediate and delayed. *Br J Plast Surg* 1972;30:676.

Grossman AR: *Augmentation Mammoplasty*. Springfield, IL, Charles C Thomas, 1974.

Heggers JP, Kossovsky N, Parson RW, et al: Biocompatibility of silicone implants. *Ann Plast Surg* 1983;11:38–45.

Horton C, Mladick R, Adamson JE, et al: The unilateral hypoplastic breasts. *Br J Plast Surg* 1970;23(2):161–164.

Jensen SR, Mackey JK: Xeromammography after augmentation mammoplasty. *AJR* 1985;144:629–633.

Johnstone FRC: Result of treatment of carcinoma of the breast based on pathological staging. *Surg Gyncol Obstet* 1972;134(2).

Kaye B; Micromastia vs. macromastia, in *Medical Aspects of Human Sexuality*, 1973.

Kissen MW, Kark AE: Late leakage of saline-filled breast prosthesis. *Arch Surg* 1983;118:769.
Koide T, Katayama H: Calcification in augmentation mammoplasty. *Radiology* 1979;130:337–340.
Koph EH, Vinnik CA, Bngiovi JJ, et al: Complications of silicone injections. *Rocky Mt Med J* 1976;73:77–80.
Leis HP Jr: Selective elective prophylactic contralateral mastectomy. *Cancer* 1971;28(4).
Leis HP Jr: Multi-disciplinary approach for the early detection of breast cancer. *Int Surg* 1971;56(3).
Martin JE: Atlas of Mammography. Baltimore, Williams & Wilkins, 1982, pp 330–340.
Morgenstern L, Gleischman SH, Michel SL, et al: Relation of free silicone to human breast carcinoma. *Arch Surg* 1985;120:573–577.
Radovan C: Breast reconstruction after mastectomy using the temporary expander. *Plast Reconstruct Surg* 1982;69:195–206.
Snider RE: Mammography: Contributions and limitations in the management of cancer of the breast. *Obstet Gynecol* 1966;9:207–220.
Strax P: Report of the New York Health Insurance Plan. *Medical World News*, 1972.
Vinnik CA: The hazards of silicone injections. *JAMA* 1976;236:959.
Wilkinson TS: Internal repair of the breast, in Owsley JO, Peterson RA (eds): *Symposium on Aesthetic Surgery of the Breast*, vol 18. St. Louis, Mosby, 1978, p 318.
Wilkinson TS: Subcutaneous mastectomy. *Ann Plast Surg* 1981;7:375.
Williams J: Silastic implants. *Plast Reconstr Surg* 1972;19(3).

8

Psychology of Breast Screening and Feminine Identity

Toni Bernay
Kathryn White

The female breast is the most primitive and evident part of the genital organs associated with a woman's body image, gender, and sexual identity. Historically, a woman's breasts have served as a sexual and cultural symbol of her physical attractiveness, femaleness, femininity, and nurturance. Western culture and the media have continued to reinforce the idea of the breast as the primary symbol of female sexuality. Because of the crucial role the breasts play in a woman's identity, any medical procedure that deals with this visible body part can be expected to arouse anxiety and fear. For a woman, a breast examination carries with it the risk of losing not only a body part but her sexual identity as well. She fears she may lose her desirability as a woman, her capacity to be a nurturing mother, her sexual attractiveness, and her capacity to be a giving wife and loving daughter .[1]

Physicians need to be aware of the psychological significance of a woman's breasts when making referrals for breast cancer screening. A woman's anticipatory fears about the threat screening poses to her body integrity, sex roles, and sexual attractiveness can be expected to greatly influence her compliance or noncompliance with referral. Yet public education campaigns encouraging women to undergo breast screening examinations have not addressed women's anxieties and psychological concerns. Rather, they have emphasized a rational approach, telling women that they can save their lives and their breasts through early detection. This "Eat your spinach, it's good for you" approach has not fared well in boosting compliance with referrals for breast cancer screening. Compliance rates hover between 47 and 55 percent nationally.[2,3]

The problem of compliance with referrals is one of perspective. For the gynecologist or other medical practitioner making the referral, further screening is a clinical tool for gathering additional data in the diagnostic investigation. For the woman, however, screening is a highly anxiety-provoking and threatening experience.[1] To increase compliance with referrals, physicians need to be aware of this gap in perspective and acquaint themselves with tactics that might be used to ease a woman's concerns. The aim of this chapter is to familiarize the reader with the psychological dynamics involved in making referrals for breast cancer screening. We will review the literature regarding the psychological meaning of breast examinations and referrals for screening, and the methods by which physicians can enhance adherence.

Incidence and Fear of Breast Cancer

Breast cancer is third only to heart disease and lung cancer as the leading cause of medical death in women. Current incidence rates indicate that almost 10 percent of American women contract breast cancer at some point in their lives.[4] Cancer tends to be the disease people worry about the most. In an American Cancer Society (ACS) survey in California, 64 percent of the respondents identified cancer as the disease they feared most, and 16 percent named heart disease as their most dreaded illness.[5] Upon learning of their cancer diagnosis, people react with fear and panic, often cloaked in initial denial. Breast cancer is an especially stressful type of cancer for women, threatening not only life but the core of sexual identity. Fearful emotional sequelae, along with other attitudes, beliefs, and behaviors, may interfere with compliance when a physician refers a woman to breast screening.[1] Yet it is well known that the most effective method for reducing breast cancer morbidity and mortality rates is through early detection, particularly via screening of asymptomatic women who meet specific National Cancer Institute (NCI) medical history and age criteria guidelines. When breast cancer is diagnosed on screening as an occult lesion, 5-year survival rates attain 89 percent. By the time the mass can be felt by hand, 5-year survival rates decrease to 66 percent.[6] In addition to life-saving effects, early diagnosis often permits the woman to save her breast, choosing available alternative treatments to mastectomy.

Evidence of Avoidance of Breast Examinations and Screening

To achieve the greater survival rates and reduce morbidity offered women by breast cancer screening, compliance with screening procedures is essential. Yet research suggests that women avoid screening procedures such as mammography as well as breast self-examination (BSE) and breast checks by physicians.[2,3,7–9] A 1979 national survey by the Opinion Research Corporation reported that about 40 percent of the 1580 adult women surveyed said they performed BSEs monthly, as recommended by both the NCI and the ACS.[10] Other studies have placed the figure for regular monthly compliance with BSEs at about 20 percent.[11,12] Not only do many women fail to perform BSE routinely, but research shows that women also do not like to have their breasts examined by physicians. In one study involving 409 female patients, women rated the breast examination, along with the traditional lithotomy position, as the most emotionally difficult aspect of the gynecologic examination.[13]

Although several reasons for avoidance of breast examinations are mentioned in the literature, none of the studies addressed reasons for noncompliance in an empiric fashion. Qualitative analysis reveals that women lack confidence in their abilities to detect lumps, fear trivialization of their concerns by physicians, find breast examinations to be anxiety-arousing in their own right, deny the reality of breast cancer as a threat to them personally, and equate breast lumps with cancer.[14] A 1973 Gallup poll indicated that 46 percent of women thought that having a monthly breast examination would make them worry unnecessarily.

Two studies sponsored by the NCI examining compliance with breast cancer screening procedures suggested that women avoid these procedures as well. The

Breast Cancer Detection Demonstration Project (BCDDP) study revealed a compliance rate of 51.7 percent for all five annual screenings.[3] Although this is a remarkable compliance rate given the grand scope of the study, the total compliance rate is still low given the risk–benefit possibilities available to screened women.[16] In addition, these estimates probably are deceptively high because many of the clinics included in these studies offered no-cost screening and were located in urban areas where it is likely that screening facilities are more readily accessible than they are in rural settings. Compliance with screenings in private practice populations and in rural areas can be expected to be lower.[17,18]

In a smaller NCI-supported study, Lane and Fine[2] reported an overall compliance rate of 44.6 percent when screening 1822 women in suburban New York. They noted that compliance rates ranged from 7.6 percent for asymptomatic women who had to pay for screening to 92.5 percent for symptomatic women with abnormal findings who had free screening. The results of this study lend further credence to the assertion that, given free choice, large numbers of asymptomatic women are not being screened. Lane and Fine suggested that researchers need to study medical practice in the private sector to better understand the reasons for avoidance of screening and to develop strategies for enhancing compliance.

Meaning of Breast Cancer Screening for Women

To understand why women avoid breast examinations and fail to comply with referrals for screening, it is necessary to consider the special meanings women attribute to their breasts. For many women, their breasts are an important aspect of their body image,[19,20] which in turn strongly affects their overall sense of personal identity.[21] Psychologically, the breasts symbolize beauty, nurturance, and femininity.[22–26] Breasts also are related to feelings of sexual attractiveness, which in turn play a crucial role in how women evaluate themselves and are evaluated by others.[27]

Research shows that many women find routine referrals to breast cancer screening to be extremely stressful.[1,2] Women often experience the procedures themselves, and anticipatorily the referral, as a "psychological mastectomy," imagining themselves going from the diagnostic examination to surgery, to breast loss, to the destruction of their attractiveness, desirability, and sexuality, to the loss of husbands or lovers and isolation from family and friends.[1,25] Research suggests that women undergoing mammography harbor negative attitudes and feelings about their bodies in general and their breasts in particular. Breast screening examinations thus represent a narcissistic injury to the sense of self, as symbolized to the breast.

One study[1] involved 109 patients undergoing one of three types of examinations (breast cancer screening, pelvic examination, or other radiologic examinations) at one of three locations (a hospital-based mammography department, a gynecologist's office, and a hospital-based radiology department). It was found that the mammography patients had significantly less favorable body concepts and self-concepts than did gynecologic patients (except those undergoing presurgery evaluations) or other radiologic patients. The women undergoing mammography experienced anxiety and insecurity about their bodies and themselves as well as threats to their sexual identity and body integrity.[1] The data suggested that the women were especially anxious and insecure about themselves and their bodies just before and during mammography. Women who had been treated for cancer experienced even more anxiety and insecurity about their bodies before and during mammography than did their counterparts who had never been treated for cancer. However, among this group of former cancer patients, employed women harbored a less negative body image than nonemployed women. Working seems to have given these women a sense of competence outside of sexual desirability. They appeared to understand that competence and femininity are not determined by genitalia alone but also by their ability to perform well on the job. Incidentally, this study also suggested that women undergoing mammography were more afraid of cancer itself than they were of the actual risks involved in the mammography procedure.

Referral to Breast Screening: Women's Decision-Making Processes

When a woman is told that she should go for breast screening by her physician, she begins an unconscious and conscious decision-making process as to whether she can tolerate the anxiety that breast screening engenders. Her inner monologue goes like this: "Oh, my gosh, if I go, they'll find something. I'll surely lose my breast. I won't be pretty, my body will be ugly, I won't be a woman." A married woman or a woman involved in a relationship thinks, "My husband [mate, boyfriend] will not want to touch me. My marriage [or relationship] will fall apart. My children will back away from me." A single woman may wonder, "How can I possibly date a man knowing that at the end of the evening I might have to expose my body to him." Concerns over the effects of radiation may serve as both a realistic fear and a defense against complying with breast screening. Fear of radiation effects are one way for the woman to concretize her anxiety and decrease her guilt over not following constructive health care routines.[1]

These psychological, interpersonal, and social concerns that are an integral part of a woman's life often far outweigh rational thoughts about the procedure. Her rational thoughts may go something like this: "If I go and they find something, and it's very small, I can just have the lump taken out and go for radiation therapy or chemotherapy, be fine, and not die," or "I can go and I know from what Dr. X said that 90 percent of all lumps are benign." This rational thinking, however, is hard-put to compete with anxious thoughts about survival, breasts, and womanhood.

The referring physician can help the patient by articulating such fears for and with her, likening the examination to a routine Papanicolaou smear and reiterating the life- and breast-saving effects of the examination. The physician also can aid the patient by providing and reviewing with her brochures and other printed materials about breast screening. The physician can ask the woman to check in with him or her to discuss the results and her impressions of the experience by phone. Providing checkpoints for further contact is a means of encouraging and reinforcing the woman for following through on the referral to breast screening. These checkpoints also may enhance her feelings of being cared about by her physician and her confidence in him or her.

Compliance-related Problems and Possible Solutions

Psychological fears may contribute to failures in compliance with referrals to breast screening, but other factors affect adherence. Reviews of patient compliance with medical instructions[29,30] make it clear that patients often do not follow instructions from their physicians, even when clearly life-threatening situations are involved. A critical review of the literature[31] reported that patient compliance with appointments is about 50 percent when initiated by health professionals. The time between the referral and the actual referral appointment appears to be an extremely important factor in adherence and compliance. In general, the longer the time, the lower are the chances of compliance.[32] In one study involving hypertensive patients, attendance rates at referral appointments rose from 50 percent with waiting times of 1 to 2 weeks to 95 percent with lag times of 1 to 2 days.[33] Thus referring patients to practitioners or clinics with short waiting times may increase compliance.

Two noteworthy controlled studies suggest that scheduling appointments for patients and continual follow-up also can increase adherence. Sackett et al.[34] found a 100 percent referral success for 115 patients when appointments were made for the patient and when missed appointments were rebooked by the physician's medical staff until the patient complied. Using a similar appointment-keeping approach, Logan et al.[35] achieved 99 percent compliance success for 225 patients referred from industrial hypertension screening to primary care physicians for follow-up. Thus physicians may boost compliance by taking an active role in scheduling screening appointments and following up to make sure their patients go for screening.

These systematic procedures of reducing waiting times and scheduling and following up patients may enhance compliance, but another factor is known to greatly influence patient adherence to medical regimens: the quality of the physician–patient relationship. In a review of 35 studies, Baekeland and Lundwall[36] reported that relationship factors affected compliance in every study. The most successful clinicians displayed a warm and empathic manner, interacted actively with patients, encouraged patients to participate in planning their regimens, and supplied both feedback and individualized instruction. Ross and Duff[37] found that positive experiences with the interpersonal aspects of the physician–patient relationship also have been found to increase patients' use of follow-up medical care. When making referrals for breast cancer screening, an empathic approach requires that physicians understand the special conscious and unconscious meanings that referrals have for women.

In addition to approaching their patients in an empathic, personable manner, evidence suggests that physicians can heighten compliance by encouraging women to participate actively in making decisions about their health care. Research indicates that increased participation is associated with increased compliance[38–41] and increased learning,[42,43] and nonreciprocal role behavior and disagreements between patient and physician may result in noncompliance.[44] Studies also show that most women prefer a participatory relationship in making decisions about their breast health.[23,42] The mutual participation model of the physician–patient relationship stands in stark contrast to the activity–passivity model of health care in which the physician is active and the patient is passive and dependent. Because most physicians are men[45] and breast cancer screening patients are women, physician–patient relationships consistent with this model recreate gender role stereotypes.[23,46] Physicians taking a paternalistic stance frequently do not provide the patient with adequate information for the kind of adult-to-adult discussion likely to enable the patient to make competent medical decisions.[47]

The mutual participation model, by contrast, involves "a mutual endeavor between two parties [physician and patient] who are dedicated to the effective management of a problem [viz., a disease or medical condition]."[47] The collaborative nature of a mutual participation model takes into account use of patient-centric technologies and an appreciation of the dual nature of health delivery, as well as human autonomy, self-responsibility, freedom of choice, and consent.[18] Research indicates that younger patients, in particular, prefer to be more informed about and to participate in their medical care.[48,49] This finding may be interpreted to suggest that the older patients tend to have more traditional values and younger patients more contemporary values. This change in values about the form the physician–patient relationship should take parallels changes in values about femininity.

Consistent with the rise in consumerism, patients in general and women (regardless of patient status) are becoming more active participants in decision making.[50,51]

To participate in health care decision making in an informed manner, patients obviously must be educated about their medical conditions and available options. Although some of these educative efforts can be undertaken by practitioners, evidence suggests that media educational packages can successfully instruct patients, reducing the burden on physicians and their staffs while enhancing compliance. One reviewer reported that patients rapidly forget nearly half of the verbal information provided by physicians and called for other means of communication to increase patient learning.[52] The reviewer concluded that the use of audiovisual aids, along with written material, increased patient adherence while reducing the average professional time spent counseling by five-sixths. Multimedia approaches have been found to be especially effective in gaining compliance. For example, Boyd et al.[53] and Clinite and Kabat[54] reported that combined visual and verbal information formats worked better than either alone. Dunbar and Agras[29] cited other studies showing the efficacy of multimedia approaches in facilitating compliance, although they emphasized that *simple* presentation of information is essential for optimal success. In addition, preliminary findings from the Stanford Heart Disease Prevention Project are encouraging of the use of multimedia approaches. However, the evidence is not yet conclusive, as Kelly[55] made clear, and more experimental tests of these educational interventions are in order.

Patient educational programs may facilitate adherence to referrals for breast cancer screening, and educational interventions for physicians should boost compliance. Educational interventions for physicians have been determined to be effective in strengthening their interpersonal skills,[56,57] increasing compliance,[58] and achieving patient satisfaction with the art of medical care received.[59] In a study by Inui et al[58] residents and staff physicians in a teaching hospital outpatient department were given tutorials about the relation of the "health belief model" to compliance and about practical methods of detecting and improving low compliance. The researchers reported that after a single teaching session tutored physicians spent a greater percentage of their time with patient teaching than did control physicians. Patients of tutored physicians also showed increased knowledge, more appropriate beliefs about their health problem (hypertension), greater compliance with drug regimens, and improved outcomes (better control of their blood pressure) than patients of untutored physicians. These results were sustained at reevaluation 6 months after the tutorials, leading the researchers to conclude that physicians were continuing to use their new skills in inducing compliance. Other studies also imply that training programs for physicians and medical students can have lasting benefit. Poole and Sanson-Fisher[57] reported that medical students who took part in an empathy training program continued to show greater skills in empathy at a 3-year follow-up than did control students. Although the instructed students' ability to empathize decreased significantly with time, their level of skills was still higher than that of students who received no training.

A study by Bernay et al.[46] evaluated the impact of physician training in sensitizing medical staffs to the women's need to participate in breast cancer screening and treatment decisions. The researchers found that physician training was associated with patients' increased sense of confidence in decision making and collaboration. In this study, a psychologist conducted a staff training program at the Woman's Breast Center in Santa Monica, California, after which 110 women who came for examinations served as subjects. Another 126 women who had come for breast screening examinations at the Santa Monica (California) Hospital Medical Center Breast Center served as controls. The training program was designed to sensitize staff to women's conscious and unconscious concerns about breast cancer screening and the patients' need to participate and collaborate in screening and treatment decisions. Staff training had a significant main effect on responses to a collaboration questionnaire developed for this study: Women who had interacted with experimentally trained staff reported a greater sense of collaboration in medical care decision making than did control participants. Neither self-reported gender-role-related personality characteristics nor preexamination anxiety level modified this effect. Thus to enhance compliance, physicians can undertake training designed to sensitize themselves and their staff to women's concerns about breast cancer screening and to encourage patient collaboration and participation in decision-making.

As clinicians involved in breast health care, it is important to work toward developing the same kind of public awareness of the need for ongoing breast health care as has been developed for the regular Papanicolaou smear examinations. To achieve this goal, physicians can use a variety of techniques to reach out to the public. These include public presentations, public service announcements on radio and television, consumer education through the schools and women's groups and organizations, scientific presentations to the medical community, and media outreach to scientific journalists who write science news for newspapers and magazines.[3]

Breast Health Specialists

In addition to their own efforts to enhance compliance, referring physicians also can take steps to ensure quality care of their patients by the screening physician and facility. It is helpful to educate the woman patient to the fact that there are now breast health specialists who perform all of the needed screening and physical examinations of the breast and who coordinate treatment with her primary care practitioner for optimal continuity of care. This clinical approach can help her believe that the breast specialist and the breast center are a person and a place she can go to for her breast health needs much as she goes to her gynecologist for gynecologic care. A well designed breast screening program provides a context in which women can think about breast screening.

Such a screening program includes the following multifaceted elements: (1) screening examinations; (2) a physician examination; (3) a caring atmosphere; (4) immediate feedback to the woman about the results of her examination; (5) a face-to-face consultation with an empathic and interested physician; (6) BSE instruction; (7) counseling on risk factors, dietary concerns, individual breast health problems, and follow-up care; and (8) patient education films and printed materials. A woman is likely to find the experience more supportive and comforting if the same technician is with her throughout her examinations, explaining the procedures and answering any questions she might have. It is preferable for the physician to do the physical examination that accompanies the procedures. In addition to providing a point of meaningful contact between patient and doctor, this examination can help the physician compare clinical and screening information, leading to a more consistent final opinion. It is also helpful for the physician to tell the patient the results of her examination in a postexamination individual consultation. Such a consultation provides the woman with information and reinforcement for compliance with the referral and fosters the continuation of a collaborative relationship between the patient and the breast health specialist.[60] It has been shown that an enhanced doctor–patient relationship increases compliance and cooperation and decreases opposition to treatment and malpractice cases.[38–41,44] Comprehensive breast screening programs such as the model presented above are consistent with the relational, affiliative, caring, and contextual qualities important to women, in contrast to the autonomous, independent, and objective stance stereotypically preferred by men.[1]

The more typical approach, of course, has been the one in which a woman appears once every year or two for a mammogram during which the technician prepares an x-ray film or does an ultrasound examination. She leaves, never knowing the results until days later when she checks back with her primary care physician for both the results and the discussion of ongoing care. This kind of experience is disconnected and anxiety-provoking, which further encourages noncompliance with follow-up care.

For a woman, a breast center can be a place where she can feel free to call with questions, such as those on BSE technique when she feels lacking in confidence about how to examine herself each week or month. The optimal center is one in which she can feel confident that she will get ready and willing answers to her questions rather than reluctant "grunts." The breast center is also a place where her records are kept on file, so that again she believes that she, her history, her concerns, and her health care are important to this physician and his or her staff.[60]

Discussion and Recommendations for Enhancing Compliance

We have considered the fear and anxiety sparked in patients by cancer in general and breast cancer in particular that may lead to noncompliance with referrals for breast cancer screening in symptomatic and asymptomatic women with sometimes tragic results. Research reviewed indicated that many women experience a breast examination or a referral for breast screening as a "psychological mastectomy" in which the screening process is equated with loss of the breast, loss of self-esteem and attractiveness, and isolation from family and friends. Research shows that simply undergoing mammography may engender in many women negative attitudes and feelings about their bodies in general and their breasts in particular. To counteract these fears and encourage compliance, we maintain that physicians must remain sensitized to the severe psychological impact that this seemingly uncomplicated referral can have on patients. The literature on patient compliance with medical regimens and referrals for screening was briefly reviewed. This review suggested that physicians can take the following steps to increase patient adherence to referrals for breast cancer screening.

1. Develop good working relationships with patients by interacting with them in a warm, empathic manner. It is especially important to remain aware of the special psychological meaning referral to breast cancer screening can have for women and to inquire about patients' reactions to and feelings about such referrals. Patients may be more likely to comply with referrals if they believe the physician empathizes with their concerns.

2. Consider undertaking training that can enhance your interpersonal and communication skills and your ability to create a mutually participatory relationship. In addition, you may want to increase your knowledge and sensitivity to the psychological issues involved in breast cancer screening and women's health and sexuality.

3. Encourage patients to participate actively in decision making about their breast health, informing them about the efficacy of various procedures as well as potential risks.

4. Provide patients with educational materials about breast health, screening procedures, and psychological issues often raised by these procedures. Multimedia packages, involving oral, written, and visual instructions, appear to have the greatest efficacy.

5. Refer patients to radiologists and breast cancer screening centers with short waiting times, preferably 1 to 2 days, between the date of referral and the actual referral appointment. You can also discuss with patients your confidence in and personal knowledge of the centers or radiologists to whom you are referring them. This helps patients recognize your personal involvement in their care, which enhances their relationship with you and increases the likelihood that they will comply with the referral.

6. It is helpful to encourage your staff to schedule referral appointments for patients and follow-up on noncompliant patients until adherence is achieved.

Although screening procedures for breast cancer have been shown to reduce mortality and morbidity, it must be remembered that the best medical technology in the world is useless unless the people who can benefit from it come in for diagnosis and treatment.

References

1. Bernay T, Porrath S, Golding-Mather JM, et al: The impact of breast cancer screening on feminine identity: Implications for patient education. *Breast* 1982;8:2–5.
2. Lane DS, Fine HL: Compliance with mammography referrals. *NY State J Med* 1983;83:173–176.
3. Baker LH: Breast cancer detection demonstration project: Five-year summary report. *CA* 1982;32:194–225.
4. American Cancer Society: *Cancer Facts and Figures, 1983.* New York, ACS, 1983.
5. American Cancer Society: What Californians think, feel and do about cancer. *Am Cancer Soc Volunteer* 1976;22:2–5.
6. Hutter RVP, Foote FW Jr, Farrow JH: In situ lobular carcinoma of the female breast 1939-1968, in *Proceedings of the 13th Annual Clinical Conference: Breast Cancer, Early and Late.* Chicago, Year Book, 1970.
7. Berkanovic E: Awareness, opinion and behavior intention of urban women regarding mammography. *Am J Public Health* 1979;69:172–174.
8. Miller AB, Bulbrook RD: Screening, detection, and diagnosis of breast cancer. *Lancet* 1982;1:1109–1111.
9. Silberfarb PM, Maurer LH, Crouthamel CS: Psychosocial aspects of neoplastic disease: 1. Functional status of breast cancer patients during different treatment regimens. *Am J Psychiatry* 1980;137:450–455.
10. *HHS News: New Cancer Study Shows Progress in Understanding of Breast Cancer.* Department of Health and Human Services, Dec 10, 1980.
11. Kegeles SS: Psychosocial research issues related to cancer screening: Some additional concerns about research issues and community cancer research, in Cohen J, Cullen JW, Martin LR (eds): *Psychosocial Aspects of Cancer.* New York, Raven Press, 1982.
12. Waters WE, Nichols S: Breast cancer: Women's knowledge and attitudes and the difficulties of influencing them. *Community Med* 1982;4:173–180.
13. Haar E, Halitsky V, Stricker G: Patients' attitudes toward gynecologic examination and toward gynecologists. *Med Care* 1977;15:787–795.
14. Hill D, Rassaby J, Gray N: Health education about breast cancer using television and doctor involvement. *Prev Med* 1982;11:43–55.
15. Frazier TG, Copleland EM, Gallagher, HS: The prognosis and treatment of minimal breast cancer. *Am J Surg* 1977;135:697–711.
16. Counte MA, Christmas LP: *Interpersonal Behavior and Health Care.* Boulder, CO, Westview Press, 1981.

17. Levy SM, Howard J: Patient centric technologies: A clinical-cultural perspective, in Millon T, Green C, Mengher R (eds): *Handbook of Clinical Health Psychology*. New York, Plenum, 1982.
18. Kelly H, Menking S: Recalled breast development experience and young adult breast satisfaction and display behavior. *Psychology* 1979;16:17–24.
19. Young M: Body image and females' sexual behavior. *Percept Mot Skills* 1980;50:425–426.
20. Secord PF, Jourard SM: The appraisal of body-cathexis: Body-cathexis and the self. *J Consult Clin Psychol* 1953;17:343–347.
21. Bard M, Sutherland A: Psychological impact of cancer and its treatment: 4. Adaptation to mastectomy. *Cancer* 1955;8:656–672.
22. Small EC: Psychosocial issues in breast disease. *Clin Obstet Gynecol* 1982;25:447–454.
23. Mead M: *Male and Female: A Study of Sexes in a Changing World.* New York, William Morrow, 1975.
24. Rosser JE: The interpretation of women's experience: A critical appraisal of the literature of breast cancer. *Soc Sci Med* 1981;15:257–265.
25. Tishler SL: Breast disorders, in Notman MT, Nadelson CC (eds): *The Women Patient: Medical and Psychological Interfaces.* Vol. 1: *Sexual and Reproductive Aspects of Women's Health Care.* New York, Plenum, 1978.
26. Dion K, Berscheid E, Walster E: What is beautiful is good. *J Pers Soc Behav* 1972;24:285–290.
27. Shainess N: Treatment of crises in the lives of women: Object loss and identity treat. *Am J Psychother* 1977;31:227–237.
28. Dunbar J, Agras WS: Compliance with medical instructions, in *The Comprehensive Handbook of Behavioral Medicine,* vol. 3. Jamaica, NY, Spectrum, 1980.
29. Becker MH, Maiman LA: Sociobehavioral determinants of compliance with health and medical care recommendations. *Med Care* 1975;13:10–24.
30. Sackett DL, Snow JC: The magnitude of compliance and noncompliance, in Haynes RB, Taylor DW, Sackett DL (eds): *Compliance in Health Care.* Baltimore, Johns Hopkins University Press, 1979.
31. Haynes RB: Determinants of compliance: The disease and the mechanics of treatment, in Haynes RB, Taylor DW, Sackett DL (eds): *Compliance in Health Care.* Baltimore, Johns Hopkins University Press, 1979.
32. Finnerty FA, Shaw LW, Himmelsback CK: Hypertension in the inner city: 11. Detection and follow-up. *Circulation* 1973;47:76–78.
33. Sackett DL, Haynes RB, Gibson ES, et al: Randomized clinical trial of strategies for improving medication compliance in primary hypertension. *Lancet* 1975;1:1205–1207.
34. Logan AS, Milne BJ, Achber C, et al: Worksite treatment of hypertension by specially trained nurses: A controlled trial. *Lancet* 1979;2:1175–1178.
35. Baekeland F, Lundwall L: Dropping out of treatment: A critical review. *Psychol Bull* 1975;82:738–783.
36. Ross C, Duff R: Returning to the doctor: The effect of client characteristics, type of patient, and experiences with care. *J Health Soc Behav* 1982;23:119–131.
37. Roter DL: Patient participation in the patient-provider interaction: The effects of patient question asking on the quality of interaction, satisfaction, and compliance. *Health Educ Monogr* 1977;5:381–315.
38. Strecher VJ: Improving physician-patient interactions: A review. *Patient Counseling Health Educ* 1983;4:129–136.
39. Gouldner AW: The norm of reciprocity: A preliminary statement. *Am Sociol Rev* 1960;25:161.
40. Peck CL, King NJ: Increasing patient compliance with prescriptions. *JAMA* 1982;248:2874–2877.
41. Feldman RJ, Driscoll CE: Evaluation of the patient-centered pelvic examination. *J Fam Pract* 1982;15:990–993.
42. Powers MJ, Woodridge PS: Factors influencing knowledge, attitudes, and compliance of hypertensive patients. *Res Nurs Health* 1982;5:171–182.
43. Davis MS: Variations in patients' compliance with doctors' advice: An empirical analysis of patterns of communication. *Am J Public Health* 1968;58:274.
44. Notman MT, Nadelson CC: The woman patient, in Notman MT, Nadelson CC (eds): *The Woman Patient: Medical and Psychological Interfaces.* Vol. 1: *Sexual and Reproductive Aspects of Women's Health Care.* New York, Plenum, 1978.

45. Bernay T, Golding J, Porrath S, et al: Women's competence in health care decision making. In progress, 1986.
46. Schain WS: Patients' rights in decision making: The case for personalism versus paternalism in health care. *Cancer* 1980;46:1035–1041.
47. Cassileth BR, Zupkis RV, Sutton-Smith K, et al: Information and participation preferences among cancer patients. *Ann Intern Med* 1980;92.
48. Lorber J: Good patients and problem patients: Conformity and deviance in a general hospital. *J Health Soc Behav* 1975;16:213–225.
49. Ruzek SB: *The Women's Health Movement.* New York, Praeger, 1979.
50. Geiger H: The causes of dehumanization in health care: Prospects for humanization, in Howard J, Strauss A (eds): *Humanizing Health Care.* Chicago, Aldine Press, 1975.
51. McKenny JM: The clinical pharmacy and compliance, in Haynes RB, Taylor DW, Sackett DS (eds): *Compliance in Health Care.* Baltimore, Johns Hopkins University Press, 1979.
52. Boyd JR, Covington TR, Stanaszck WE, et al: Drug defaulting: 1. Determinants of compliance. *Am J Hosp Pharmacol* 1974;31:362–364.
53. Clinite JC, Kabat HF: Improving patient compliance. *J Am Pharmacol Assoc* 1976;16:74–76.
54. Kelly A: A media role for public health compliance, in Haynes RB, Taylor DW, Sackett DS (eds) *Compliance in Health Care.* Baltimore, Johns Hopkins University Press, 1979.
55. Farsad P, Galliguez P, Chamberline R, et al: Teaching interviewing skills to pediatric house officers. *Pediatrics* 1978;61:384–388.
56. Poole AD, Sanson-Fisher RW: Long-term effects of empathy training on the interview skills of medical students. *Patient Counseling Health Educ* 1980;2:125–127.
57. Inue T, Yourtee E, Williamson J: Improved outcomes in hypertension after physician tutorials. *Ann Intern Med* 1976;84:646–651.
58. DiMatteo MR, Taranta A, Friedman HS, et al: Predicting satisfaction from physician nonverbal communication skills. *Med Care* 1980;18:376.

9

Diagnosis and Treatment of Breast Pain and Tenderness

Saar Porrath

Breast pain and tenderness are very common complaints. They are seen far in excess of the numbers of breast cancers or benign lesions removed at surgery. Most women with breast pain or tenderness are anxious and frightened. To simply tell the patient that "It's normal, it will go away, don't worry about it" is insufficient and does not provide the reassurance and relief the patient is looking for. It behooves the physician to try to determine the cause of the pain or tenderness and, if possible, to undertake measures to alleviate the problem.

Most breast pain occurs in cyclic patterns that correlate with the menstrual cycle. It is easiest to diagnose in the patient who is still having a regular menstrual cycle. It becomes more difficult to correlate posthysterectomy, or in the postmenopausal patient who is on hormone replacement therapy. Cyclic breast pain is always of breast origin. Some patients report breast pain unrelated to the menstrual cycles. This noncyclic breast pain can be of either breast or nonbreast origin, e.g., originating in the chest wall.

A careful breast history and physical examination are basic in determining the cause of the tenderness or pain and should precede diagnostic imaging procedures. As with pain or tenderness elsewhere in the body, the onset, duration, distribution, and timing of the symptoms can be determinates in deciding the etiology of the symptoms.

Cyclic Pain and Tenderness

On a monthly basis there is hormonal stimulation with a proliferation of the glandular elements and ducts. It is thought that cyclic breast pain may be due to an imbalance of the estrogen–progesterone relation. This imbalance can occur because of an overabundance of estrogen with a normal progesterone level, a normal estrogen level with a diminished progesterone level, or an overabundance of both, with more estrogen than progesterone. When the pregnancy fails to occur, the breast undergoes a regressive process that is repeated the following month with a new cycle.

There is similar stimulation of glandular tissue in the postmenopausal woman who is on hormone replacement therapy. Many studies have shown that if the uterus has not been removed, both estrogen and progesterone should be given to decrease the incidence of endometrial carcinoma that occurs with the administration of estrogens only. Although unproved, it is currently thought that progesterone may have a slight preventive effect on the occurrence of breast cancer.

Although cyclic pain and tenderness can occur anywhere there is glandular tissue, the usual distribution is in the upper outer aspect of the breast. The pain is usually of a dull aching variety, seldom sharp or sudden. It may be exaggerated by exercise. The tenderness may be associated with glandular lumps, or it may be generalized. It can sometimes be alleviated or decreased by wearing a brassiere. The duration and amount of the pain and tenderness may vary tremendously from patient to patient, or even in the same patient from cycle to cycle. If there is glandular tissue in the axilla or ectopic breast tissue anywhere along the milk line, there may be pain and tenderness in these areas.

Noncyclic Pain and Tenderness

In addition to cyclic pain there may be noncyclic pain and tenderness. Noncyclic pain can occur at anytime and is unrelated to the menstrual cycle. Its onset can be sudden or insidious, and its duration very short or prolonged. The distribution can be anywhere within the breast area and depends on its etiology. The pain may be sharp, stabbing, dull aching, or nondescript. The tenderness varies from minimal to marked, again depending on the cause.

The discussion of noncyclic pain and tenderness is more involved than that of cyclic origin. The first question that must be answered is what is the location of the pain? Is it really in the breast, or is it referred to the breast? Sometimes this question is relatively easy to answer, and sometimes it is necessary to make a diagnosis by exclusion.

Not of Breast Origin

Examples of noncyclic pain or tenderness not of breast origin, but with the pain being referred to the breast, include cardiac, pulmonary, chest wall, rib, costal cartilage, shoulder, brachial plexus, or neurologic pain secondary to cervical nerve root involvement and axillary and muscular disorders.

It is important when obtaining the history to pinpoint the location of the pain or tenderness, as well as determining the duration, type of symptoms, radiation of pain, and circumstances that may add to or minimize the symptoms. When examining the patient's breast, is it important to accurately locate the site of the pain or tenderness.

With the increasing interest in health and exercise there has been an increase in muscle pain. The pectoralis muscles are located behind the breast. On physical examination the breast can be pulled forward and the tenderness elicited by palpating the muscle. It can occur anywhere along the muscle but is commonest behind the upper outer portion of the breast. The patient often relates either engaging in an increased exercise program or performing a chore where the upper arms were used. Chest wall syndrome, severe pain caused by an inflammation of the chest wall muscles, can present with the same symptoms. In both of these circumstances the pain or tenderness is seen on physical examination to be outside the breast if the technique of physically pulling the breast away from the chest wall and then palpating is used.

There are other examples of noncyclic breast pain, not of breast origin. Tsetse syndrome—pain and tenderness in the costochondral junction, usually the junction of the second or third rib with its cartilage—is one. The pain may be increased by moving the upper extremities. On palpation the tenderness or pain can be elicited by palpating the cartilage junction.

Occasionally a chondral sternal separation or a slight tear in the attachment can elicit the same symptoms and signs. A fracture or tumor of an underlying rib can reflect as breast pain.

Pleural or pulmonary involvement such as with pulmonary infarction, pneumonia, or pleuritis can produce a sharp or dull pain in the breast area. Not infrequently the patient describes the pain worsening with a deep breath or cough. There may also be radiation to the back, a very unusual finding with true breast pain.

Radiation of cardiac pain occasionally produces chest wall or breast pain. In patients with severe congestive failure the lymphatic drainage to the breast may be impaired, with the breast swelling. This may be accompanied by some pain and tenderness.

Neurologic pain referred from the brachial plexus, cervical nerve roots, or more commonly upper thoracic roots can also result in breast pain. Shingles, or the involvement of a thoracic nerve root by herpes virus, may manifest as breast pain. On occasion shoulder injury or inflammation can produce breast symptoms by referred pain.

In women with large, pendulous breasts that extend over the upper abdomen, there may be gallbladder, liver, stomach, or splenic pain in rare circumstances that reflects symptoms which the patient may initially interpret as breast pain but which on examination the physician finds not to be of breast origin.

Of Breast Origin

Breast infections can cause pain or tenderness. The type of pain and tenderness, duration, location, and severity differ depending on the area involved.

Breast infections may be accompanied by some axillary lymph node involvement, and there may be localized heat; however, there are seldom generalized signs of temperature, malaise, or weakness. The signs and symptoms are almost always confined to the breast.

Mastitis often presents suddenly, producing a constant dull aching pain. It is usually confined to a segment of the breast, seldom involving more than one-fourth of the glandular area. There may be skin redness if the area is relatively superficial, and there may be a mass effect. A breast abscess or infected cyst presents with a mild ache to sharp pain. If located deep in the breast there may be little tenderness and few signs. Infected ducts can cause an itching sensation in the area of the nipple and a pulling sensation behind it. A slight nipple discharge may be present. Duct pain from a deep area can be reflected through the ductal system and present with nipple symptoms, but it lacks the signs of a nipple infection.

Infections of the nipple and areolar area are very tender. Inspection of the area usually reveals redness and swelling. Montgomery's glands are sebaceous cysts with blind-ending ducts which surround the nipple and help lubricate the nipple area. When infected they can quickly form an abscess that is painful and very tender.

Because the breast is encased in skin, any lesion that presents on the skin elsewhere can present on the skin of the breast. There may be infections of the hair follicles, sebaceous cysts can become infected, and skin cancers with a localized infection can occur. These problems are easily identified with inspection of the breast.

Dermatitis of the skin or nipple area is not uncommon; it can present with some discomfort or tenderness, and the involved area is usually reddened. This condition can be contact dermatitis or exzema.

The breast is very vascular. Whereas arterial abnormalities are unusual, venous problems are not uncommon. Thrombophlebitis or thrombosis of the lateral thoracoepigastric vein with an overlying skin retraction is termed Mondor's disease, named after the physician who described it. As the inflammation of the vein subsides, the overlying tissues may be pulled in toward the previously swollen area, causing in some cases a retraction. This retraction can mimic that seen with carcinoma of the breast. Thrombophlebitis can occur in any vein, not just in the lateral location. It is not uncommon in the inferior portion of the breast following surgery. The area presents as a ropey, painful mass that regresses over a 6- to 8-week period. The pain may disappear, but the ropey area may persist. The entity is more common than appreciated but is usually not considered in the differential diagnosis. The skin retraction is an unusual finding.

Cysts are the most common benign lesions of the breast. They can develop quickly and attain the size of a few centimeters within a short time. The sudden distention may present as a painful area. Whereas most cysts are fluctuant or soft, the distended cyst may be firm and tender. It is rare for a cyst to become infected following needle aspiration, but it can occur. A more common finding is the refilling of the cyst by fluid or occasionally blood, causing a painful mass; this recurrence is seen less than 2 percent of the time.

Acute obstruction of the ducts of the breast with dilatation is a common cause of sharp pain, especially in the upper portion of the breast, often with radiation to the nipple. It is usually of short duration. Such obstruction is not uncommon during late pregnancy and while the patient is nursing. The condition is usually self-limiting and regresses.

Breast trauma with the development of hematomas is also a cause of pain or tenderness. It is very common for a small amount of trauma to result in a small, tender hematoma, and the patient may be unaware of the episode of trauma. An example is the relative frequency that women who garden bruise their breasts and are unaware of the episode.

Most benign tumors of the breast, e.g., adenomas, fibroadenomas, hemangiomas, lipomas, and papillomas, do not cause breast pain or tenderness. Most painful or tender areas that are palpated are glandular. This is not an absolute rule, however, and any lump must be investigated, painful or not. Not infrequently when the patient palpates a lump, psychologically it begins to be painful. This pain must be dealt with by determining the origin of the mass and reassuring the patient.

Cancers of the breast are usually painless, although there may be some tenderness on palpation. Again this is not an absolute rule, and it is a dangerous old wife's tale that cancer never causes pain. Paget's disease, an involvement of the nipple by an underlying intraductal carcinoma or invasive ductal cancer, may present with nipple itching, and the nipple is often raw. If a cancer becomes necrotic or invades the underlying chest wall, pain can occur. Inflammatory carcinoma, caused by plugging of the lymphatics by tumor cells, results in skin thickening, redness, and a peau d'orange effect. The breast is swollen and may be painful or tender.

Scars and postsurgical defects can be painful, probably owing to transected nerves or skin pulling. This pain or tenderness usually stabilizes within a few months after surgery. If changes occur after this time interval, other causes should be sought, although late fibrosis can occur.

With the increased use of lumpectomy and radiation therapy to treat breast cancer, physicians will be following more patients who have opted for this therapy. Although the postsurgery and irradiation changes usually stabilize by 6 months, the late development of radiation fibrosis is not uncommon. It is extremely important to obtain baseline studies on these patients within 6 months of the cessation of radiation therapy and to follow them closely so that later changes, if they do occur, can be compared and an early recurrence not missed. In older patients who underwent mastectomy and radiation therapy on the megavoltage therapy units, before cobalt or linear accelerators were available, there can be osteonecrosis of the underlying ribs that presents with pain. Metastatic lesions to the breast are usually insidious.

In men, gynecomastia can be painful, especially in the older patient who is on hormone therapy for prostatic cancer. Some authors advocate the use of radiation therapy to the male breast prior to the institution of hormones in order to decrease the pain.

Imaging Procedures

The history and physical examination form the base for the diagnosis and treatment of the causes of breast pain and tenderness. The use of diagnostic imaging procedures, including mammography, ultrasound, diaphanography, and thermography, as well as specialized procedures such as ductography (also known as galactography) can be extremely helpful in differentiating the entities that cause the breast symptoms, but they should be used in an expeditious fashion. [The reader is referred to the specific chapters dealing with mammography (Chapter 2), thermography (Chapter 5), diaphanography (Chapter 4), ultrasound (Chapter 3), and ductography (Chapter 6), and to the case reports dealing with the use of these procedures for a specific disease in Section II.]

In the patient who has noncyclic pain not of breast origin, the imaging procedures are used primarily to rule out a nonpalpable breast lesion, rather than to establish a reason for the pain. The diagnosis is made with a careful history and physical examination.

When dealing with the patient who has cyclic pain, which is almost always of breast origin, the imaging procedures are primarily used to establish that the tender or painful areas are probably glandular tissue and that no other lesion is present.

Evaluation of a symptomatic patient is different and often more difficult than screening for breast malignancy in the asymptomatic patient. It is not enough to establish with an accuracy of 82 to 95 percent (figures quoted for the accuracy of mammographic screening for malignancy) that cancer is not present. The cause of the problem must be defined.

The use of the imaging procedures should be selective, based on their need. It is not necessary to do all procedures in every patient.

Treatment

Once the etiology has been established in patients with noncyclic pain and tenderness, whether of breast origin or not, treatment can be directed at the offending cause. If there is a lesion, surgery is indicated; if there is an infection, antibiotics are instituted; and if thrombophlebitis is present, warm packs and reassurance suffice.

Most patients presenting with breast pain and tenderness fall into the category of cyclic pain of breast origin. Most of these patients simply need reassurance that their pain or tenderness is "normal," not from cancer, and that it will vary with the cycles, usually disappearing with menopause.

Minton during the 1970s advocated abstention of caffeine and methylxanthines in the treatment of these patients. Although a number of double-blind studies have shown no conclusive evidence that this dietary exclusion is significant, my own personal experience with more than 2,000 such patients has shown that in more than 70 percent of these women there is a diminution in symptoms as well as a decrease in the nodularity of the breast with abstention. Not infrequently the patient has given up coffee but is ingesting large doses of caffeine through medication such as Cafergot and Fiorinal for migraines, or diet pills.

It is probable that caffeine abstention has no effect on true fibrocystic disease as determined by pathology. The effects appear to be due to a decrease in glandularity. Most of the women described clinically as having fibrocystic disease on physical examination do not have a disease but have a nodularity better described as fibrocystic syndrome, or normal cyclic variations in the breast.

The addition of vitamin E, 400 to 800 units a day, and of vitamin B_6, 100 mg a day, has been helpful in my practice, although again no blind study has demonstrated their efficacy. A trial of the exclusion of caffeine and methylxanthines and the administration of vitamins should be tried before resorting to the use of hormones. Progesterone can be very successful in diminishing pain and tenderness. When using vaginal suppositories of progesterone, 200 to 400 mg per day is usually sufficient. This author has had relative success in the use of progesterone cream to the breast. It is administered in the form of a topical cream containing 100 mg of powdered progesterone per ounce of unibase. It is used twice daily. Its usage has been reported in the French literature as well. Progesterone cream is sold over the counter in parts of Europe.

In postmenopausal patients on estrogen, the addition of low doses of Provera, 2.5 mg per day, may suffice. Occasionally cycling the patient on birth control pills for a few months may "break the pain cycle." Loestrin may be helpful. The administration of testosterone by injection is helpful in some cases, but it should be used very carefully as the side effects may not be reversible. Tamoxifen, an antiestrogen, can be effective, although its use is not widespread. If these methods are unsuccessful, and they are in more than 95 percent of cases, the administration of danazol may be tried. The dosage for breast symptoms is less than that used for the control of endometriosis and seldom exceeds 200 mg per day. Bromocriptine is very successful in the treatment of pituitary adenomas and in addition, diminishes breast pain in patients who have elevated prolactin levels, even without an adenoma being present. The use of subcutaneous mastectomy for the treatment of breast pain is confined to the rare patient who has not responded to any of the above regimens of therapy.

The purpose of treatment in these patients is to decrease the symptoms, which can usually be accomplished with a limited treatment schedule. It should then be possible to stop the therapy, hopefully without the resumption of symptoms.

Bibliography

The Fibrocystic Breast: A Multidisciplinary Approach. Proceedings The Society for the Study of Breast Disease, Boston, 1983.

Fibrocystic breast disease and danocrine. Clinical papers presented at a symposium on fibrocystic breast disease, Washington, DC, 1979.
Blichert-Toft M, Andersen AN, Henriksen OB, et al: Treatment of mastalgia with bromocriptine: A double-blind cross-over study. *Br Med J* 1979;1:237.
Huber CJ, Pons JY: Breast fibrocystic disease and thermography. *Acta Thermogr* 1980;5(1):48–50.
London RS, Sundaram GS, Goldstein PJ: Medical management of mammary dysplasia. *Obstet Gynecol* 1982;59(4):519–523.
Montgomery ACU, Palmer BU, Biswas S, et al: Treatment of severe cyclical mastalgia. *J R Soc Med* 1979;72:489–491.
Ouimet-Oliva D, Van Campenhout J, Hebert G, et al: *J Can Assoc Radiol* 1981;32:159–161.
Porrath S: Hormone mastitis. Presented at a meeting of the Society for the Study of Breast Disease, San Fancisco, 1984.

Section II

Benign Disease

10

Cysts

Saar Porrath

Cysts are the most common lesions in the breast, varying in size from microcysts of 1 to 2 mm to large cysts of many centimeters. They are almost always benign. Malignant degeneration in the form of the unusual intracystic carcinoma seldom occurs. Cysts can develop very suddenly, attaining a considerable size almost virtually overnight. The patient who presents with a suddenly occurring lesion usually has a cyst, less often an infection.

It is thought that when a duct or portion of a duct becomes plugged with debris the resulting accumulation of secretions and back-pressure causes formation of a cyst. Cysts are hormonally related, but that alone does not explain their existence. Cysts are commonest in the actively menstruating woman who is in her thirties and forties. They occur less often in women in their twenties and only occasionally in teenagers, appearing most often in teenagers who drink large amounts of caffeinated soda. Cysts are not unusual in the postmenopausal woman on estrogen replacement therapy. When seen in the postmenopausal woman who is not on hormones, the possibility of a cancer with excitation of the adjacent tissue should be considered (see case studies, below).

Physical examination plays a role when the cysts become large enough to be palpated. Cysts are often soft and fluctuant but may be firm and even hard. Depending on their location and the amount of surrounding glandular tissue, they may be well defined and discrete or ill-defined, blending into the surrounding area.

They are commonly multiple. Interestingly, their distribution and number in each breast may be very unequal, as may be their physical appearance. It is possible for some cysts in the same breast to be soft and others hard; there may be multiple gross cysts in one breast but only microcysts or no cysts in the other. Cysts can also be multiloculated, conglomerate, or single.

Thermography seldom plays a diagnostic role. When a cyst grows large enough to distort normal anatomy, it may appear as a cold, avascular area on the thermogram. If a cyst becomes blood-filled or infected, the thermogram is usually positive, with increased heat, vascularity, or both.

Mammography does not show microcysts. The lesion must be large enough to be defined, usually at least 5 mm or greater, depending on the surrounding glandularity. Obviously, in a fatty-type breast (Wolfe N1) a smaller lesion can be more clearly defined than in a dense glandular breast (Wolfe DY). (The use of the Wolfe classification does not mean that the author subscribes to this classification, but uses it as a common descriptive "visual" term.) Cysts usually have well defined, smooth borders on mammography unless a portion of the cyst is obscured by overlying tissue. Cysts may be circular or ovoid in shape. If lobulated, the outline is smooth or somewhat irregular, reflecting the composite mass. The diagnosis cannot be made on mammography alone; it can only be suggested that the lesion is probably benign and that it may be a cyst. Accurate differentiation from fibroadenomas, medullary and colloid carcinomas, and other well defined solid tumors cannot, and should not, be made on the basis of an x-ray examination alone.

Diaphanography can be very helpful depending on the size of the mass, its depth in the breast, the thickness of the cyst wall, and its contents. Usually there is increased light transmission through a cyst, especially if the cyst is superficial and large enough to be imaged. If there has been a recent bleed, the cyst appears as an area of increased light absorption. If the cyst is chronic and thick-walled, it may also appear as an area of decreased light. The deeper the cyst, the poorer is the definition. Small cysts or even large cysts deep in the breast, especially a dense glandular breast, may not be visible.

Ultrasound is the most definitive procedure, exclusive of needle aspiration or biopsy. Its accuracy approaches 99 percent. It can visualize microcysts of 1 to 2 mm, as well as much larger lesions. The configuration of the internal cyst wall can be seen with relative clarity. Ultrasound can also show if there is clear fluid or small filling defects, often caused by epithelial debris, old hemorrhage, or concretions of cystic fluid. Internal filling defects can be identified and should be investigated further.

Cyst fluid when aspirated can be clear, serous, or colored light yellow to greenish to dark brown. Hemorrhage, if it has occurred in the cyst, may cause darkening of the fluid, with brownish colors. Most surgeons recommend that if clear fluid is obtained the fluid be discarded as the analysis of cyst fluid is usually normal, often acellular, and occasionally misleading. The pathologic diagnosis even with intracystic lesions is often incorrect.

Tabár et al. have recommended that pneumocystography be done on any questionable cystic area to be sure the cyst is normal. They found a 1.3 percent incidence of intracystic carcinoma in their series. This incidence is much greater than is usually found. Other series have cited an incidence of less than 0.5 percent. Tabár speculated that the air may cause sclerosis and drying of the cyst wall, which would account for the decreased incidence of cyst recurrence following pneumocystography in their series.

In my practice large cysts, cysts that appear abnormal on ultrasound, or any cysts the patient can feel are aspirated. Care is taken to be sure that the mass disappears following aspiration. If it does not, biopsy is done, unless it can be shown that there is incomplete removal of the fluid. In this circumstance reaspiration is done and again care is taken to be sure that the mass is gone. Removal of a palpable mass makes the patient feel much better. Aspiration and pneumocystography are performed on any cyst that has unclear margins or internal echoes on ultrasound. On pneumocystography, a clear wall should be seen with no internal defects. If all the fluid has not been removed, the air tends to form bubbles, making the evaluation difficult. If care is not taken during the injection, the air tends to leak out of the cyst into the tissues.

The radiologist who seldom aspirates cysts is usually unaware that about 2 percent of cysts recur, some of them rapidly. If a cyst tends to recur quickly and often, further investigation such as biopsy may be indicated. Occasionally the cyst fills with blood or, rarely, becomes infected following aspiration. The blood-filled cyst is dark on diaphanography and warm on thermography; if the blood clots, ultrasound may show a filling defect. These cysts should be followed until resolution to be sure that the blood was due to the aspiration and not a lesion in the cyst wall.

Infected cysts are seldom caused by aspiration; they occur not infrequently, and the etiology of the route of infection is unknown. The infected cyst is tender; the thermogram is hot; diaphanography is positive; and ultrasound may show multiple filling defects in the fluid. Aspiration may reveal pus. These cysts can usually be treated with antibiotics, surgery seldom being necessary.

There are many medications and substances in the diet that may facilitate cyst formation. Propranolol (Inderal), antidepressives, hormones, birth control pills, caffeine, xanthines, and herbs such as ginsing (which contains estrogen) have been linked to breast nodule and cyst formation. This list is not complete but is included here to make the physician aware of the cyst-related potential of these substances. A fair amount of success in decreasing the incidence of cyst formation has been achieved by decreasing or removing drugs or materials such as caffeine from the diet.

Haagensen et al. have shown a relation between the presence of gross cystic disease and the development of carcinoma. Interestingly, their large series showed a prevalence of cystic disease in the left breast and the subsequent development of carcinoma in the right breast. Haagensen et al. thought that cysts do not cause the carcinoma but that there may be a biochemical relation between the two. DuPont and Page in an excellent article on risk factors concluded that although "cysts alone do not elevate the risk, women with both cysts and a family history of breast cancer had a risk 2.7 times higher than that for women without either of these risk factors."

Case Studies

Case 1

E.B. is a 14-year-old girl who presented with a 2 cm firm nodule just above the left nipple. A very slight, sticky, clear nipple discharge was noted on the left. Thermograms were normal. There was increased light transmission through the nodule (Fig. 10-1).

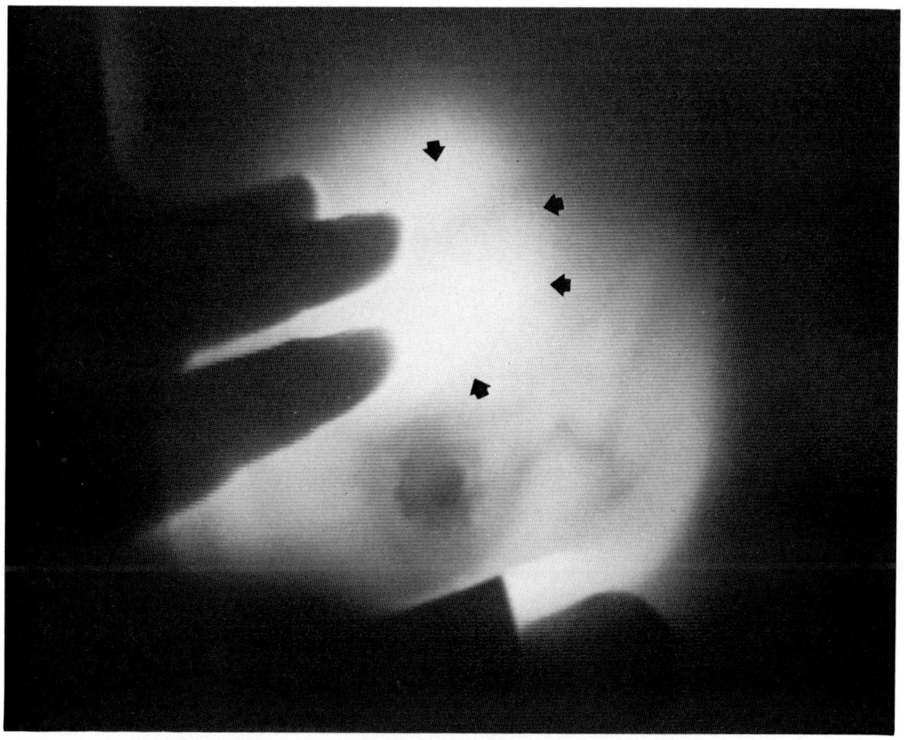

Fig. 10-1 Diaphanography. The area of increased light transmission is outlined by arrows. As the light probe pushes from behind, the area of increased light appears larger than the cyst dimension, as the compression tends to flatten the cyst.

Mammography was not performed. On ultrasound a 2 cm cyst was identified. The cyst regressed over the next few menstrual cycles.

Case 2

D.B. is a 39-year-old woman who presented with a 2 cm mass just above the left nipple. There was marked nodularity of the breasts. Liquid crystal thermograms were normal. Diaphanography showed some decrease in light transmission through the mass. There was marked glandularity on the mammograms (DY pattern), with no discrete mass identified. On ultrasound there were many cysts bilaterally. The mass palpated was a 2 by 3 cm cyst (Fig. 10-2). The palpable cysts were aspirated, but no attempt was made to aspirate the nonpalpable smaller cysts. The mass disappeared following the aspiration. There has been no recurrence.

Case 3

B.G. is a 68-year-old woman who during a screening mammogram elsewhere was noted to have a 1 cm density in the right breast. There was nothing palpable. She was on estrogen replacement therapy. Thermograms and diaphanography were normal. The mammograms were not repeated. On ultrasound there was a well defined 1 cm cyst present (Fig. 10-3). A recheck of the ultrasound 6 months later showed a slight decrease in the size of the cyst.

Case 4

E.S. is a 42-year-old woman who presented for a checkup. On physical examination there was a 2 by 3 cm ridge in the outer aspect of the right breast. Thermograms were normal, as was diaphanography. On mammography there was a well defined 2 by 3 cm mass in the outer right breast, without calcification (Fig. 10-4). On ultrasound there were diffuse low-level echoes throughout the mass. Because of the echo pattern on

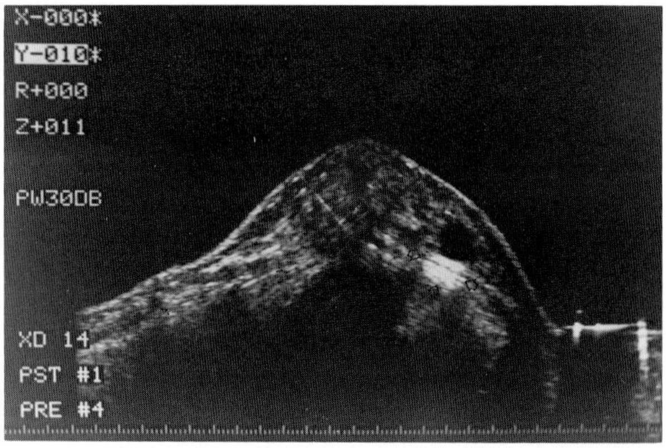

A

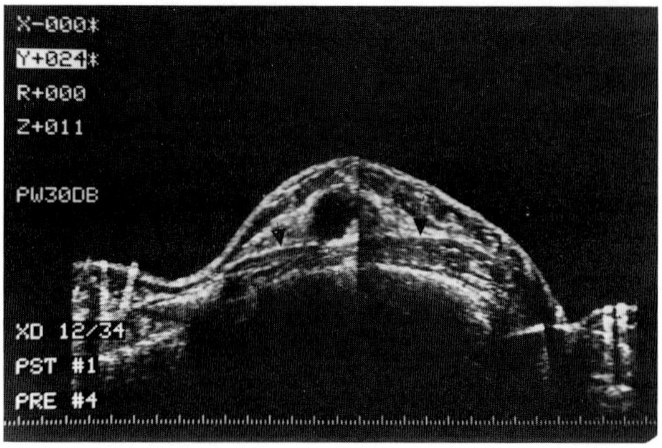

B

Fig. 10-2 **A:** Transverse scan through the midbreast. The cyst appears as a well defined anechoic area with increased through transmission (arrows). **B:** Transverse scan. Use of a split screen does not show the increased through transmission as it is voided by the computer. There is a good demonstration of the fat (F) echo pattern and the pectoralis muscles (arrows).

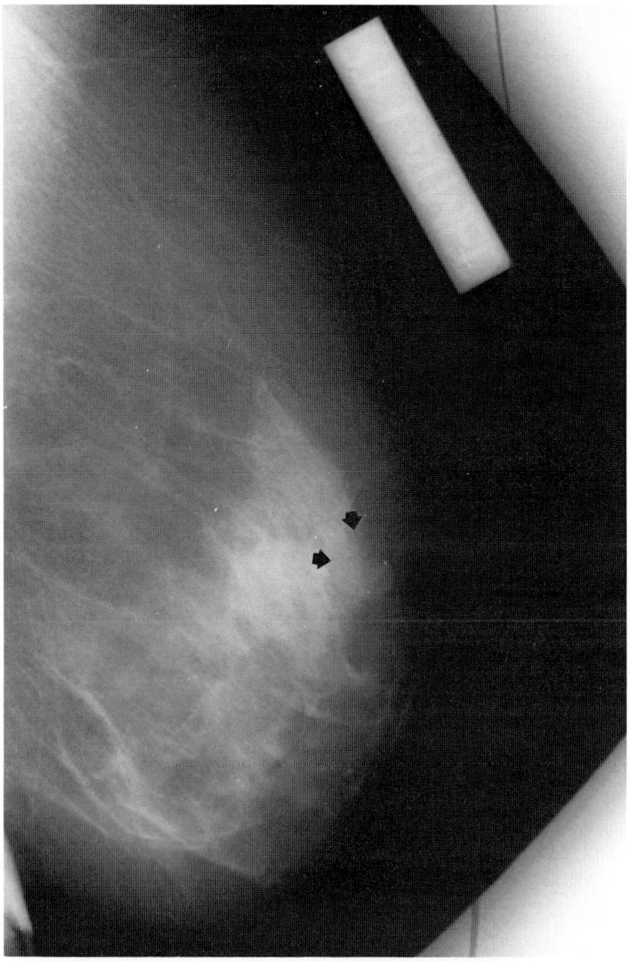

A

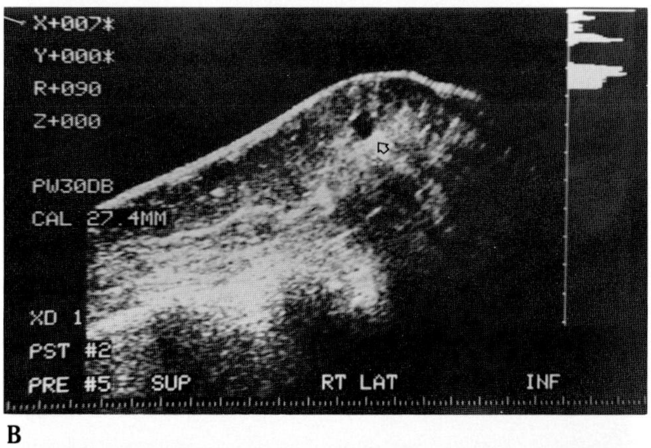

B

Fig. 10-3 **A:** Well defined mass extending into the fatty area (arrows). **B:** Anechoic area with well defined walls and increased through transmission (open arrow). Note the anechoic area on A-mode ultrasound.

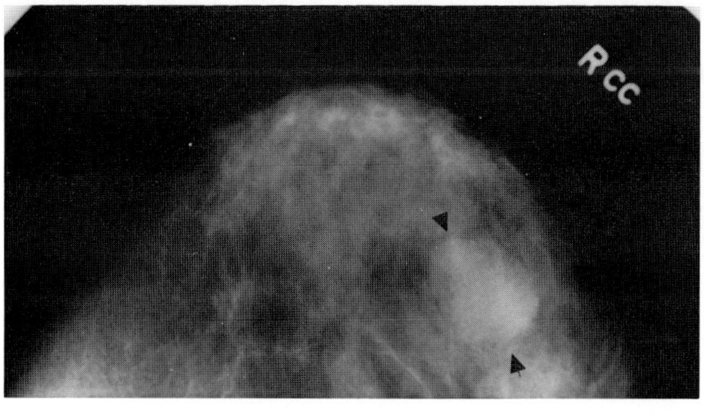

Fig. 10-4 Cephalocaudad (CC) view with smooth borders and increased density (arrow).

ultrasound the mass was thought to represent a fibroadenoma. A surgeon aspirated fluid, and the mass disappeared.

Case 5

C.G. is a 36-year-old woman who presented with a firm, tender 5 cm mass behind the left nipple. Liquid crystal thermograms showed markedly increased nipple heat, peri-areolar heat, and vascularity on the left (Th IV thermogram). There was decreased light transmission through the mass. On mammography there was marked glandularity (P2 pattern), and a poorly defined density behind the left nipple. The mass on ultrasound was cystic with some internal echoes and the suggestion of a thick wall (Fig. 10-5). On aspiration 3 cc of clear fluid was obtained. The fluid revealed class II cells and large numbers of polymorphonuclear leukocytes, consistent with an infection. The cyst did not recur. The thermogram was normal on a follow-up examination.

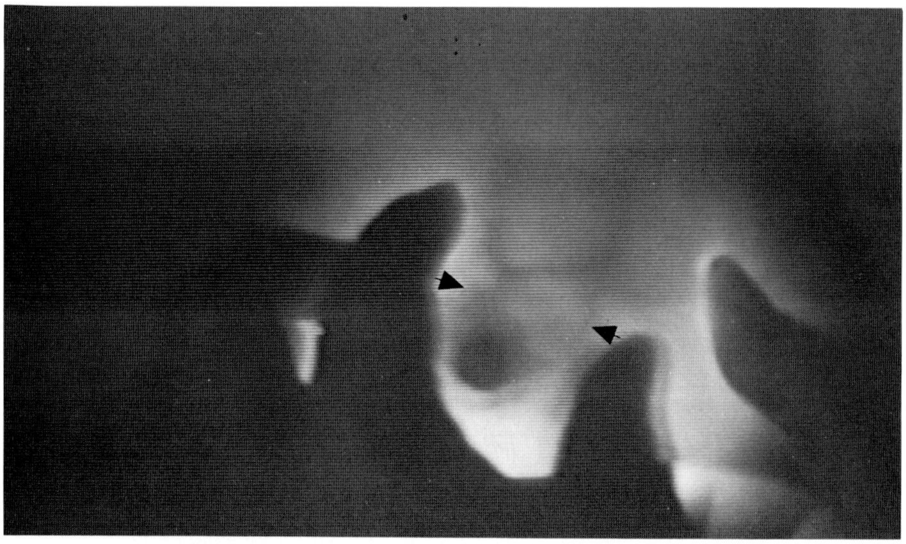

A

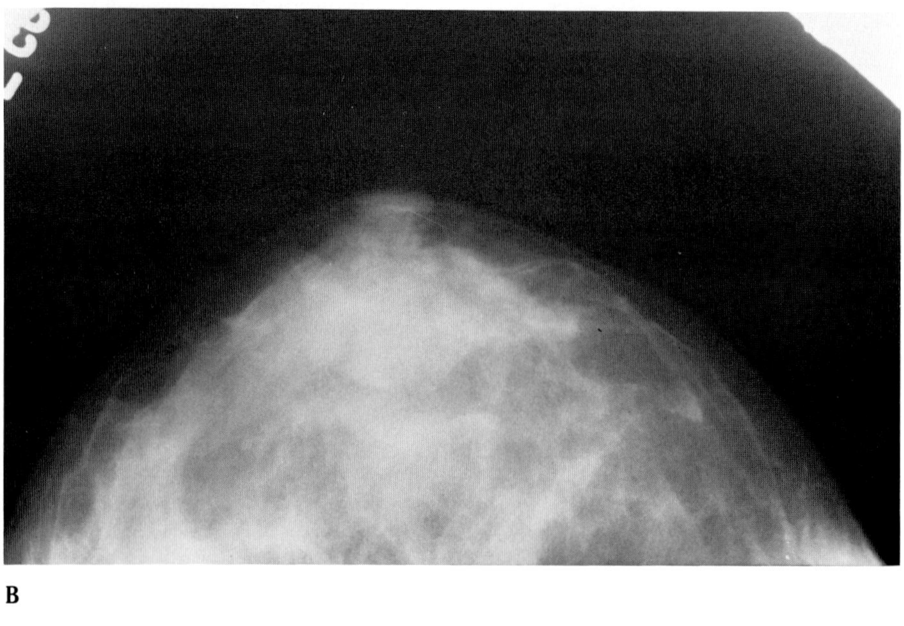

B

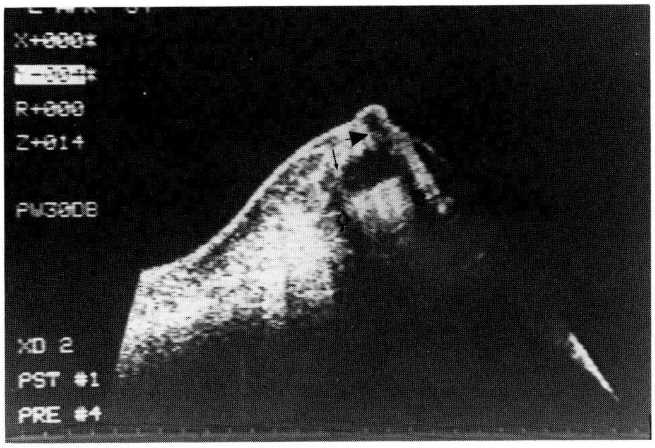

C

Fig. 10-5 **A:** Diaphanography shows decreased light transmission above the nipple area (arrows).
B: Mammogram, CC view. Note the poorly defined mass behind the nipple.
C: Ultrasound, single transducer. There is a well defined anechoic area with minimal increased through transmission. Note the shadowing from the edges of the mass (open arrows) and nipple (closed arrow). The thick wall (thin arrow) and a few scattered internal echoes suggest an infected cyst.

Case 6

M.S. is a 46-year-old woman who presented with a 5 cm nontender, movable mass at 12 o'clock in the right breast of 5 days' duration. Thermograms were normal. There was increased light transmission through the mass. The mass was moderately well defined on mammography, with not all the borders seen. On ultrasound there was a lobulated mass with a somewhat peculiar posterior wall formation and some internal echoes (Fig. 10-6A, B). On aspiration 22 cc of yellowish fluid was obtained. Cytology of the fluid was class I. Air was injected and a pneumocystogram performed. There was a multiloculated cyst with large and small components; the peculiar posterior wall seen on ultrasound was due to septation of the cyst (Fig. 10-6C).

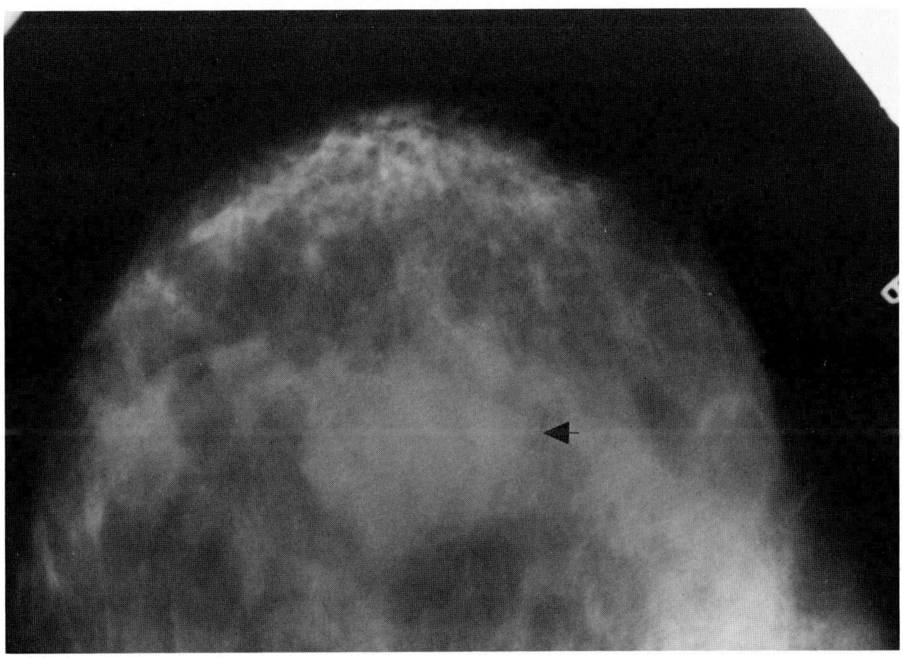

A

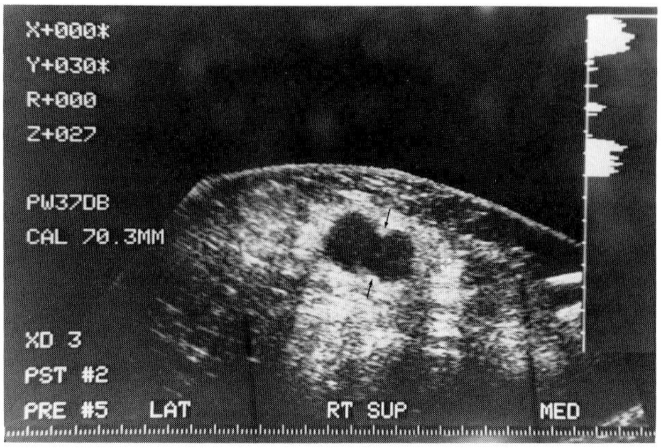

B

Fig. 10-6 A: Mammogram, CC view. The mass with borders is partially obscured by adjacent glandular tissue (arrow). **B:** Ultrasound, single transducer, transverse scan. Note the internal echoes and irregular anterior and posterior walls (arrows). There is increased through transmission. Internal echoes are seen on A-mode ultrasound also. **C:** Pneumocystogram. Note the marked cystic loculation causing irregularity on ultrasound.

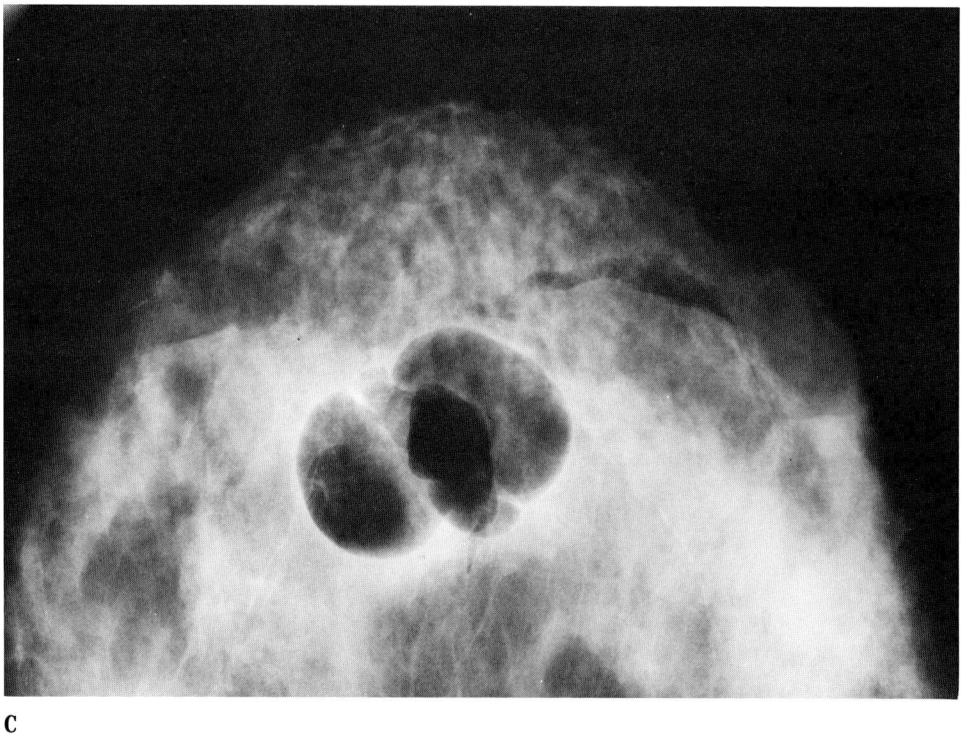

C

Case 7

M.B. is a 41-year-old woman who was referred because of a left breast mass of unknown duration. On physical examination there was a firm 2 cm mass in the lower outer left breast and a 2 by 4 cm oblong soft mass in the inner aspect of the right breast. Thermograms were normal. There was increased light transmission through both masses. On mammography there was marked glandularity (DY pattern). There was the suggestion of a density in the lower left breast, but it was inconclusive. On ultrasound there was a 2 by 3 cm cyst in the inner right breast, a smaller cyst in the lateral right breast, a large cyst in the lower left breast, and a smaller cyst elsewhere on the left (Fig. 10-7A). On aspiration the palpable cysts revealed 9 cc of brownish fluid on the right and 5 cc of yellowish fluid on the left. The cytology of the fluid was class I. The lower cyst on the left recurred within a week. Reaspiration obtained 2 cc of yellowish fluid. A pneumocystogram demonstrated smooth walls (Fig. 10-7B).

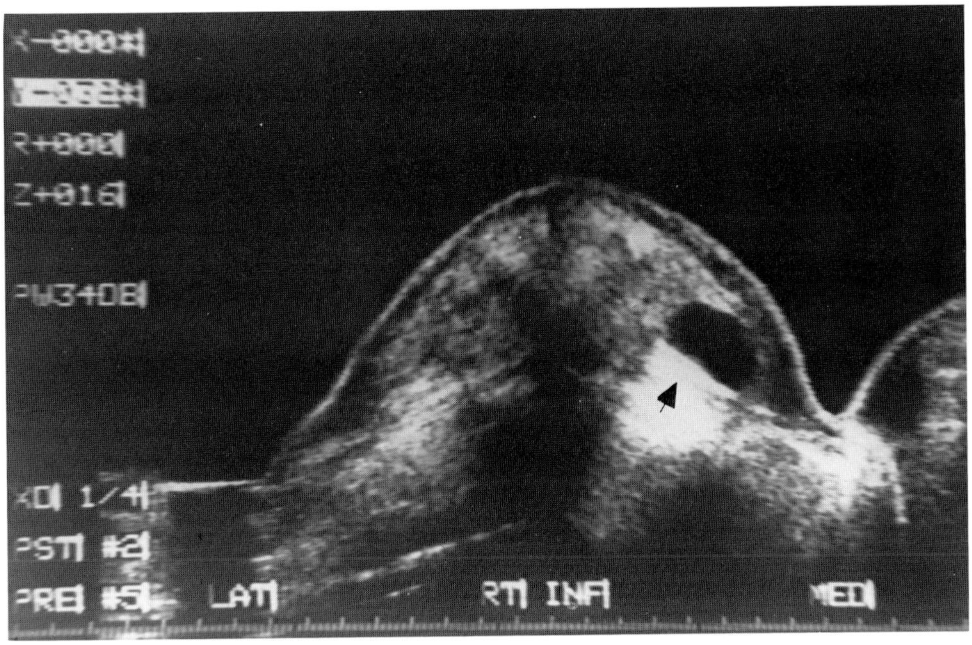

A

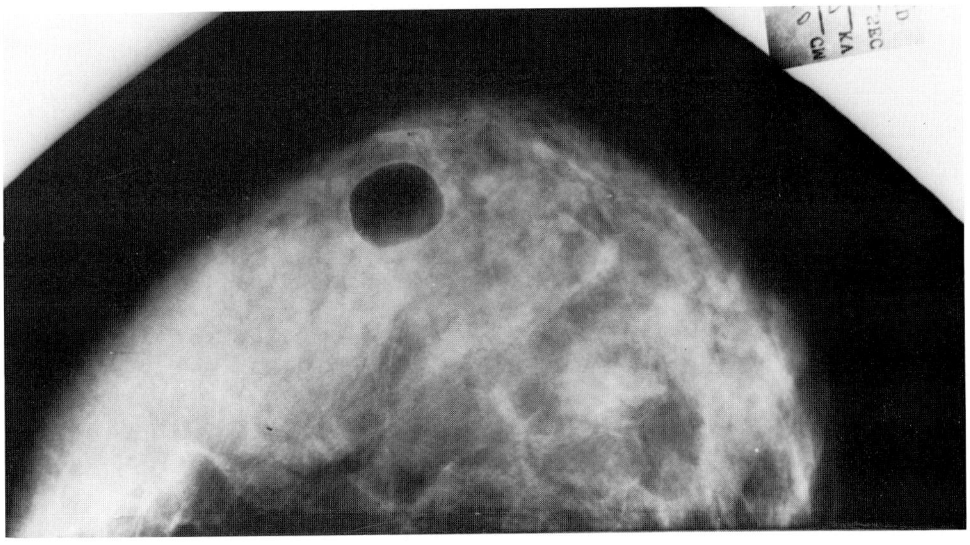

B

Fig. 10-7 **A:** Transverse ultrasound. Note the smooth-walled anechoic cyst with increased through transmission (arrow). **B:** Pneumocystogram. The cyst was smaller after recurrence. Note the air defining the smooth walls.

Discussion

Cysts usually occur in the actively menstruating woman in her thirties and forties, as in cases 2, 4, 5, 6, and 7. Case 1 is a teenager, an unusual but not rare occurrence. Case 3 is the opposite end of the age scale, a 68-year-old, who probably developed the cyst secondary to her estrogen therapy.

Thermography is usually normal unless the fluid is infected, as in case 5, where it reverts to normal once the infection has been cured. Diaphanography usually demonstrates increased light transmission through the cyst unless it is too deep to be seen. In case 5 the decreased light transmission was probably due to the thickened walls associated with an infected cyst. It is unsure why the cyst in case 2 demonstrated decreased light transmission.

It is not unusual for many cysts to be present and not palpated. In the dense glandular breast many cysts are not demonstrated on mammography, but they are seen on ultrasound.

In case 4 the cyst was incorrectly diagnosed on ultrasound as solid. Although this mistake is often due to incorrectly assigning a TGC curve with a resultant poor image quality, it must be remembered that ultrasound is not 100 percent accurate even in the diagnosis of cyst versus solid tumor. With any cyst that shows internal echoes or an irregular wall, cyst puncture and pneumocystography are indicated. Most often, as in case 6, the irregular walls are due to a multiloculated cyst.

About 2 percent of cysts recur following cyst aspiration, as they did in one of the above cases (case 7).

Bibliography

Barth V: *Atlas of Diseases of the Breast.* Stuttgart, Georg Thieme, 1979.

Cooke CG, Grant EG, Ciglay OS: Ultrasound demonstration of giant malignant breast cyst undetected by xeromammography. *J Clin Ultrasound* 1981;9:461–462.

Dupont WD, Page DL: Risk factors for breast cancer in women with proliferative breast disease. *N Engl J Med* 1985;312:146–151.

Egan R, McSweeney MB: Breast sonography—interpretative criteria, in Jellins J, Kobayashi T (eds): *Ultrasonic Examination of the Breast.* London, Wiley, 1983, pp 307–318.

Gautherie M, Kotewicz A, Gueblez P: Accurate and objective evaluation of breast thermograms: Basic principles and new advances with special reference to an improved computer-assisted scoring system, in Gautherie M, Albert E, Keith L (eds): *Thermal Assessment of Breast Health.* Lancaster, MTP Press, 1984, pp 74–97.

Haagensen CD, Bodian C, Haagensen DE: *Breast Carcinoma: Risk and Detection.* Philadelphia, Saunders, 1981.

Jellins J, Kossoff G, Reeve TS: Detection and classification of liquid-filled masses in the breast by Gray scale echography. *Radiology* 1977;125:205–212.

Kasumi F, Tanaka H: Diagnosis of intracystic tumors by ultrasound, in Jellins J, Kobayshi T (eds): *Ultrasonic Examination of the Breast.* London, Wiley, 1983, pp 283–291.

Martin JE: *Atlas of Mammography.* Baltimore, Williams & Wilkins, 1982.

Page DL, Vander Zwaag R, Rogers LW, et al: Relation between component parts of fibrocystic disease complex and breast cancer. *J Natl Cancer Inst* 1978;61:1055–1063.

Porrath S, Sandhu R, McNeil J: Thermography and benign breast disease. Proceedings American Academy of Thermology, Los Angeles, 1984.

Reuter K, D'Orsi CJ, Reale F: Intracystic carcinoma of the breast: The role of ultrasonography. *Radiology* 1985;153:233–234.

Sickles EA, Abele JS: Milk of calcium within tiny breast cysts. *Radiology* 1981;141:655–658.

Tabár L, Dean DB: *Teaching Atlas of Mammography.* Mammography. New York, Thieme-Stratton, 1983.

Tabár L, Pentek Z, Dean PB: The diagnostic and therapeutic value of breast cyst puncture and pneumocystography. *Radiology* 1981;141:659–663.

Wolfe JN: Breast patterns as an index of risk for developing breast cancer. *AJR* 1976;126:1130–1139.

11

Fat and Fatty Tumors

Saar Porrath

The accumulation of fat within the breast varies with age, menstrual or hormonal status, and of course weight. The greater a person's weight the more likely is it that the breast contains fat. The amount tends to increase with the degree of obesity.

Male breasts are usually fatty, except when there is gynecomastia. The prepubescent female breast contains fat and a small nubbin of glandular tissue. After the onset of menses, if the teenager is not heavy, there is an increase in glandularity, with little fat seen. During her twenties the amount of fat surrounding the glandular tissue increases. This is especially true if the patient has been pregnant and has nursed. The amount of fat in the breast varies in patients in their twenties, thirties, and forties.

The fat variation in the breast is evident with the Wolfe mammographic classification. There is little glandular tissue in N1 breasts, with primarily fat present. In the P1 category there is less fat and more glandularity, and in P2 even less fat and more glandularity. Finally in the DY breast there is very little fat, the breast being composed mostly of dense glandular tissue. The fat in the younger breast and in the DY breast is primarily on the outside, an insulating layer, and in the retroglandular area in front of the pectoralis muscle, whereas in the N1, P1, and P2 breasts fat is everywhere, around and throughout the glandular tissue.

In the postmenopausal women there is a general decrease in the glandular tissue, with fatty replacement. Unless there is hormone replacement therapy, the breast of the older woman and man is usually (but not always) fatty.

Fat occasionally appears in the middle of a glandular region as a distinct area. It is poorly defined, having no borders of its own but using that of the surrounding glandular tissue. If superficial, it may feel similar to a distinct mass; more commonly it is deep and seen only on mammography and ultrasound. On mammography the lobulated fat appears as a lucent (fatty) area surrounded by glandular tissue. On ultrasound it is seen as an area of low-level echoes or is almost echo-free, with rather distinct borders. If it is followed on serial ultrasound scans, it is usually seen to break up into subcutaneous fat. This accumulation of fat is known as a fatty lobule. It is not a tumor or pathologic condition.

In older patients and in women who have lost weight, there is often palpated on physical examination a superficial area, well defined, that can be soft or rather firm. This area may represent a fatty region between fibrous bands or Cooper's ligaments. It shows increased light transmission, as do most fatty areas. Thermography plays no role in its diagnosis. Mammography shows fat in the area of the palpable density, but there are no borders or capsule to the fatty area. Ultrasound shows low-level echoes consistent with fat. These areas do not change with the menstrual cycle. No treatment is necessary if the diagnosis is established with any certainty; however, if there is any question, biopsy may be indicated.

The fat lobule and the "trapped fat" pseudotumor described above are very different from the true fatty tumor, the lipoma. The lipoma is a well defined mass of fat cells surrounded by a distinct, thin-walled capsule. It can vary in size from a few millimeters to many centimeters. It usually feels soft and pliable, much like a partially water-filled balloon, although on occasion it feels firm and hard (see case 2, Chapter 23). It is rare that the lipoma creates symptoms or signs other than those seen with a mass. Malignant degeneration into a liposarcoma is very unusual. If large and relatively superficial, the lipoma can present as an area of decreased heat and vascularity on thermography. On light scanning there is usually increased light transmission, simulating a cyst. Ultrasound shows a well defined area of diffuse low- to moderate-level echoes. Mammography usually establishes the diagnosis, demonstrating a well defined fatty area with a thin capsule.

Angiolipoma and fibrolipoma are additional benign tumors of mixed content, containing fat and other tissue. Their clinical presentation may be similar to that of the lipoma, but more often they are firmer and more distinct. The thermogram may be positive, depending on the vascularity. Diaphanography may be positive owing to the increased vascularity. Mammography shows a distinct tumor with well defined borders, demonstrating a mixture of fat and other tissue. The ultrasound also demonstrates a well defined lesion with a mixed echo pattern.

Fat necrosis is caused by the release of enzymes into the fat, resulting in an area of acute liquefaction and inflammation. Fat necrosis has a myriad of presentations. It can be innocuous and asymptomatic, or it can simulate a cancer. It usually occurs after trauma or surgery. On occasion it is secondary to a medical disease such as pancreatitis. Usually the involved area is tender, occasionally painful. A mass may be present. Retraction occurs occasionally. The thermogram is usually normal. Diaphanography may show some decreases in light transmission or be normal. The mammogram may show a mass with somewhat ill-defined borders, a well defined area, or some increase in density, or it may be normal. Later there may be spiculization as the area retracts, forming a scar-like lesion that may simulate carcinoma. There may be punctate calcifications or more commonly, rounded or irregular calcifications. The ultrasound may show shadowing, with or without a low-level echo mass. The diagnosis is established on biopsy but can be suspected by the clinical findings.

Case Studies: Lipomas

Case 1

P.F. is a 34-year-old woman who was evaluated by mammography 3 months earlier for a soft, movable, 4 cm mass in the lower outer aspect of the right breast. The mass had not been appreciated on outside xeromammograms (Figs. 11-1A, B). Repeat mammography with attention to the mass showed a 4 cm well defined lipoma (Fig. 11-1C). It was thought that because of the softness and the mobility of the lesion it had slipped on previous films and was not visible.

Case 2

T.W. is a 38-year-old woman who had a soft, movable, 4 by 5 cm mass in the upper outer aspect of the right breast for years. Thermograms and diaphanography were normal. There was a well defined lipoma present on mammography (Fig. 11-2). On ultrasound an area of low-level echoes was defined.

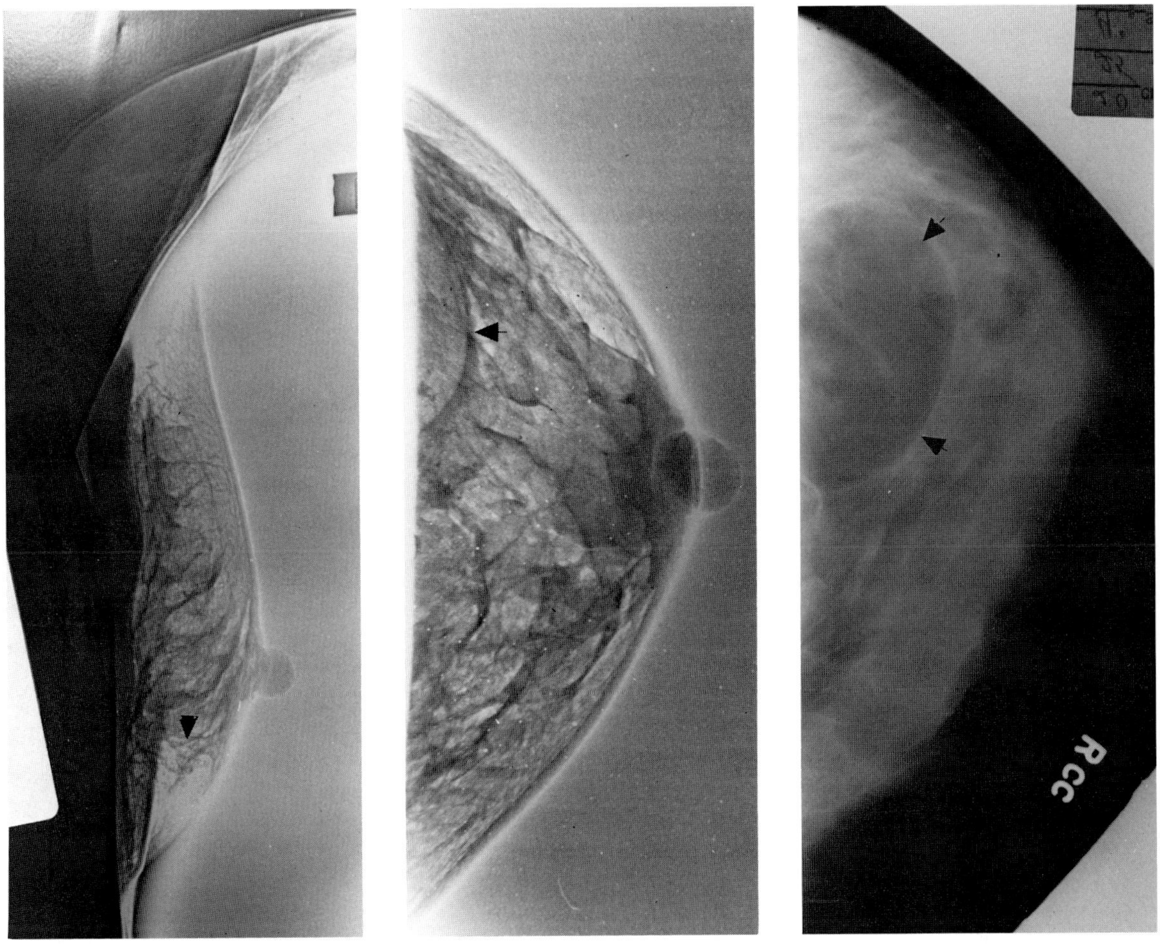

A B C

Figure 11-1 **A:** Xeromammogram, lateral view. Note the fat area in the inferior breast (arrow). **B:** CC view. Note the anterior edge of the lipoma (arrow). The lipoma should have been appreciated from these films. **C:** CC view. This is a well demarcated lipoma (arrows).

Case 3

F.P. is a 64-year-old woman who was referred because of a lateral left breast mass. On physical examination there was a 3 by 4 cm firm mass just lateral and inferior to the breast itself, overlying the ribs. The breast examination was normal. X-ray films over the mass demonstrated a scalloping fatty defect of the muscle overlying the ribs. At surgery a lipoma was excised.

Discussion

On physical examination most lipomas are soft and movable. The diagnosis can usually be made with great accuracy on mamography. As in case 1, attention must be directed to be sure that the lesion does not slip off the plate when compression is applied. Usually on diaphanography there is increased light transmission through the lipoma. (The reader is also referred to case 2 in Chapter 23.)

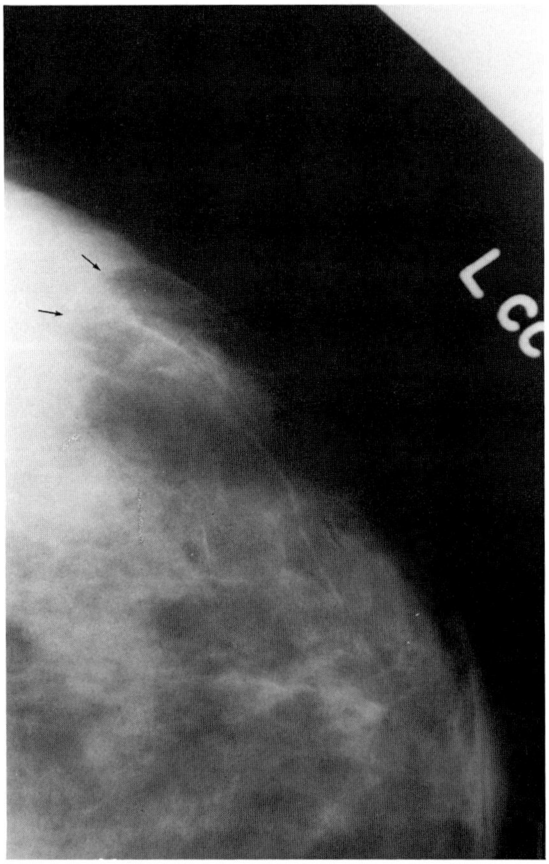

Fig. 11-2 CC view. Note the fat area with a well defined capsule (arrows).

Case Studies: Fat Necrosis

Case 4

V.H. is a 63-year-old woman who was referred because of slight dimpling of the left breast at 9 o'clock. There were tender areas within the left breast but no discrete mass. Thermography and diaphanography were normal. Mammography revealed a well defined 2 cm mass without calcification. Ultrasound showed the mass to be solid with diffuse echoes. A needle biopsy was attempted and revealed adipose tissue. A biopsy was advised.

At surgery an organizing hematoma of recent duration was found with some surrounding fat necrosis. There was also ductal ectasia and focal atypical cribriform intraductal hyperplasia. This finding did not correlate with the mammographic picture, and the patient was requested to return for postoperative mammography.

She was seen 2 months later. There was a scar just medial to the left nipple, and nodular density was felt adjacent to the scar. Mammography again showed the well defined 2 cm mass. There was a 2.5 cm area of disorganized fat just medial to the well defined lesion (Fig. 11-3A) that had not been present on the earlier mammograms. A needle was inserted into the nodular mass that had been felt clinically, and a repeat mammogram showed the needle to be present in the encapsulated poorly defined fat area. The lesion was interpreted as postoperative fat necrosis. A biopsy of the well defined lesion was again suggested. After preoperative localization a fibroadenoma was removed. The nodular area thought to be fat necrosis was left in the breast.

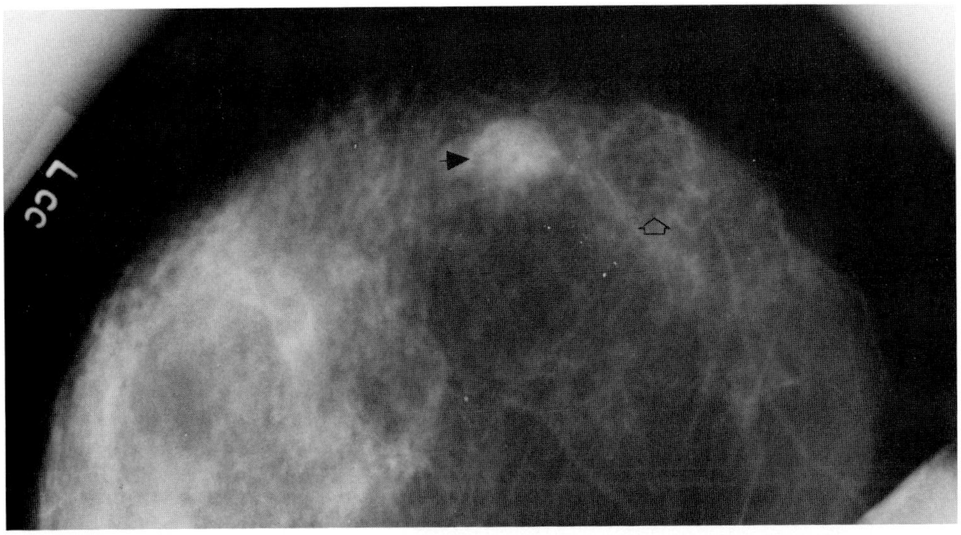

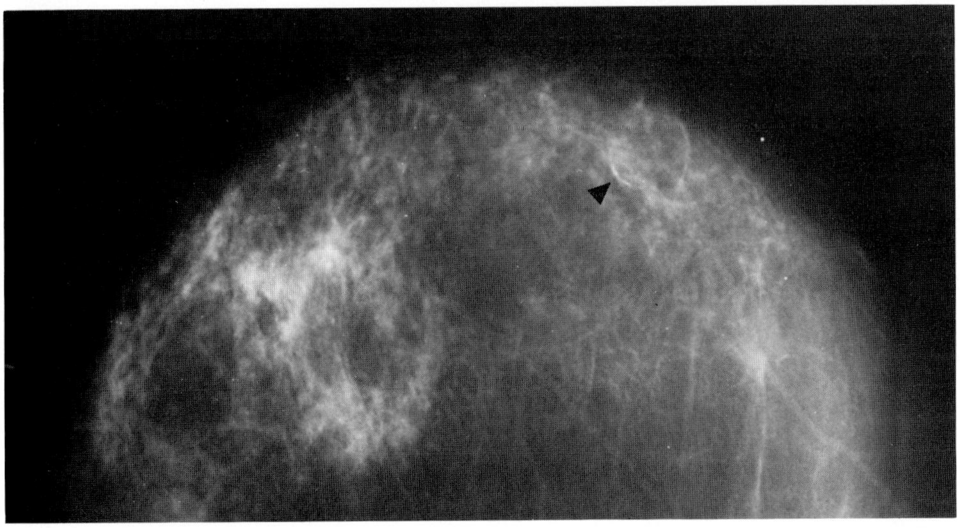

B

Fig. 11-3 **A:** CC view. Note the well defined area of slightly increased density (solid arrow) and the disorganized fatty area (open arrow). **B:** CC view. The mass is gone. The rim of calcification partially surrounding the fatty area which is now smaller and less disorganized (arrowhead).

Repeat mammography 8 months later showed the well defined area to be absent. There was a fine rim of calcification now partially surrounding the encapsulated area of disorganized fat (Fig. 11-3B). Incidentally, the dimpling was no longer present.

Case 5

M.J. is a 74-year-old woman who was referred because of a painful right breast mass of 4 months' duration. Mammograms done elsewhere were reported as "fatty, no lesion." On physical examination there was a tender, poorly defined, 2 cm mass in the outer aspect of the right breast.

Liquid thermograms were normal. There was a slight decrease in light transmission over the mass. A repeat single-view mammogram demonstrated fat (N1 pattern), with no lesion. There was a poorly defined low-level echo density with some shadowing seen on ultrasound (Fig. 11-4).

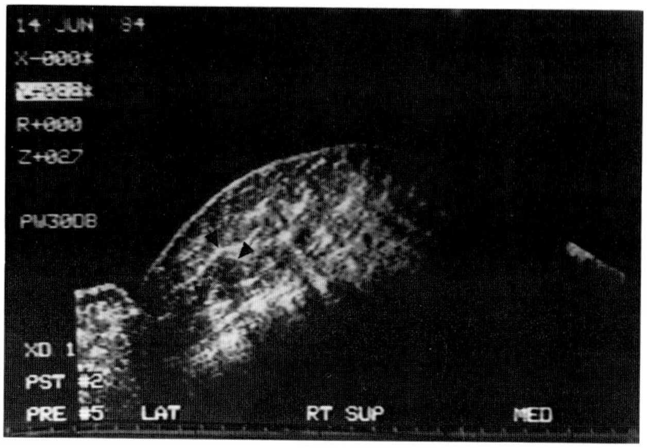

Fig. 11-4 Ultrasound. There is a poorly defined low-level echo density with slight posterior shadowing (arrows).

Because of the presence of a mass, the positive diaphanography, and the ultrasound findings, biopsy was suggested, with a diagnosis of probable fat necrosis. An area of fat necrosis was found at surgery.

Discussion

In case 4 the needle biopsy caused a hematoma and minimal fat necrosis. A normal report of a needle biopsy in the face of a well defined lesion on mammography may imply that the lesion was missed by the needle, and a formal biopsy is indicated.

The surgery done without localization did not find the lesion described on mammography. Any lesion that is not palpable deserves preoperative localization, as was done on the second attempt.

It is important that the mass palpated corresponds to the mass seen on mammography. By inserting a needle into the palpable mass and repeating the mammogram, it was apparent that the palpable mass was new, probably fat necrosis, and that the lesion seen on mammography was not the lesion being felt.

If the pathology report does not correspond to the mammographic findings, further investigation is necessary. The repeat mammogram in case 4 revealed that the lesion seen initially had not been resected. It is imperative for the breast imager to obtain pathology reports and to correlate them with the studies that have been performed, both to improve his or her learning curves and statistics and to be sure that the correct area was removed at surgery.

The density felt 2 months after the initial surgery and seen as a new area of encapsulated poorly defined fat, which later had a partially calcified rim, was due to fat necrosis caused by the first surgery. It is probable that this patient for some reason is particularly susceptible to fat necrosis.

As in case 5, a mass found clinically in a patient who has a normal "fatty" mammogram must be investigated further. When diaphanography and ultrasound showed the mass to be real in case 5 and not a fatty area, the probable diagnosis of fat necrosis was made. There are no other lesions that would cause these findings. A lipoma would be seen on the mammography and show increased light transmission on diaphanography, whereas a 2 cm cancer would be seen on mammography in a fatty breast.

Bibliography

Lipomas

Barth V: *Atlas of Diseases of the Breast.* Stuttgart, Georg Thieme, 1979.

Beham M, Kazam E: The echographic characteristics of fatty tissues and tumors. *Radiology* 1978;129:143–151.

Egan RL, McSweeney MB: Breast sonography—interpretative criteria, in Jellins J, Kobayashi T (eds): *Ultrasonic Examination of the Breast.* London, Wiley, 1983, pp 307–318.

Martin JE: *Atlas of Mammography.* Baltimore, Williams & Wilkins, 1982.

Tabar L, Dean DB: *Teaching Atlas of Mammography.* New York, Thieme-Stratton, 1983.

Wolfe JN: Breast patterns as an index of risk for developing breast cancer. *AJR* 1976;126:1130–1139.

Fat Necrosis

Barth V: *Atlas of Diseases of the Breast.* Stuttgart, Georg Thieme, 1979.

Egan RL, McSweeney MB: Breast sonography—interpretative criteria, in Jellins J, Kobayashi T (eds): *Ultrasonic Examination of the Breast.* London, Wiley, 1983, pp 307–318.

Martin JE: *Atlas of Mammography.* Baltimore, Williams & Wilkins, 1982.

Nielsen BB, Fenger C, Kjeldsen H: Massive bilateral fat necrosis of the male breast. *Breast* 1984;10(4):2–4.

Orson LW, Cigtay OS: Fat necrosis of the breast: Characteristic xeromammographic appearance. *Radiology* 1983;146:35–38.

Sonnefeld M, D'Orsi CJ, Sadowsky NL, et al: Mammographic patterns of unusual breast lesions. *JCE Radiol* 1979;1:13–30.

Tabár L, Dean DB: *Teaching Atlas of Mammography.* New York, Thieme-Stratton, 1983.

12

Fibroadenomas

Saar Porrath

Fibroadenomas are the second most common benign tumor of the female breast, cysts being the commonest. Fibroadenomas are most prevalent during the teenage years through the thirties. There may be a resurgence during the postmenopausal decades.

There is a division of the broad category of adenomas into juvenile adenomas, adenomas, adenomas of pregnancy or gestational adenomas, giant fibroadenomas, cystosarcoma phylloides, and fibroadenomas.

On rare occasions there is a malignant degeneration into fibrosarcoma. More commonly there is replacement of the adenoma by a ductal carcinoma, which may arise from the glandular elements of the adenoma. Except for the growth that may occur, there is nothing which signifies this change into malignancy. There may be some pain, but it is unusual. An example is the cystosarcoma phylloides. Most of these tumors are benign, although on occasion there are sarcomatous tissues present.

On physical examination the adenoma in teenagers presents as a small, firm mass. Usually superficial, that does not change with the menstrual cycle. It seldom shows any significant growth, the growth being slow and difficult to measure over short time spans. Often if left alone the adenoma regresses as the woman enters her twenties. The lesions are often multiple.

The adenoma seldom calcifies and on mammography may not be seen in the background of the dense glandularity of the young breast. If seen, it is well defined with smooth borders and occasionally a halo of lucency due to compressed fat surrounding the lesion. Because the younger breast tends to have less fat, this sign is more common in the older patient than in the teenager.

Diaphanography may show the adenoma as an area of decreased light transmission. Often it is not visible in the dense, glandular young breast, which in itself may show a generalized decrease in light transmission. The degree of differentiation depends on the size of the adenoma, the density of the surrounding tissue, and most independently the depth of the adenoma in the breast.

Thermography plays no active role in the diagnosis, usually being normal unless a large size is obtained. Ultrasound allows identification of the mass as a solid structure, usually with homogeneous low-level echoes throughout. The borders are well defined, and a strong anterior echo is seen. There is often edge shadowing from the posterior corners, resulting in a "tadpole" sign posteriorly as originally reported by Kobayashi. Harper thought that the findings are virtually pathognomonic. Although the ultrasonic picture is almost diagnostic and at the age encountered there are few other tumors present, it is not possible to have an accurate diagnosis without a pathologic specimen.

This author is willing to watch small, well defined adenomas in young patients. If is thought that the patient will be lost to follow-up biopsy is usually recommended. If any growth occurs, a biopsy is mandatory at that time.

The same principles are true for fibroadenomas in women in their twenties and thirties except that calcifications are more common. The calcifications may be "typical" with gross clumps of calcium measuring 2 mm or more, although occasionally small punctate calcifications are seen not unlike those of malignancy. In this age group there is no waiting if there is the slightest doubt about the diagnosis, biopsy is recommended in all but those with gross calcifications.

The postmenopausal fibroadenoma usually presents as a well defined mass with gross calcification. Not infrequently there are only calcifications, without a mass.

Sartorius has shown that on ductography a pattern of duct ramifications are seen throughout the adenoma. This pattern is virtually pathognomonic of the entity (see Chapter 6).

The adenoma of pregnancy, also known as a gestational adenoma, shows accelerated growth owing to the hormonal influence of pregnancy. It presents as an enlarging mass that usually regresses after pregnancy unless the patient nurses, and then it regresses after lactation ceases. Because of the markedly increased density of the breast seen on mammography during pregnancy and lactation the lesion may not be apparent. The thermogram is diffusely vascular during pregnancy and lactation, and hence there may be no apparent difference. On the light scan there is a very dense area seen, although the breast itself is diffusely light-absorptive during pregnancy and lactation. If deep, the lesion may be impossible to identify. Ultrasound shows a well defined lesion with many internal echoes. If a needle biopsy shows a well defined acinar pattern, the lesion should be followed to see if regression occurs.

A giant fibroadenoma usually presents during the late teens and twenties. It is an arbitrary decision that adenomas over 3 cm are called giant. For the most part the giant adenoma is and acts like other fibroadenomas with the exception that there may be accelerated growth compared to the usual fibroadenoma. The presentation on physical examination is mass often 6 cm in diameter. There is a history of the mass having enlarged. It may be smooth or lobulated and is usually well defined. It usually feels firm, although it may be soft.

Mammography shows a dense mass, well defined. Calcification is unusual. Because of its size some of the borders may be obscured by overlying glandular tissue and hence poorly defined. Diaphanography shows a decrease in light transmission. Thermography may show an increase in both heat and vascularity due to the size of the mass. Ultrasound demonstrates a solid mass with low-level echoes and well defined borders. There is a strong anterior echo, with some shadowing posterior to the lesion.

Cystosarcoma phylloides presents much like the giant fibroadenoma; it is a smaller but different lesion. It may have sheets of tissue with some clefts. The tumor is sometimes seen on ultrasound as diffuse low-level echoes with a variation in density reflecting the clefts. The other tests are usually the same as those for the giant fibroadenoma. There is a propensity for the lesion to recur, so there should be careful postoperative follow-up. If there is sarcomatous degeneration, it may be difficult to detect.

Surgery is the treatment of choice for fibroadenomas. Simple excision is usually all that is necessary. In the case of cystosarcoma phylloides, if there has been sarcomatous degeneration mastectomy may be indicated. Lumpectomy and radiation therapy are not advocated for these lesions. If there is a malignant growth such as a ductal carcinoma that has replaced all or part of a fibroadenoma, these lesions are treated as if they were the cancer, ignoring the fibroadenoma portion. Cystosarcoma phylloides has a propensity to recur, and hence these patients are followed carefully. If adenomas are allowed to grow, there can be a pressure necrosis of the adjacent tissues necessitating simple mastectomy for a benign condition.

There is nothing to indicate that fibroadenomas are premalignant. The coexistence of a fibroadenoma and a malignancy in the same breast is not unusual. For this reason a preoperative mammogram should be done in patients over thirty who have a mass that is clinically an adenoma.

Case Studies: Fibroadenomas

Case 1

A.V. is a 33-year-old woman who presented with a 1 by 2 cm bilobed, discrete, firm mass in the upper inner aspect of the left breast. Thermograms showed increased nipple heat on the left. Diaphanography showed glandular tissue with no change in light absorption over the mass. Mammograms showed a P2 pattern with a poorly defined, somewhat smooth-bordered 2 by 3 cm mass without calcifications. Ultrasound demonstrated a low-level echo mass, well defined, with slight shadowing from the edges (Fig. 12-1). A fibroadenoma was removed at surgery.

Case 2

C.S. is a 31-year-old woman who presented with a firm, well defined nodule at 9 o'clock in the right breast of unknown duration. There was no pain or tenderness. Thermog-

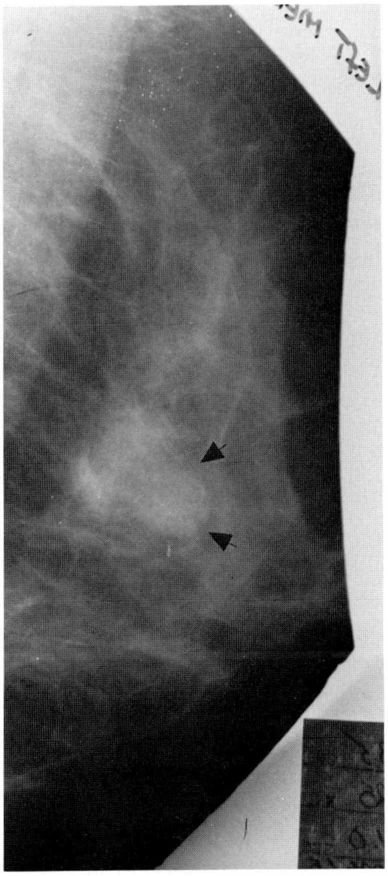

A

Fig. 12-1 **A:** Medial lateral view. Note the mass with some borders well defined (arrows) and others obscured by glandular tissue. **B:** Ultrasound. There is a moderately defined mass with internal echoes and a strong anterior echo (arrow). Note the slight shadowing from the posterior edge (thin arrows).

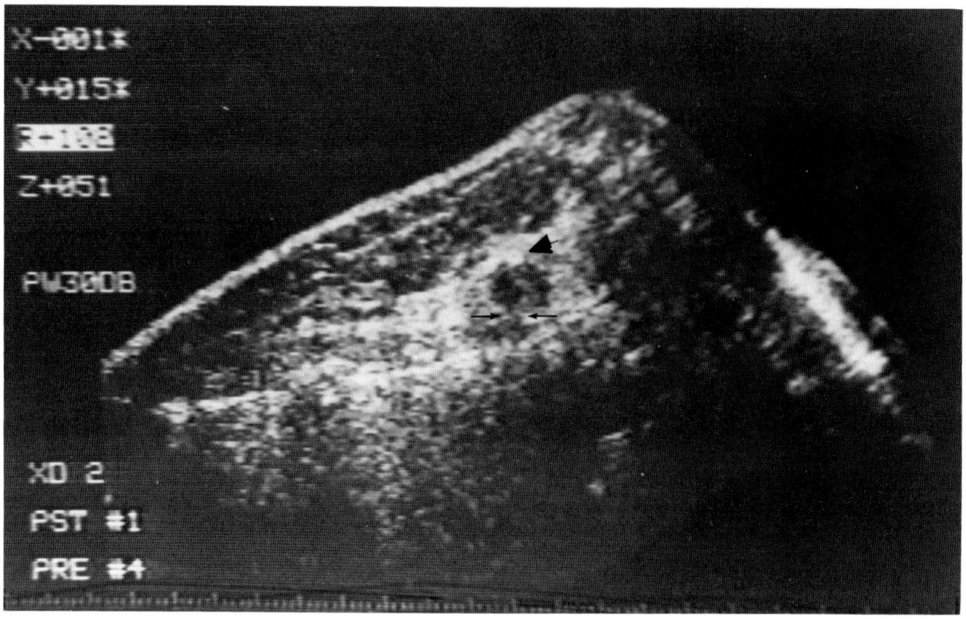

B

raphy and diaphanography were normal. Mammography showed markedly glandular tissue (Wolfe DY), with the mass not evident. Ultrasound demonstrated a moderately defined lesion with diffuse low-level internal echoes and no shadowing. A juvenile fibroadenoma was removed at surgery.

Case 3

C.A. is a 37-year-old woman who was referred after an aspiration attempt of a breast mass revealed no fluid. The mass had been present for about 2 months. On physical examination there was a slight hematoma from the recent aspiration. Below this was a freely movable, well defined, firm, 2 cm mass in the outer aspect of the left breast.

Liquid crystal thermograms showed increased nipple heat on the left (Th III thermogram). Diaphanography demonstrated markedly decreased light transmission over the hematoma and a slight decrease in light transmission over the nodule (Fig. 12-2A). Mammograms showed a 2 cm nodule with most of the borders seen and well defined. Glandular tissue obscured part of the borders (Fig. 12-2B). Ultrasound revealed diffuse low-level echoes throughout the mass (Fig. 12-2C). A fibroadenoma was removed at surgery. A repeat thermogram 2 months later was normal. Diaphanography revealed a very slight decrease in light transmission consistent with resolving postoperative changes.

Case 4

E.H. is a 29-year-old woman referred because of multiple bilateral breast masses. On physical examination she was noted to have extremely large breasts. There were more than 10 masses felt, the largest almost 8 cm in diameter, in the outer aspect of the left breast. The masses varied from firm and well defined to soft and less defined.

Thermograms were normal. Diaphanography showed diminished light transmission through the masses. Mammography showed moderate glandular tissue (Wolfe P1 pattern). There were many well defined masses present bilaterally, measuring from 0.5 to 8 cm. Behind the right nipple was a well defined 4 cm mass containing many diffuse microcalcifications (Fig. 12-3A, B, C). Automated breast ultrasound showed all the masses to be solid with varying degrees of internal echoes, from very minimal echogenicity to diffuse low-level internal echoes (Fig. 12-3D, E).

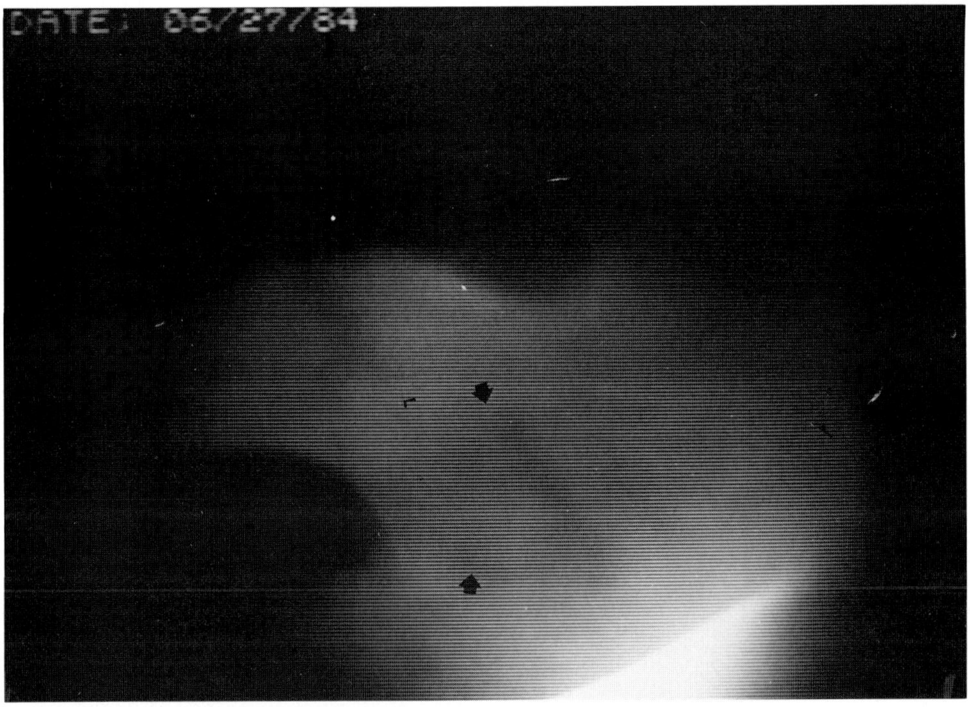

A

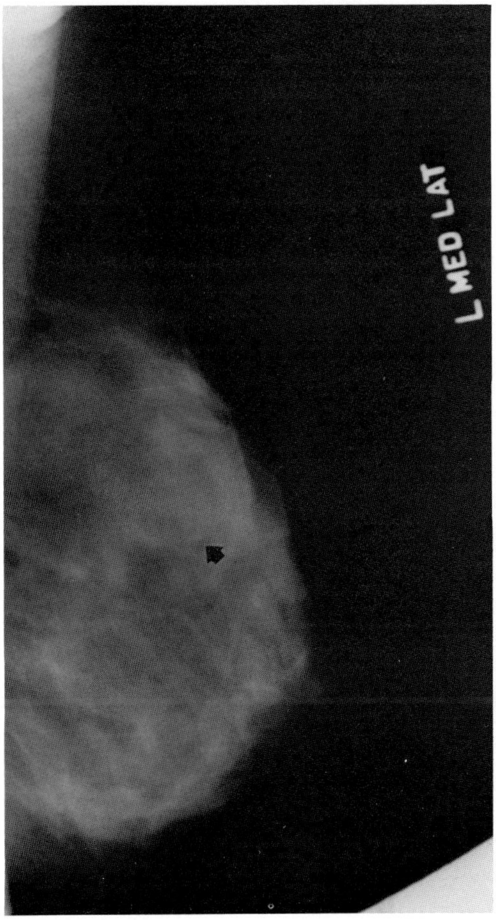

B

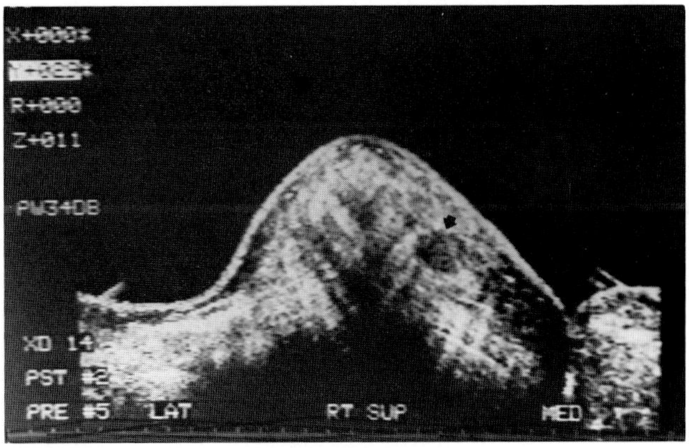

C

Fig. 12-2 **A:** Diaphanography. Note the area of decreased light transmission (arrows). **B:** Mammmography, lateral view. There is a mass with some borders well seen and others obscured by glandularity (arrow). **C:** Ultrasound. There is a moderately defined mass with diffuse internal echoes (arrow) and minimal posterior shadowing.

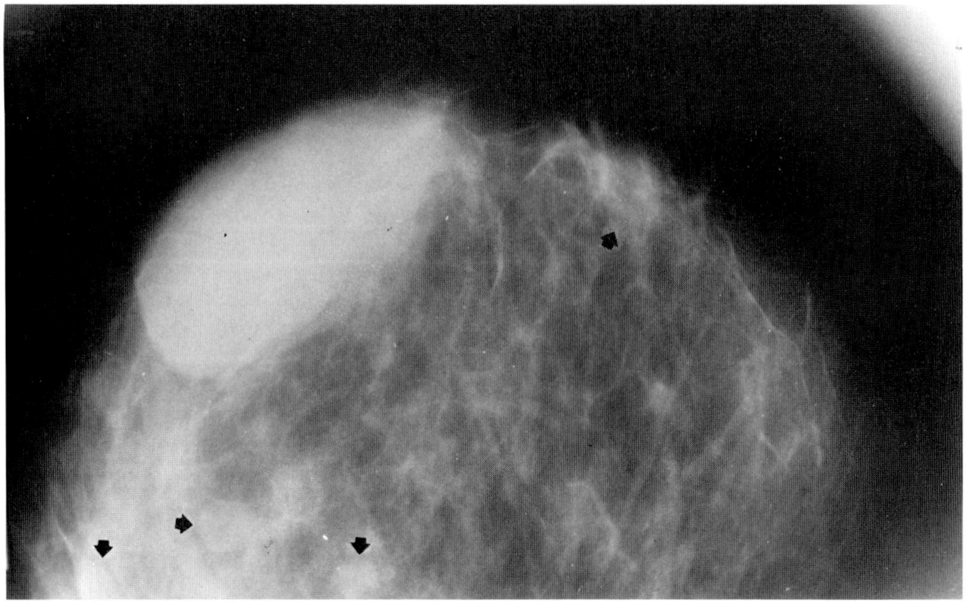

A

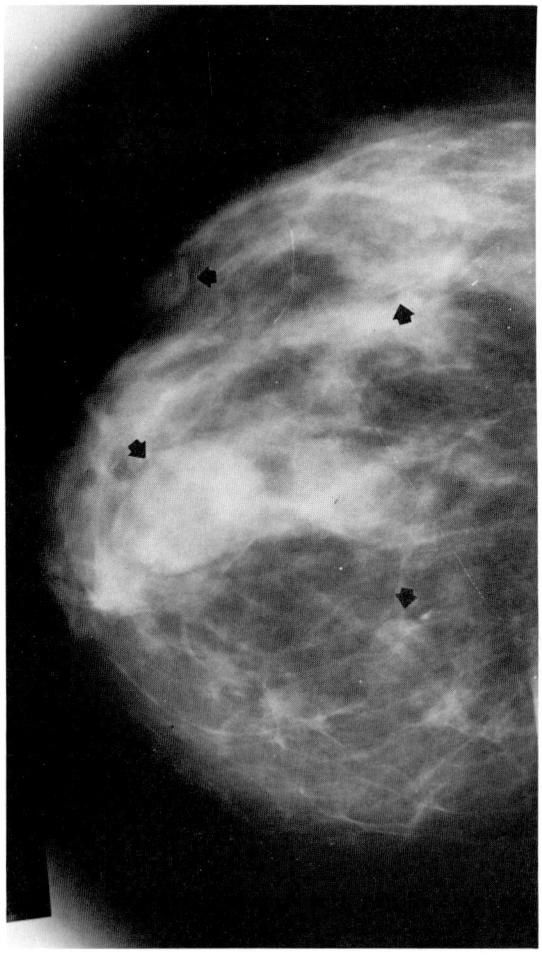

B

Fig. 12-3 **A:** Mammograph, left CC view. There is a large (8 cm) well defined mass. Four additional fibroadenomas are also seen (arrows). **B:** Mammograph, right CC view. Note the well defined masses (arrows). **C:** Higher magnification of an anterior mass on the right. There are diffuse small calcifications within the mass; two are indicated by thin arrows. (*Figure continues.*)

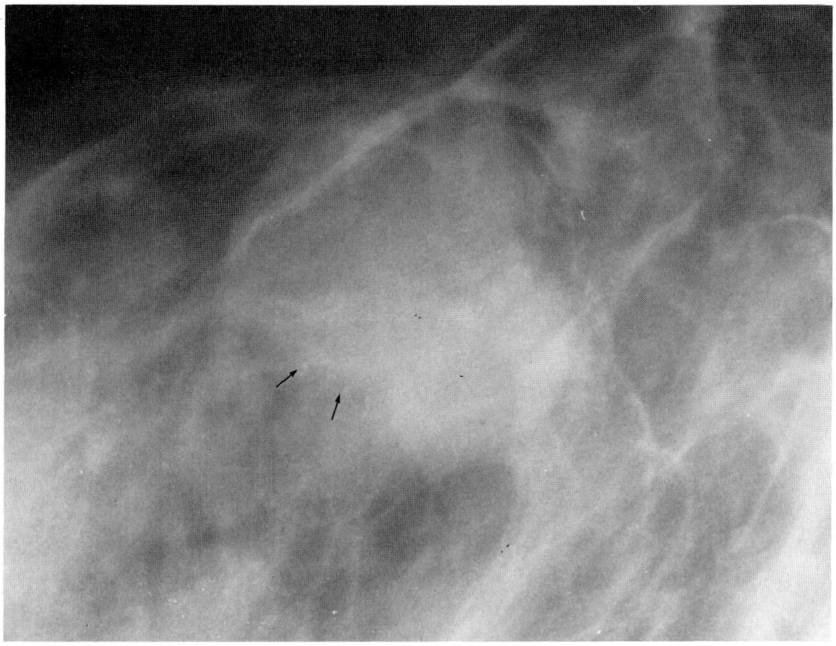

C

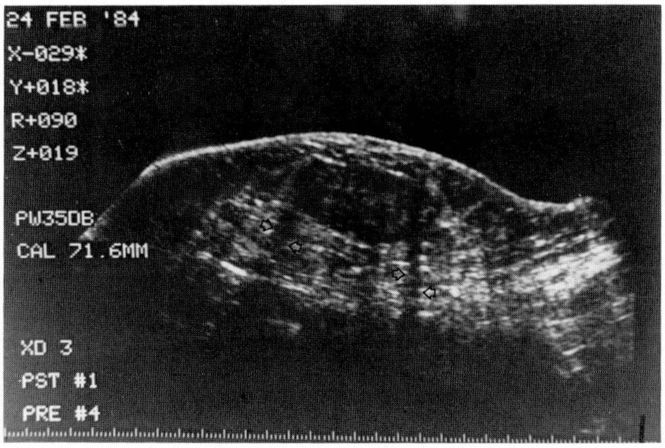

D

Fig. 12-3 D: Ultrasound. There is a well defined low-level echo mass with diffuse internal echoes and posterior edge shadowing (open arrows). E: Ultrasound. Open arrows outline the compression band. (This is not a double line of skin thickening.) There is a well defined mass with a few internal echoes. Compare Figs. D and E with Figs. 10-2A, 10-5C, and 10-6B of cysts and note the lack of through transmissions and internal echoes which differentiate fibroadenomas from cysts.

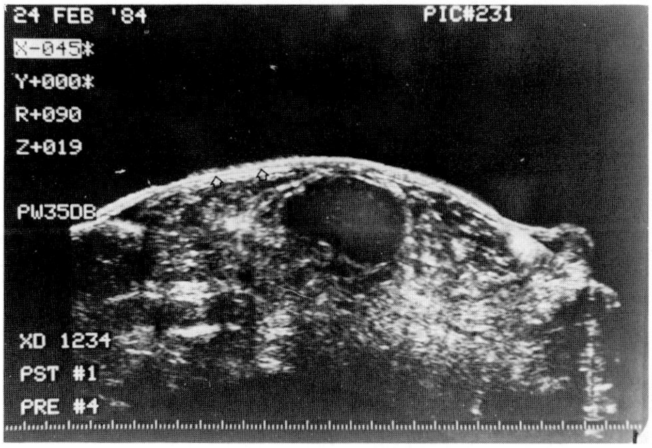

E

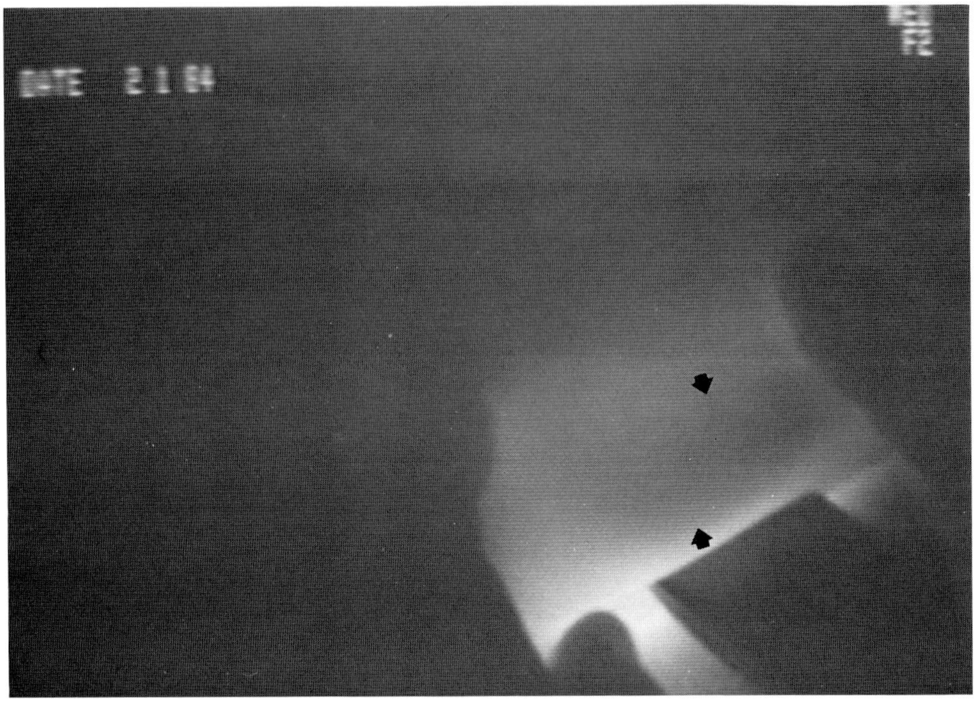

A

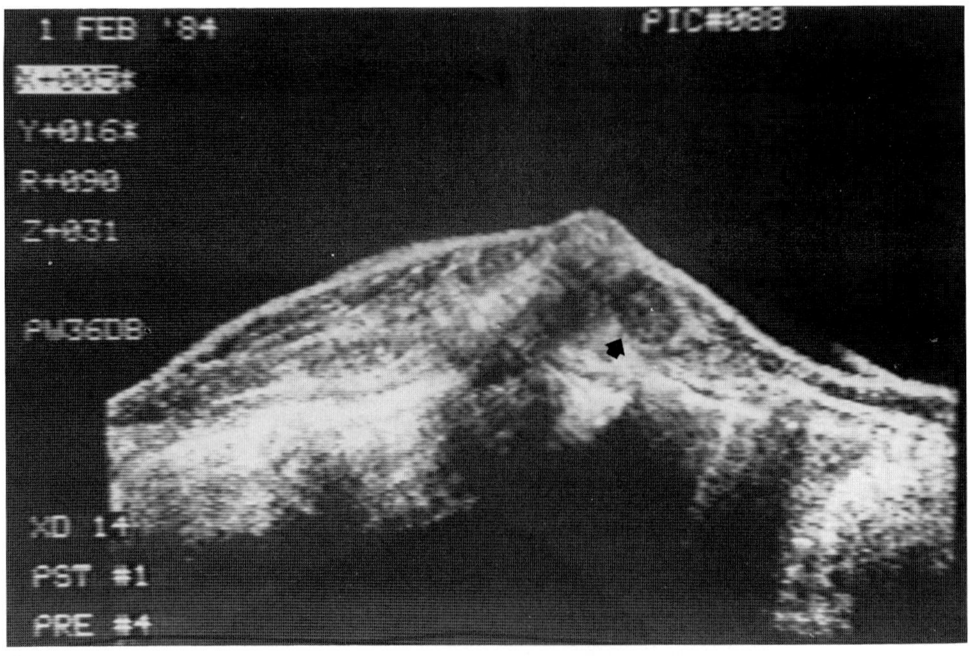

B

Fig. 12-4 A: Diaphanography. Note the area of decreased light transmission. **B:** Ultrasound. Note the well defined area of low-level echoes with no increased through transmission (arrow).

At surgery multiple fibroadenomas were removed. There were also areas of adenofibrosis. The mass with the calcifications was a fibroadenoma. Eighteen months later the patient presented with seven new fibroadenomas that had not been evident on review of the previous imaging studies.

Case 5

G.K. is a 19-year-old woman who presented with a 4 cm freely movable firm mass in the lower aspect of the right breast. Thermograms were normal. Light scanning showed a diffuse decrease in light transmission throughout the breast due to glandular tissue, with a further decrease in light transmission over the nodule itself (Fig. 12-4A). A mammogram showed marked glandularity (DY pattern), with the mass poorly defined and indistinguishable from the underlying tissue. Ultrasound demonstrated a well defined area of diffuse low-level echoes (Fig. 12-4B). At surgery a giant fibroadenoma was removed.

Case 6

S.L. is a 14-year-old girl who presented with a 5 cm firm mass behind the right nipple causing moderate distortion of the breast contour. She had been seen at a local health maintenance organization (HMO) where after physical examination she was told that she had a benign lesion and surgery was unnecessary.

Liquid crystal thermograms showed increased vascularity on the right (Th III thermogram). There was marked decrease in light transmission through the mass (Fig. 12-5A). A single-view mammogram demonstrated a large homogeneous mass without calcifications. On ultrasound there was a well defined mass with low level echoes (Fig. 12-5B).

Because the mass was enlarging, which presented a danger of tissue necrosis owing to pressure on the adjacent tissue, removal was suggested. At surgery a giant fibroadenoma was found.

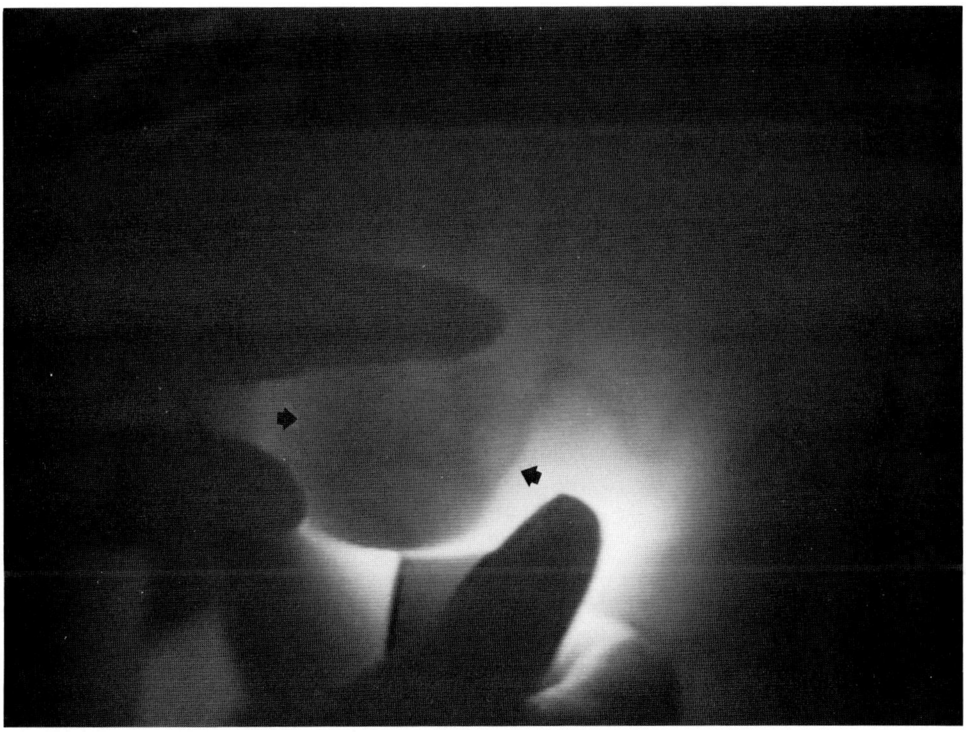

A

Fig. 12-5 A: Diaphanography. Note the markedly decreased light transmission behind the right nipple (arrows).

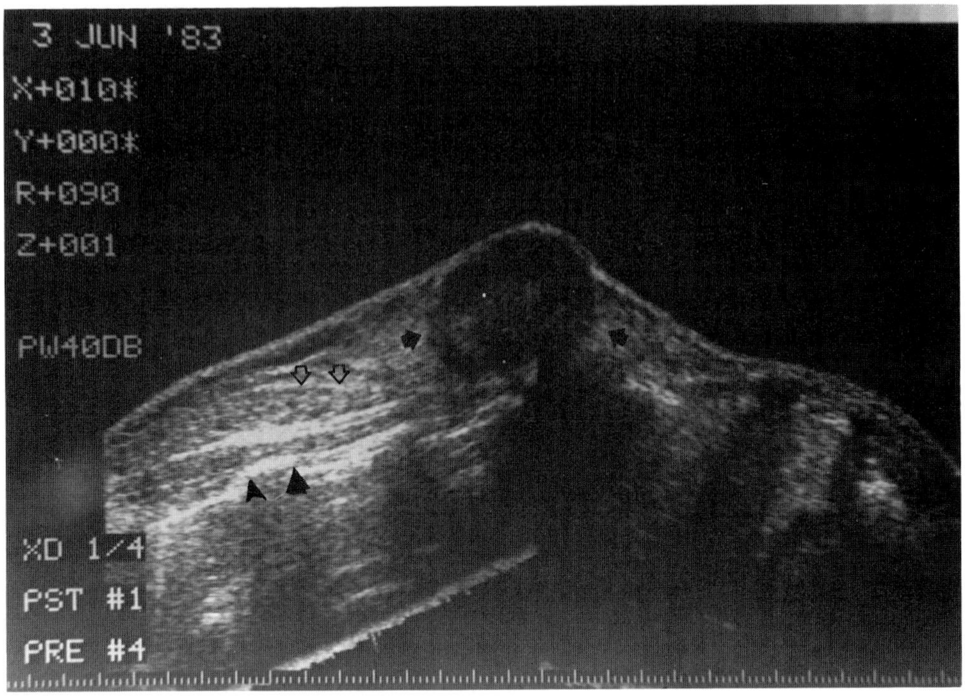

B

Fig. 12-5 B: Longitudinal ultrasound. Note the well defined mass with diffuse low-level echoes and no increased through transmission (solid arrows). Note the pectoralis muscle (open arrows) and intercostal muscle. Arrowheads flank the rib echo area indenting the intercostal muscle.

Case 7

L.J. is a 44-year-old woman who 2 years previously had had a left mastectomy. On physical examination there was mild glandularity and multiple scars on the right breast; no masses were felt.

Thermograms and diaphanography were normal. On mammograms there were four nodular densities containing gross calcifications, consistent with fibroadenomas. There were three other poorly defined densities, one of which contained a very small amount of calcification thought to also be a fibroadenoma; the other two masses did not contain calcifications (Fig. 12-6C). Ultrasound demonstrated two cysts, consistent with the two noncalcified densities and shadowing from some of the other calcified lesions. A review of previous mammograms showed a changing pattern of calcifications, with minimal findings 2 years earlier (Fig. 12-6A), to more calcification a year later (Fig. 12-6B), to much more calcification on the present mammograms (Fig. 12-6C).

Discussion

A variety of fibroadenomas are presented to show the variation of imaging examinations. The thermogram was positive in some cases but not all. When seen on diaphanography there was a decrease in light transmission from moderate to relatively marked as with the giant fibroadenoma. In the dense glandular breast the fibroadenoma, unless surrounded by a halo of fat, may not be visible, as in cases 2 and 5. If all the borders are not well defined, as in case 3, there may be some doubt as to the nature of the lesion. Ultrasound demonstrated the lesion most

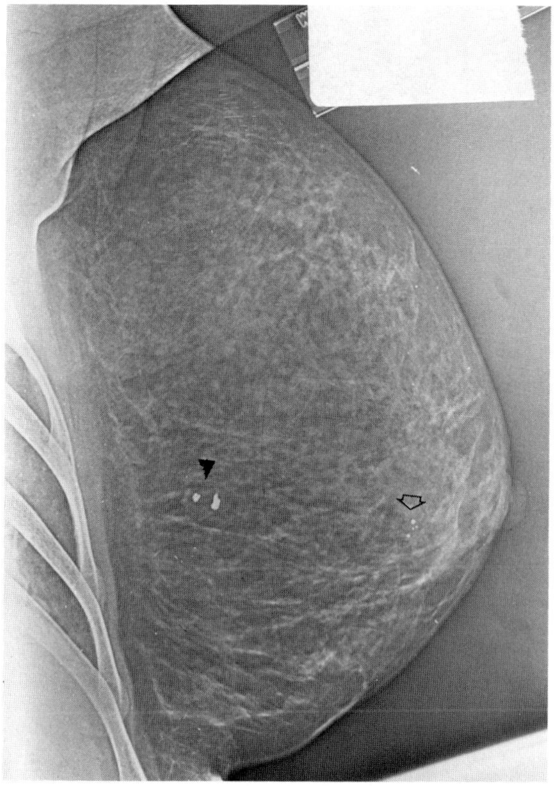

A

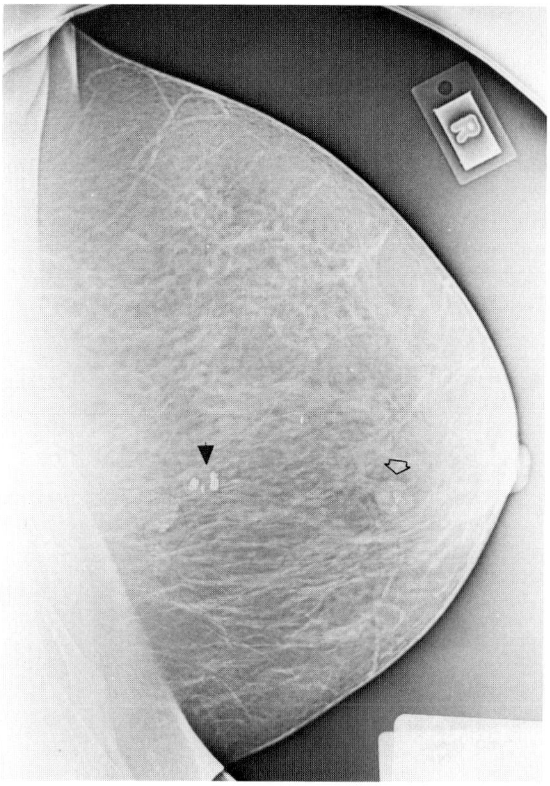

B

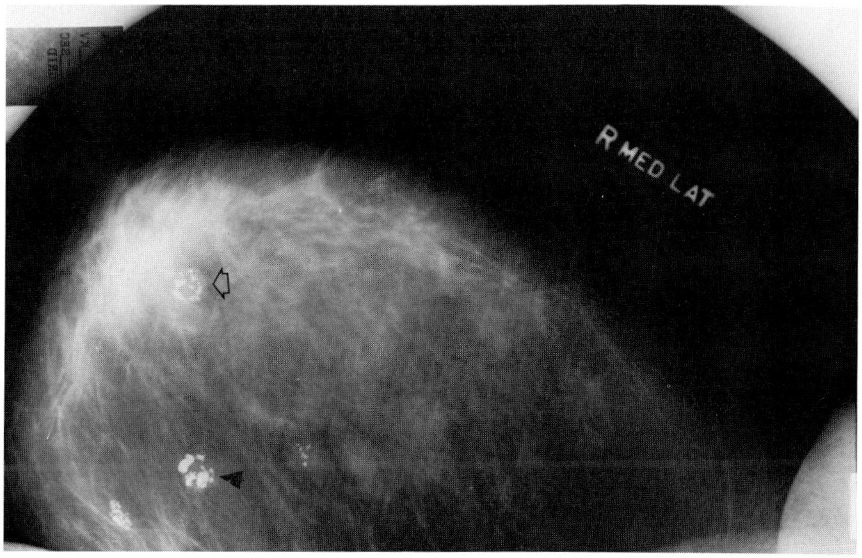

C

Fig. 12-6 Note the changing pattern of calcifications (arrows) in right lateral views. The two areas of calcification seen in 1983 **(A)** defined by the solid arrowhead and open arrow, are also seen in 1984 **(B)** and 1985 **(C)**. New areas appeared in 1984 and 1985 as well as change in the calcifications.

consistently and with the best definition. There are usually low-level echoes seen throughout the lesion that are highly suggestive of the diagnosis, although as mentioned in the text on fibroadenomas these echoes are not definitive. The rapid growth of fibroadenomas after surgical removal of other fibroadenomas, as in case 4, is very unusual.

In case 7 there was a changing pattern of calcification in the fibroadenomas over a 3-year period. Often we think of a calcified fibroadenoma as a stagnant lesion, but is is not. It depends at which point in its course of progression the fibroadenoma is first recognized.

Case Study: Gestational Adenoma

Case 8

T.W. is a 30-year old woman who developed a mass in the inner aspect of the right breast during the last trimester of her second pregnancy. Mammography done elsewhere was reported as inconclusive owing to the marked density of the breast. Ultrasound done at the same time revealed the mass to be solid. The patient was referred to us for further evaluation.

On physical examination there was a firm, ovoid 2 by 4 cm mass in the inner lower aspect of the right breast. Liquid crystal thermograms showed an extremely vascular pattern bilaterally consistent with pregnancy. Light scanning revealed a diffuse decrease in light transmission throughout both breasts, with a marked decrease in light transmission through the lesion (Fig. 12-7A). Limited ultrasound of the right breast showed a smooth, well defined solid density with a diffuse pattern of low-level echoes highly suggestive of an adenoma (Fig. 12-7B).

A needle biopsy showed lobules of proliferating acinar tissue situated in a compact fashion with one another and displaying epithelium with secretory activity. This finding was consistent with the clinical impression of gestational adenoma.

The patient was seen 2 months later, a month after her delivery. She related that the lesion enlarged slightly just before nursing and diminished in size after nursing. (This is not surprising considering that gestational adenomas have secretory activity as does the normal lactating breast.) The size of the lesion had not changed appreciably on physical examination. Four months later the same findings were still evident as the patient continued to nurse. It was expected that the lesion would regress when she discontinued nursing.

Six months later the patient stopped nursing on the right breast, continuing to nurse on the left. On physical examintion there was marked fullness on the left, with a milky discharge. The right breast was smaller, with no milk. The lesion was much smaller and softer, about 1.5 by 3 cm. The patient related that the decrease in size occurred during the 2 weeks since she had stopped nursing on the right. Thermograms demonstrated marked vascularity on the left consistent with nursing and a normal pattern on the right. There was a marked decrease in light transmission over the left breast and normal light transmission on the right with the exception of decreased light over the lesion. A single-view right mammogram demonstrated moderate glandularity, much less than in her previous mammograms done elsewhere, and the anterior border of the lesion, which was of glandular density. On ultrasound the size of the lesion was decreased and the echogenicity of the mass diminished.

Discussion

Although any lesion discovered during pregnancy must be viewed with suspicion and cancer ruled out, if the diagnosis of gestational adenoma can be made with confidence the patient can be allowed to deliver and nurse normally without surgical

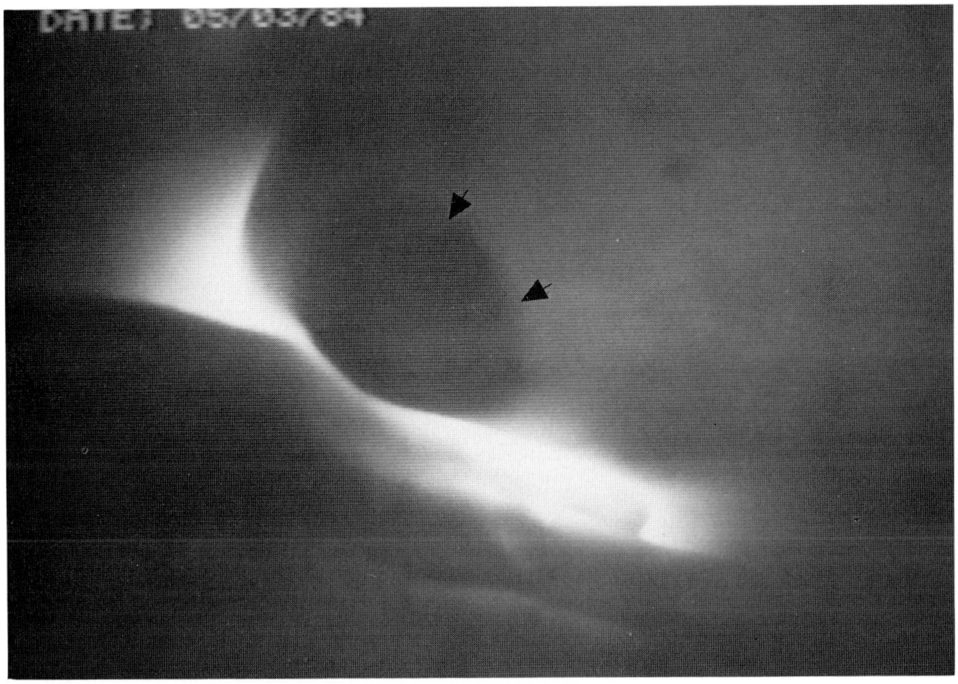

A

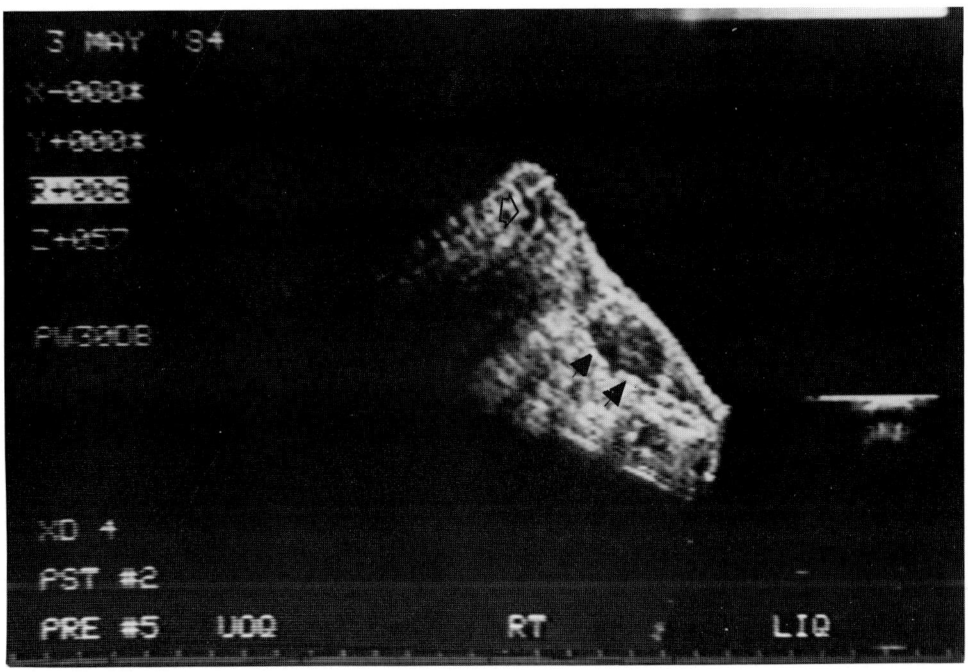

B

Fig. 12-7 **A:** Diaphanography. Note the marked decrease in light transmission in the anterior inferior breast (arrows). The hand under the breast is used to shield the excess light. **B:** Ultrasound. There is a well defined mass with diffuse internal echoes and no increased through transmission (arrows). Note this dilated ampulla of ducts under the nipple in this lactating breast (open arrow).

intervention. Surgery may produce a draining area owing to the continued milk production.

The usual scenario when evaluating a lactating patient with a mass is to have the patient stop nursing to see if the mass resolves. In this case it was possible to allow the patient to continue nursing, something desirable to many mothers.

Case Study: Cystosarcoma Phylloides

Case 9

D.D. is a 22-year-old woman who presented with an enlarging mass in the right breast. On examination elsewhere 4 months earlier, there was a 2 cm mass in the inferior portion of the right breast that was seen on mammograms as a well defined mass.

On the current physical examination there was a 6 by 7 cm hard firm mass occupying more than one-third of the breast with deformity of the inferior lateral aspect of the breast. Because of the large size of the mass it was impossible to determine if it was fixed to the chest wall.

Liquid crystal thermograms showed increase heat over the lateral and inferior aspects of the right breast, with increased vascularity (Th III thermogram). There was an inability to penetrate the mass with light on diaphanography. A single-view mammogram demonstrated an inability to adequately penetrate the mass with no delineation from the surrounding glandular tissue. On ultrasound there was a moderately well defined mass of 6 cm with low-level echoes throughout, except for a degree of lucency in the center of the mass (Fig. 12-8).

It was thought that this represented either a giant fibroadenoma with rapid growth and central necrosis or a cystosarcoma phylloides with possible malignant degeneration. At surgery a cystosarcoma phylloides with a central cyst was found.

Discussion

It may be impossible to differentiate a cystosarcoma from a giant fibroadenoma or from a tumor with central malignant degeneration. The rapid growth of the described tumor in the above case is very disturbing and necessitates surgery and adequate pathologic correlation for an answer. There may be areas of cystic change on cystosarcomas, but these have been described as forming sheets. In this case there apparently was cystic degeneration in the center of the tumor that probably accounted for its rapid increase in size, although the fact that the cyst had a thin wall is unusual for cystic degeneration.

There may be a recurrence after surgery that is more likely to be incomplete removal of the tumor than a true recurrence.

Bibliography

Fibroadenomas

Barth V: *Atlas of Diseases of the Breast.* Stuttgart, Georg Thieme, 1979.

Egan RL, McSweeney MB: Breast sonography—interpretative criteria, in Jellins J, Kobayashi T (eds): *Ultrasonic Examination of the Breast.* London, Wiley, 1983, pp 307–318.

Gautherie M, Kotewica A, Gueblez P: Accurate and objective evaluation of breast thermograms: Basic principles and new advances with special reference to an improved computer-assisted scoring system, in Gautherie M, Albert E, Keigh L (eds): *Thermal Assessment of*

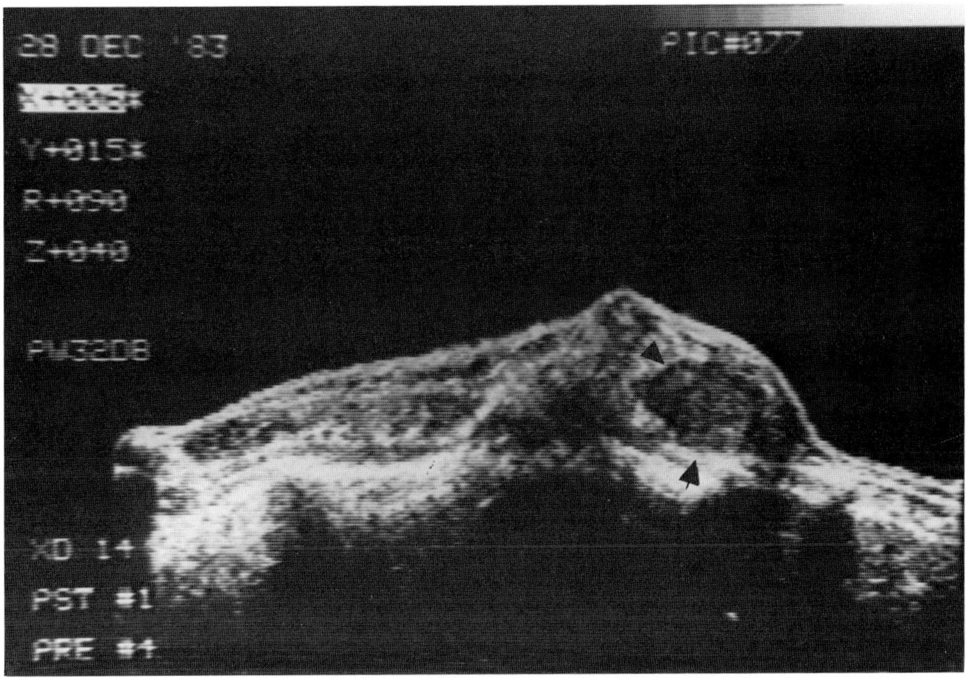

A

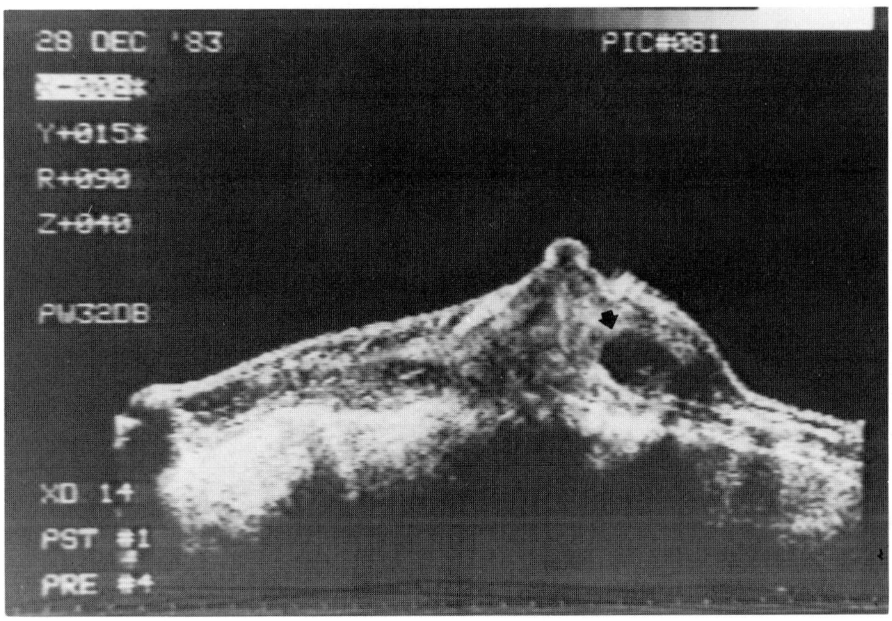

B

Fig. 12-8 A: Longitudinal ultrasound. There is a well defined low-level echogenic mass with some increased through transmission (arrows). Compare to cysts in Figs. 10-2A and 10-3B, and fibroadenomas in Figs. 12-1B, 12-2C, 12-3D, and 12-3E. **B:** Longitudinal ultrasound. Note the cystic area with slightly increased through transmission (arrow).

Breast Health. Lancaster, MTP Press, 1984, pp 74–97.
Haagensen CD, Bodian C, Haagensen DE: *Breast Carcinoma: Risk and Detection.* Philadelphia, Saunders, 1981.
Harper P, Kelly-Fry E: Ultrasound visualization of the breast in symptomatic patients. *Radiology* 1980;137:465–469.
Hutchinson WB, Thomas DB, Hamlin WB, et al: Risk of breast cancer in women with benign breast disease. *J Natl Cancer Inst* 1980;65:13–20.
Kobayashi T: *Clinical Ultrasound of the Breast.* New York, Plenum, 1978.
Martin SE: *Atlas of Mammography.* Baltimore, Williams & Wilkins, 1982.
Ozzello L, Gurney FE: The management of patients with carcinomas in fibroadenomatous tumors of the breast. *Surgery* 1985;160(2):99–104.
Patchen GA, Schiller I: The multimodal approach to detecting breast disease. *RNM Images* Sept/Oct 1984, pp 34–39.
Porrath S, Sandhu R, McNeil J: Thermography and benign breast disease. Proceedings American Academy of Thermology, Los Angeles, 1984 (in press).
Sandison AT, Walker JC: Diseases of the adolescent female breast. *Br J Surg* 1968;55(6):443–448.
Schwartz GF: Benign neoplasms and "inflammations" of the breast. *Clin Obstet Gynecol* 1982;25(2):373–385.
Tabár L, Dean DB: *Teaching Atlas of Mammography.* New York, Thieme-Stratton, 1983.

Gestational Adenoma

Egan RL, McSweeney MB: Breast sonography—interpretative criteria, in Jellins J, Kobayashi T (eds): *Ultrasonic Examination of the Breast.* London, Wiley, 1983, pp 307–318.
Martin JE: *Atlas of Mammography*. Baltimore, Williams & Wilkins, 1982.

Cystosarcoma Phylloides

Agnantis NJ, Apostolikas N: Histologic classification of cystosarcoma phyllodes: A study of 33 cases. *Breast* 1981;7(4):24–28.
Barnhart GR, DeBlois GG, Kay S, et al: Management of cystosarcoma phylloides: A reassessment. *Breast* 1985;11(2):17–23.
Barth V: *Atlas of Diseases of the Breast*. Stuttgart, Georg Thieme, 1979.
Cole-Beuglet C, Soriano R, Kurtz AB, et al: Ultrasound, x-ray mammography and histopathology of cystosarcoma phylloides. *Radiology* 1983;146:481–486.
Gautherie M, Kotewica A, Gueblez D: Accurate and objective evaluation of breast thermograms: Basic principles and new advances with special reference to an improved computer-assisted scoring system, in Gautherie M, Albert E, Keith L (eds): *Thermal Assessment of Breast Health*. Lancaster, MTP Press, 1984, pp 74–97.
Gittleman MA, Horstmann JP: Cystosarcoma phyllodes and concurrent infiltrating ductal carcinoma. *Breast* 1983;9(1):15–17.
Jellins J, Hughes C, Ryan J, et al: A comparative evaluation of a case of cystosarcoma phylloides: Ultrasound, xeroradiography, and thermography. *Radiology* 1977;124:803–804.
Kobayashi T: *Clinical Ultrasound of the Breast*. New York, Plenum, 1978.
Martin JE: *Atlas of Mammography*. Baltimore, Williams & Wilkins, 1982.
Schwartz AN, Dalton JC, Szyfelbein WM, et al: Diagnosis of metastatic cystosarcoma phylloides via percutaneous aspiration biopsy of a lung mass. *Appl Radiol* Mar/Apr 1983, pp 99–100.
Schwartz GF: Benign neoplasms and "inflammations" of the breast. *Clin Obstet Gynecol.* 1982;25(2):373–385.
Sonnefeld M, D'Orsi CJ, Sadowsky NL, et al: Mammographic patterns of unusual breast lesion. *JCE Radiol* 1979; 1(4/5):13–30.
Tabár L, Dean DB: *Teaching Atlas of Mammography.* New York, Thieme-Stratton, 1983.

13

Fibrocystic Disease

Saar Porrath

The term fibrocystic disease, as it is presently being used in clinical medicine, is a misnomer. In its strictest form it refers to a discrete pathologic condition; however, in common usage it describes a clinical condition of lumpy, sometimes painful, often tender breasts seen most commonly in menstruating women. It is a common "normal" finding in younger women and at best should probably be referred to as fibrocystic "syndrome," not "disease."

The breast can vary markedly during the cycle. It is not uncommon to find large, tender, painful nodules premenstrually, which when reexamined a week later postmenstrually have almost disappeared. With the admonition of "beware calling something normal a disease," the discussion here centers on the pathologic entity.

Fibrocystic disease is a catch-basket diagnosis that includes a variety of benign breast conditions of epithelial origin. Among these diagnoses are terms in current usage and some no longer in use, including cystic disease, chronic mastitis, cystic mastitis, cystic mastopathy, fibrocystic disease, epithelial dysplasia, blunt duct disease, adenosis, papillomatosis, fibrous disease, hyperplasia, and fibrosis.

Because of the confusion of terms it is somewhat difficult to discuss the clinical and radiographic findings. The descriptions here are therefore general when possible. [Papillomatosis is discussed in the chapter on papillomatous lesions (Chapter 17), and cystic disease is discussed under cysts (Chapter 10).]

The physical findings may vary from normal to a well defined nodule, firm and often several centimeters in size. The firmness may increase as the amount of fibrotic tissue or sclerotic component increases. It is very difficult, if not impossible, to evaluate clinically. A cystic area surrounded by fibrosis may feel rock hard, and a discrete glandular nodule made up almost entirely of normal tissue may also feel firm. Not infrequently, but by no means always, the nodularity is two-dimensional, without a depth that is discrete. The fibrocystic area has a greater tendency than cancers to appear clinically to blend into the surrounding tissue.

Diaphanography may show some decreased light transmission but more often than not is normal. There is a relative inability of the light scan to differentiate glandular tissue changes from normal. Unless the area has marked sclerosis, fibrosis, or inflammatory changes, there may be no changes visualized.

Thermography is usually normal. If the tissue is active metabolically, there may be increased heat seen. Troicore has demonstrated a change in the vascular appearance and distribution of the breast in fibrocystic disease (FCD). He described sharp, pencil-like vessels ending almost abruptly, with a change in their distribution. This finding is not accepted by all thermographers, however. In general, the thermogram, like the light scan, is unable to differentiate FCD from normal glandular tissue.

Ultrasound, like the two above tests, has not reached a stage capable of differentiating. FCD from normal glandularity with any regularity. There are changes, however, that can be seen. Any cystic formation or duct dilation can be seen. As the amount of fibrosis and sclerosis increases, often the amount of shadowing, or deflection of sound waves, also increases. It becomes a difficult point of differentiation, as marked glandularity can and often does cause similar shadowing.

Mammography demonstrates the microcalcifications that are often present, especially in sclerosing adenosis. These objects cannot be seen by any other imaging technique. Not infrequently similar calcifications are seen, although in lesser amounts, in other forms of FCD. At times these calcifications cannot be differentiated from those of a malignancy, and biopsy may be necessary. The area may show up as asymmetry of glandular tissue or as an increased density. The tissue density seen with most types of FCD is equal to that of the surrounding glandularity, whereas cancer usually appears as increased tissue density. Duct dilatation may be evident, especially in the less glandular breast.

If all of the above tests are combined, the best hope of differentiating FCD from malignancy is achieved. Even then, however, it is not totally accurate.

According to Haagensen et al., the presence of adenosis and gross cystic disease indicates an increased incidence of carcinoma. The subsequent development of the cancer in gross cystic disease can be in either breast, whereas in adenosis it usually occurs on the same side as the adenosis. Dupont and page found that women who had a proliferative form of breast pathology (atypical lobular hyperplasia, atypical "ductal" hyperplasia, moderate and florid hyperplasia of the usual type, papillomas, ductal involvement with cells of the atypical lobular hyperplasia, and sclerosing adenosis) had a moderate to marked increased risk of developing breast cancer. Their findings indicated that a diagnosis of nonproliferative breast disease does not significantly increase the patient's subsequent risk. The exception they found was that in patients who had cysts and a family history of breast cancer the risk was more than double the risk found with a family history only.

Fibrocystic disease is a disorder of the menstruating woman, often changing as the cycles change and decreasing with the onset of menopause. It is not known if the increased use of estrogens in the postmenopausal woman also results in an increase in FCD in these women as well.

Minton et al., in studies on the decreased intake of caffeine and methylxanthines, showed that there was a diminution of nodularity in the women they observed. These results have been questioned by other studies. (The reader is referred to the discussion concerning caffeine and breast nodularity in Chapter 9.) It has been speculated that if the prevalence of FCD in the breast can be decreased by reducing caffeine intake and by other methods, the incidence of subsequent cancer will also be decreased. Because only proliferative changes appear to influence the subsequent development of breast cancer, it is probable that these dietary methods will have no real effect on the cancer risk. The one measure that may have an effect on is if the subsequent risk of cancer is if cyst formation can be reduced in patients with a family history of cancer.

Bromocriptine (which inhibits prolactin) and danazol (Danocrine), tamoxifen (used extensively in breast cancer chemotherapy), and testosterone—all of which decrease the amount of estrogen—have been advocated for the treatment of FCD. These agents produce a decrease in the nodularity of the breast and even a visible change on the mammogram as well as a decrease in the clinical symptoms of pain and tenderness. It is questionable if these medications exert a real effect on true fibrocystic changes or, more realistically, a decrease in the glandularity.

There is currently controversy about the use of the terms fibrocystic disease and dysplasia on radiology reports of breast imaging. Wolfe believed that he was justified in describing the increased density and nodularity seen as dysplasia, as it corresponds to the pathologic description. (This corresponds to the P2 and DY terms.) Others, this author included, believe that the use of these terms should be confined to the pathology report and that they do not belong in the radiologic impression. It is thought that the terms increase the anxiety of the patient, confuse the primary physician who ordered the examination, and are used by some insurance companies to rate the patient or place riders on the policy, an unfortunate circumstance.

There have been conflicting reports in the literature about the risk factors of cancer that accompany the use of the Wolfe classification, especially the P2 and DY categories. Because the term dysplasia is used by many pathologists to signify a variety of FCDs and there appears to be no increased incidence of cancer with many forms of FCD, it is recommended to the readers that they review the original articles so as to form their own opinion.

Case Studies

Case 1

D.S. is a 44-year-old woman who was referred because of a questionable lump in the left breast of 2 months' duration. On physical examination there was marked glandularity to the upper portions of both breasts with hard, movable, glandular areas. There was a ridge of tissue just above the left nipple.

Thermography and diaphanography were normal. On mammography there was marked glandularity, a DY pattern. There were multiple benign-appearing calcifications present bilaterally, more on the left, that were thought to represent sclerosing adenosis (Fig. 13-1A). On ultrasound there was glandularity bilaterally with shadowing in the upper outer aspects. On the left, just above the nipple in the area of the ridge felt clinically, there were two small cystic areas and marked shadowing, the overall area about 1.5 cm in size (Fig. 13-1B).

Preoperative localization utilizing ultrasound was done. The area on biopsy was found to contain small cysts, apocrine metaplasia, focal blunt duct adenosis, and focal intraductal papillomatosis.

Case 2

G.M. is a 31-year-old woman who was referred because of a right breast lump. On physical examination there was a poorly defined ovoid density measuring about 1.5 cm.

Liquid crystal thermograms were normal, as was diaphanography. On mammography there was some increase in glandularity in the upper outer right breast; no masses or calcifications were noted. There was a poorly defined area with low-level echoes seen on ultrasound. At biopsy there was marked fibrocystic disease with apocrine metaplasia as well as sclerosing adenosis with focal intraductal calcifications.

Case 3

H.S. is a 66-year-old women who was self-referred for a second opinion. On a mammogram 1 month earlier a well defined 1 cm density thought to represent a cyst was seen that did not correspond to a 1.5 cm nodule felt clinically. On our physical examination there was no nodule palpated.

Thermograms and diaphanography were normal. On mammography there was a moderately defined 1 cm nodule without calcifications in the right breast (Fig. 13-2A). There was no cyst evident on ultrasound, but some shadowing was present. After preoperative mammographic localization (Fig. 13-2B) an area of adenofibrosis with mild atypical hyperplasia was noted.

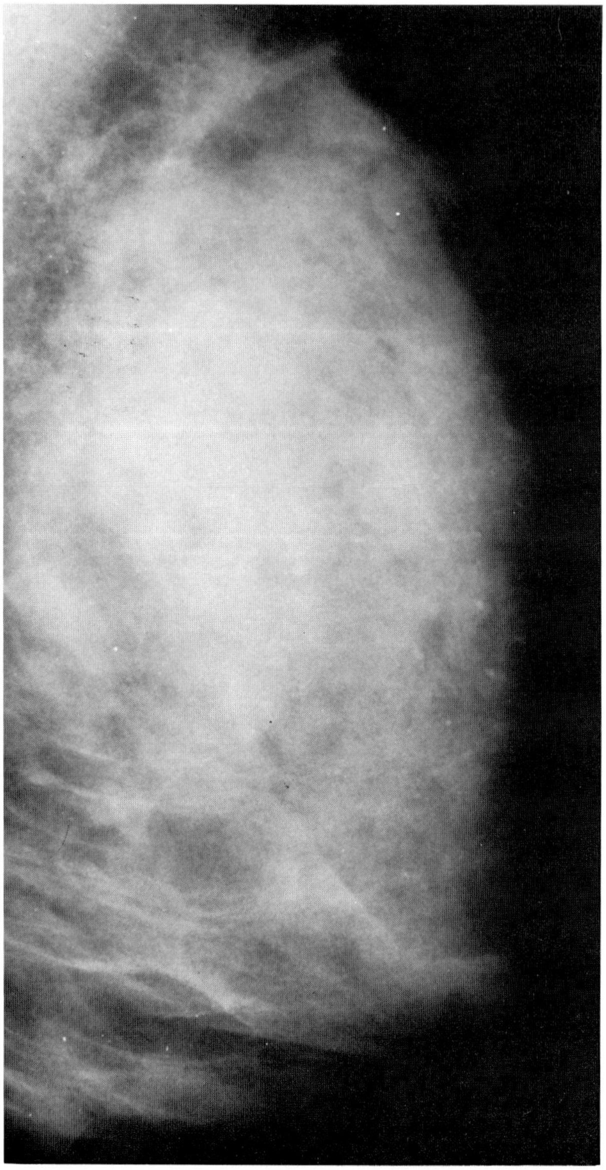

A

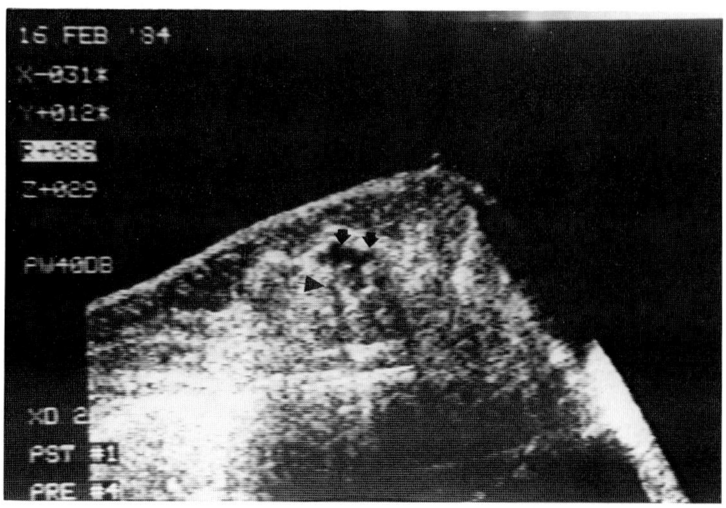

B

Fig. 13-1 A: Mammogram, lateral view. Note the diffuse small calcifications superimposed on marked glandularity. **B**: Ultrasound. There is an irregular echo-free area (arrows) with some posterior shadowing (arrowhead).

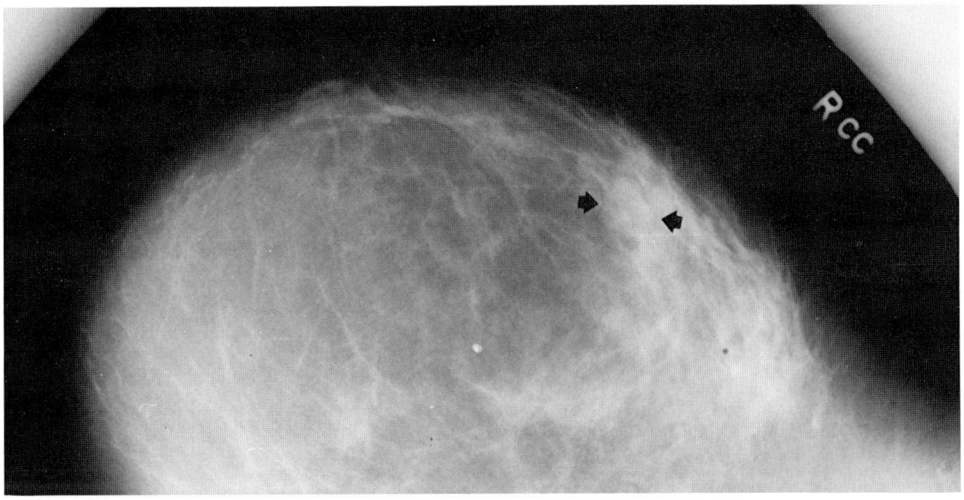

A

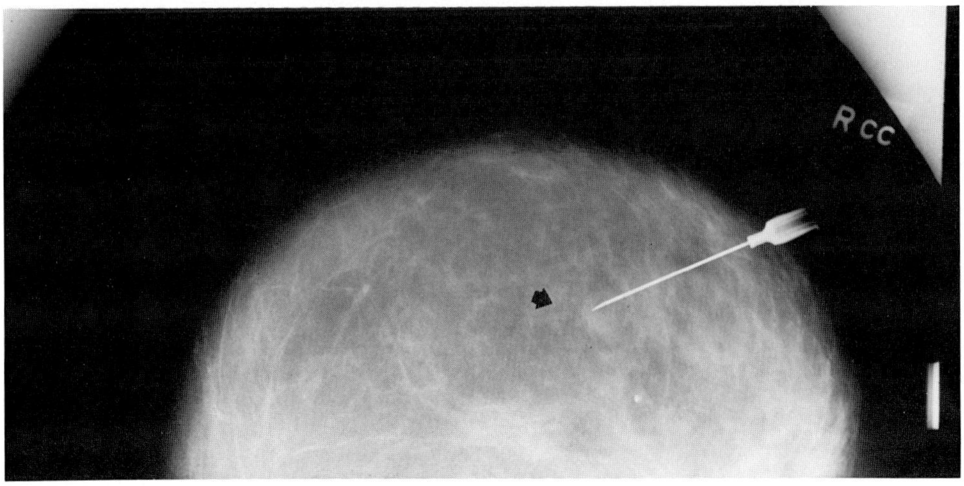

B

Fig. 13-2 A: Mammogram, CC view. Note the well defined nodule (arrows) with normal density. **B:** Localization mammogram. The nodule is more medial in location because of the need to position the breast somewhat differently because of the needle (arrow).

Case 4

J.E. is a 69-year-old woman who 10 days prior to this examination had had a mass in the left breast aspirated, with fluid obtained. A small mass remained after the aspiration. On physical examination there was a 3 cm mass behind the left nipple.

Thermograms demonstrated increased periareolar and nipple heat on the left, consistent with a Th IV thermogram. There was a decrease in light transmission through the mass. Mammography showed mild glandularity (P1 pattern) and a well defined 3 cm mass. On ultrasound there was a cystic lesion with slight irregularity of the lateral borders (Figs. 13-3A,B,C).

Aspiration of the mass obtained 3 cc of yellowish fluid, the cytology of which was class II. A pneumocystogram showed air in a small area with a large portion of the mass unfilled with the air (Fig. 13-3D). It was apparent that there was a small multiloculated cyst that had been aspirated but that occupied only a portion of the larger mass. Biopsy was recommended, at which many small cystic structures were found; the largest was 1.5 cm and contained an organizing clot. There was adjacent FCD and intraductal papillomatosis.

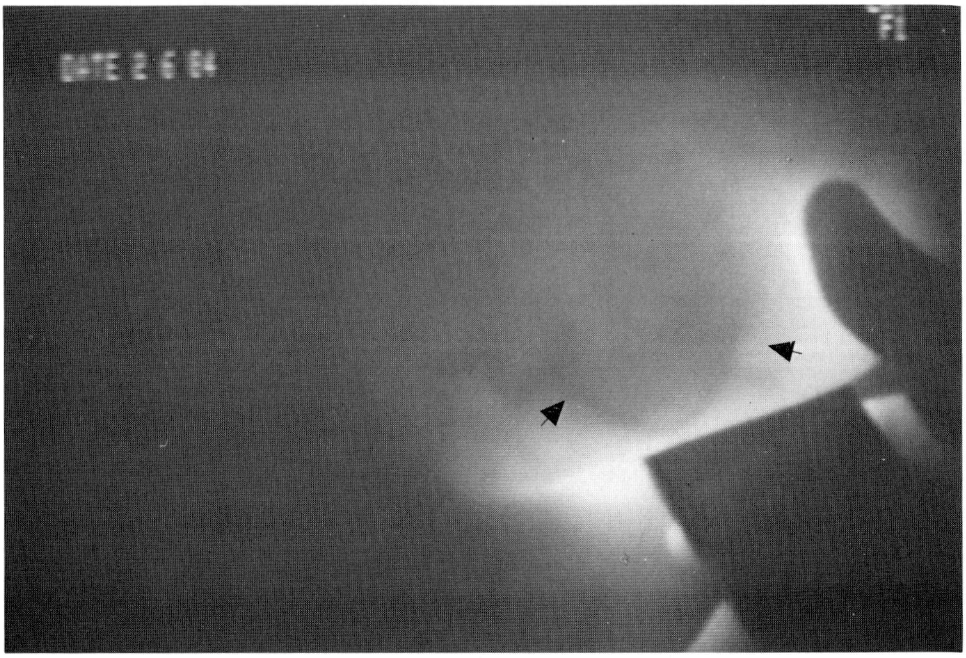

A

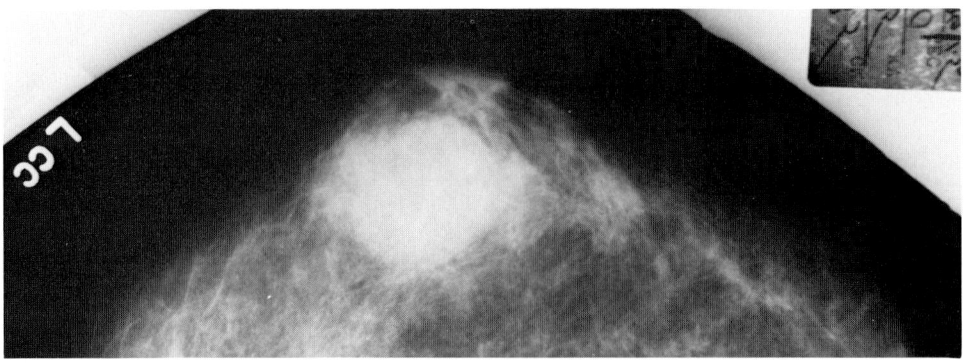

B

Fig. 13-3 **A:** Diaphanography. Note the area of decreased light transmission (arrows). **B:** Mammogram, CC view. There is a dense, well defined mass. **C:** Ultrasound. There is an anechoic area with edge shadowing (arrows) and no increased through transmission. *(Figure continues.)*

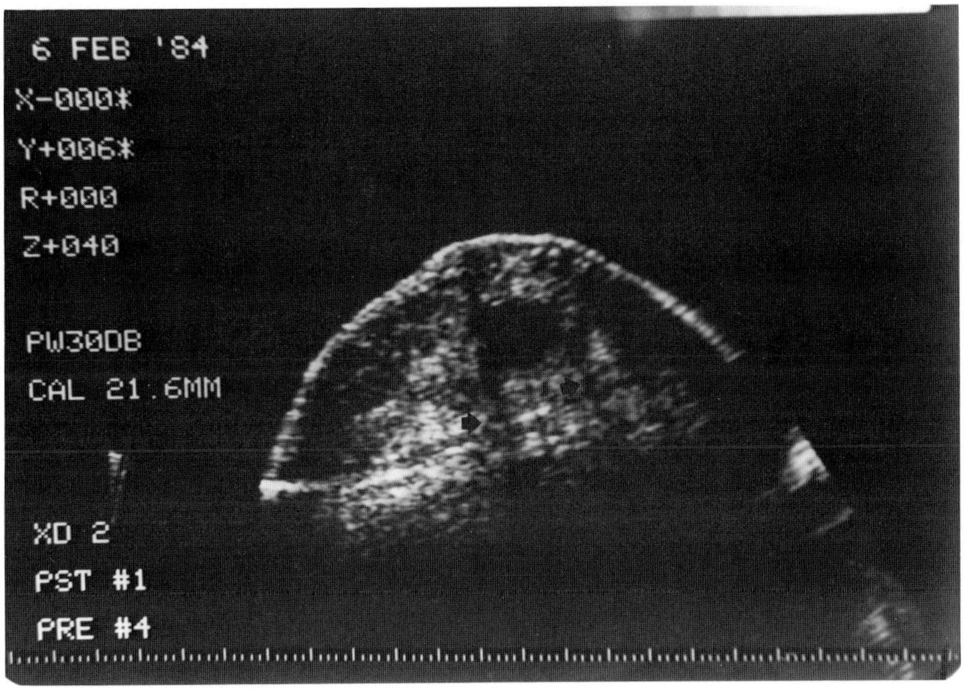

C

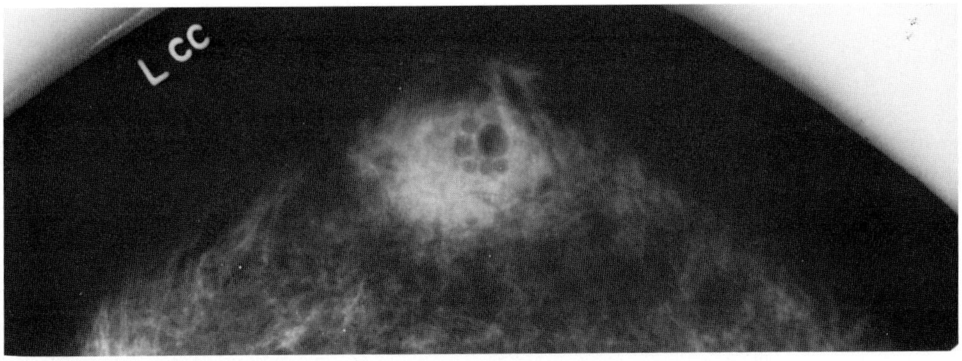

D

Fig. 13-3 D: Pneumocystogram. Small air bubbles surround a slightly larger air bubble within a multiloculated cystic structure. Note that the air bubbles do not occupy the entirety of the mass.

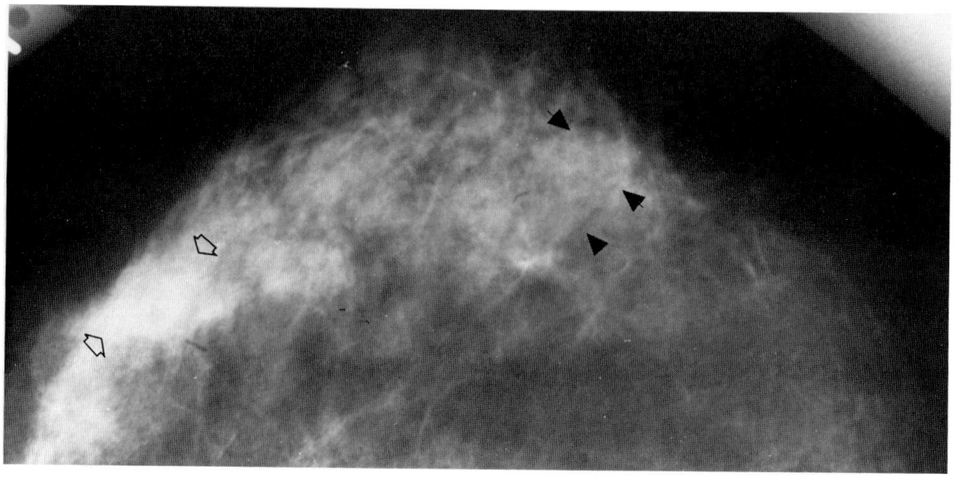

Fig. 13-4 Mammogram, CC view. There is a well defined mass in the anterior breast (arrows) and an area of increased density in the outer breast (open arrows).

Case 5

P.H. is a 46-year-old woman who was referred for screening. Physical examination, thermograms, and diaphanography were normal. On mammography three masses were seen, two of which were shown to be cysts on ultrasound. The third mass was a poorly defined area of increased density (Fig. 13-4), which on ultrasound demonstrated decreased echogenicity and shadowing. Preoperative mammographic localization was done followed by biopsy. Sclerosing adenosis with focal apocrine metaplasia and cystic change was found.

Case 6

E.G. is a 70-year-old woman who was referred for evaluation of breast pain. On physical examination there was a tender 2 cm nodular density in the outer right breast. Thermograms were normal. There was decreased light transmission on diaphanography through the density. On mammograms there was an increase in the amount of tissue with a punctate calcifications present (Fig. 13-5). Ultrasound demonstrated glandular

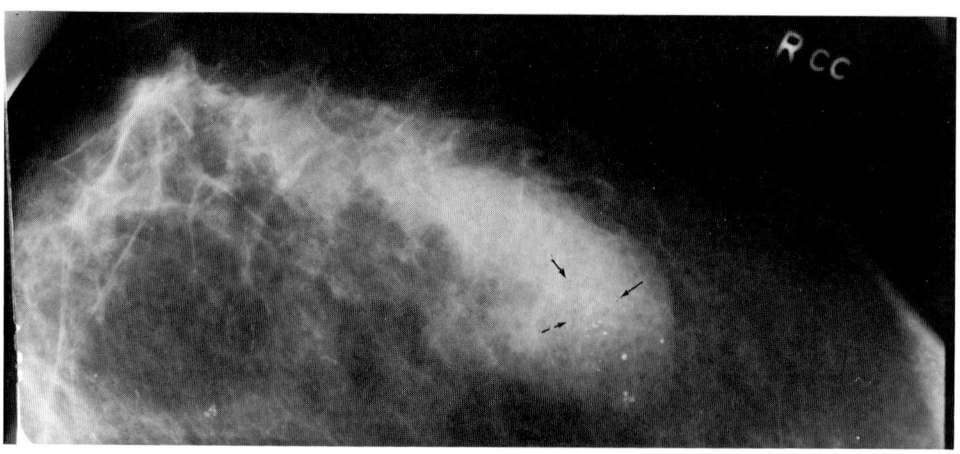

FIG. 13-5 Mammogram, magnification, CC view. A glandular density with punctate and other calcifications of varying size (arrows) are seen.

tissue and no mass. Preoperative mammographic localization was done. Adenofibrosis was found at biopsy. The breast pain was thought to be due to the patient's estrogen therapy.

Case 7

L.G. is a 31-year-old woman who was found to have a 0.5 cm firm nodule adjacent to the right nipple and a popcorn-like 2 cm nodule in the outer aspect of the left breast. The right nodule has been needled a year earlier and was reported as benign tissue.

Thermograms and diaphanography were normal. On mammography there was mild glandularity with a smooth, well defined nodule on the left, larger than on the mammograms of a year earlier (Fig. 13-6). The right nodule could not be seen. On ultrasound there was marked shadowing from the nodule on the left; no lesion seen on the right. At biopsy the nodule on the right was reported as nodular stromal fibrosis and on the left as fibroadenomatous nodular sclerosis.

Case 8

H.C. is a 68-year-old woman referred for screening. On physical examination no masses were felt. Thermograms and diaphanography were normal. On mammography there was mild glandularity (P1 pattern). On the right there was a spiculated lesion 1 cm in size containing small, somewhat irregular calcifications, not truly malignant in character (Fig. 13-7). Preoperative mammographic localization was done. Marked atypical hyperplasia in a background of stromal sclerosis was found.

Discussion

The variation in the presentation of FCD is demonstrated in the above cases. Some lesions present clinically, whereas others show up as microcalcifications, areas of cystic change, or shadowing on ultrasound. Some of these lesions mimic carcinoma. Biopsy is indicated if there is any question of the diagnosis, as it is impossible to be totally accurate with the present imaging modalities.

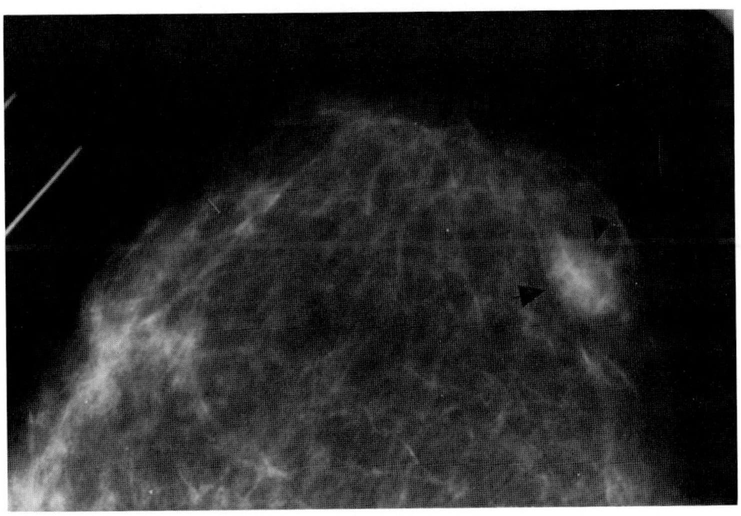

Fig. 13-6 Mammogram, CC view. Note the well defined normal-density mass (arrowheads).

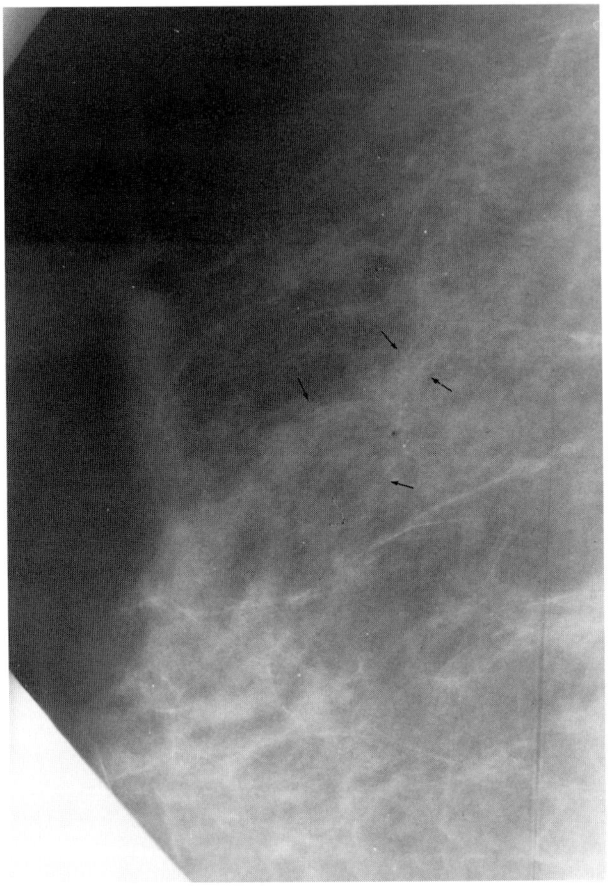

Fig. 13-7 Mammogram, magnification. Note the spiculated lesion (arrows) with irregular nonmalignant-type calcifications.

Bibliography

Barth V: *Atlas of Diseases of the Breast*. Stuttgart, Georg Thieme, 1979.

Dupont WD, Page DL: Risk factors for breast cancer in women with proliferative breast disease. *N Engl J Med* 1985;312:146–151.

Haagensen CD, Bodian C, Haagensen DE: *Breast Carcinoma: Risk and Detection*. Philadelphia, Saunders, 1981.

Huber CJ, Pons TY: Breast fibrocystic disease and thermography. *Acta Thermogr* 1980;5(1):48–50.

Hutter RVP: Goodbye to "fibrocystic disease." *N Engl J Med* 1985;312:179–181.

Leis HP, Cammarata A, La Raja RD: Nipple discharge: Significance and treatment. *Breast* 1985;11(2):6–12.

Martin JE: *Atlas of Mammography*. Baltimore, Williams & Wilkins, 1982.

Martinac P, Romic-Stojkovic R, Gamulin S: Estrogen and progesterone receptors in fibrocystic breast disease. *Breast* 1983;9(1):24–25.

Meeting of the Society for the Study of Breast Disease. The Fibrocystic Breast, A Multidisciplinary Approach, Boston, May 21, 1983.

Minton JP, Foecking MK, Webster DJT, et al: Caffeine, cyclic nucleotides, and breast disease. *Surgery* 1979;86(1):105–109.

Moskowitz M, Fox SH, Brundel Re R, et al: The potential value of liquid-crystal thermography in detecting significant mastopathy. *Radiology* 1981;140:659–662.

Page DL, Vander Zwaag R, Rogers LW, et al: Relation between component parts of fibrocystic disease complex and breast cancer. *J Natl Cancer Inst* 1978;61:1055–1063.

Patchen GA, Schiller I: The multimodal approach to detecting breast disease. *RNM Images* Sept/Oct 1984, pp 34–39.

Porrath S, Sandhu R, McNeil J: Thermography and benign breast disease. Proceedings American Academy of Thermology, Los Angeles, 1984 (in press).
Rosenberg L, Miller DR, Helmrich SP, et al: Breast cancer and the consumption of coffee. *Am J Epidemiol* 1985;122(3):391–399.
Tabár L, Dean DB: *Teaching Atlas of Mammography.* New York, Thieme-Stratton, 1983.
Tabár L, Dean DP, Pentek Z: Galactography: The diagnostic procedure of choice for nipple discharge. *Radiology* 1983;149:31–38.
Tricoire J: La thermographie in plaque: Technique nouvelle d'utilisation des cristaux liquides. *Presse Med* 1970; 78:2481–2482.

14

Hemorrhage

Saar Porrath

The amount of trauma and resultant hemorrhage into the breast has an effect on the presenting signs and symptoms. It is not infrequent to find a patient who has had a slight trauma to the breast, enough to cause a minimal bruise, that is unknown to the patient until it is pointed out to her. It usually shows up on the undersurface or lateral aspect of the breast and is superficial in nature.

During the evaluation of slight hemorrhage palpation may elicit a small amount of tenderness. Occasionally there is a small mass present from the localized bleed that usually resolves within 4 to 6 weeks. Thermography and mammography are normal. Ultrasound may show some light skin thickening or slight disruption of the subcutaneous tissues. Diaphanography is very positive, out of proportion to the other tests but in keeping with the physical findings. The light scan remains positive at least until the physical signs clear and sometimes longer. The light absorption reflects the presence of unobserved blood beneath the skin. Care must be taken not to biopsy these areas based on diaphanography only. Follow-up is indicated to be sure that there is not another cause for the bleed, e.g., an underlying mass, hidden by the hemorrhage.

More extensive trauma presents with more extensive findings. The greater the trauma, the more bleeding there is and the greater the resultant effect on the breast. This trauma may occur with an injury such as a fall or a blow to the breast, and it may be induced by a physician attempting a needle aspiration or biopsy, especially if a cutting edge needle is used. This is not to imply that any or all needle aspirations or biopsies cause significant trauma but that the findings vary depending on the technique used and the problems encountered. For example, if the wall of the cyst is slightly lacerated by the tip of the needle during a simple cyst aspiration, the cyst may fill with blood. On ultrasound this appears as a fluid mass with some internal echoes. There tends to be a change in the ultrasonic picture: As the blood clots there are more echoes than were seen initially. Later, as the clot liquefies, the echogenicity diminishes. The blood-filled cyst shows up as a rounded mass on mammography, thermography may be positive, and the light scan shows an area of marked light absorption.

If the bleeding has not been confined to a circumscribed area, e.g., a cyst, but is within the tissue, the resultant findings vary. On physical examination there may be a mass or "pseudomass" with induration of the tissues. If the trauma is deep, there may be no skin changes or palpable mass; however, if the trauma has affected the skin, ecchymoses are present. The area is usually tender and may be painful. The findings have been discussed above.

Surgery causes significant traumatic changes to the breast, depending on the amount of surgery done. Usually there is extensive blood in the tissues, with a very positive diaphanography. Thermography is positive with a diffuse increase in heat and vascularity. Ultrasound shows diffuse, increased tissue echoes, possibly with small fluid areas. There is some distortion of the subcutaneous area and possibly slight skin thickening. The mammogram also shows marked changes, reflecting, as do all the tests, the increased density in the subcutaneous and deeper tissues. The ducts may be transected during the surgery, and occasionally there is a bloody discharge. Diaphanography in these cases may show the darkened, blood-filled ducts. It may take months before the changes resolve and the tests become normal.

Case Studies: Hemorrhage

Case 1

R.C. is a 71-year-old woman who was referred because of a bruise on the lateral aspect of the right breast. She denied any trauma. On physical examination there was a large bruise occupying the lateral periareolar area and adjacent breast with a 2 cm mass in the center of the ecchymotic area.

Thermograms were positive bilaterally, with a warm nipple on the left and increased vascularity on the outer portion of the right breast. Diaphanography showed markedly increased light absorption over the area of the bruise, with even more light absorption in the area of the mass and nipple (Figs. 14-1A, B). Mammograms showed moderate glandularity with a well defined 1.5 cm mass (Fig. 14-1C). Ultrasound demonstrated a 1 cm cystic area and increased echogenicity surrounding it (Fig. 14-1D). On aspiration of the mass, 0.5 cc of blood was obtained. The patient was told to use warm packs on the breast.

Follow-up examination 1 month later showed that the hematoma had almost totally resolved, with just a yellowish tint to the skin and minimal nodularity in the area of the mass. Light scanning demonstrated slightly increased light absorption in the area. The thermograms were normal. A single-view mammogram showed that the mass had almost completely resolved. A year later all findings were normal except for a slight yellowish tinge remaining in the skin area.

Case 2

H.G. is a 43-year-old woman who presented with a bloody left nipple discharge of 3 weeks' duration. The patient denied any trauma. On physical examination there was a 6 by 6 cm ill-defined tender mass without a good third dimension of depth. It was present at 12 o'clock on the left. A bloody discharge was noted from a single duct, which when examined microscopically revealed blood and macrophages but no abnormal cells.

Thermograms were normal. On diaphanography there was marked absorption of light over the area of the mass, which was present in a triangular orientation (Fig. 14-2A). On the lateral view the light absorption was noted to be superficial. Mammograms revealed mild glandularity bilaterally (P2 pattern), with marked asymmetry. There was an increase in density in the upper mid-portion of the left breast, the density, like diaphanography, indicating a lobule of the breast (Fig. 14-2B, C). On ultrasound there was shadowing present and a dilated duct. On ductography the area defined on mammography was seen to be a lobule, with dilatation of the distal ducts. No discrete mass or filling defects within the ducts were demonstrated (Figs. 14-2D, E).

The area of the mass was milked and a large amount of reddish brown material consistent with new and old blood obtained. Repeat diaphanography demonstrated a moderate decrease in the amount of light absorption. On repeat examination 3 weeks later there was a moderate decrease in the size of the mass. Repeat diaphanography demonstrated an overall diminution in light absorption. It was thought that this case represented a bleed into a ductal system and lobule with partial resolution of the blood accumulation. The primary physician decided that there was a need for surgical inter-

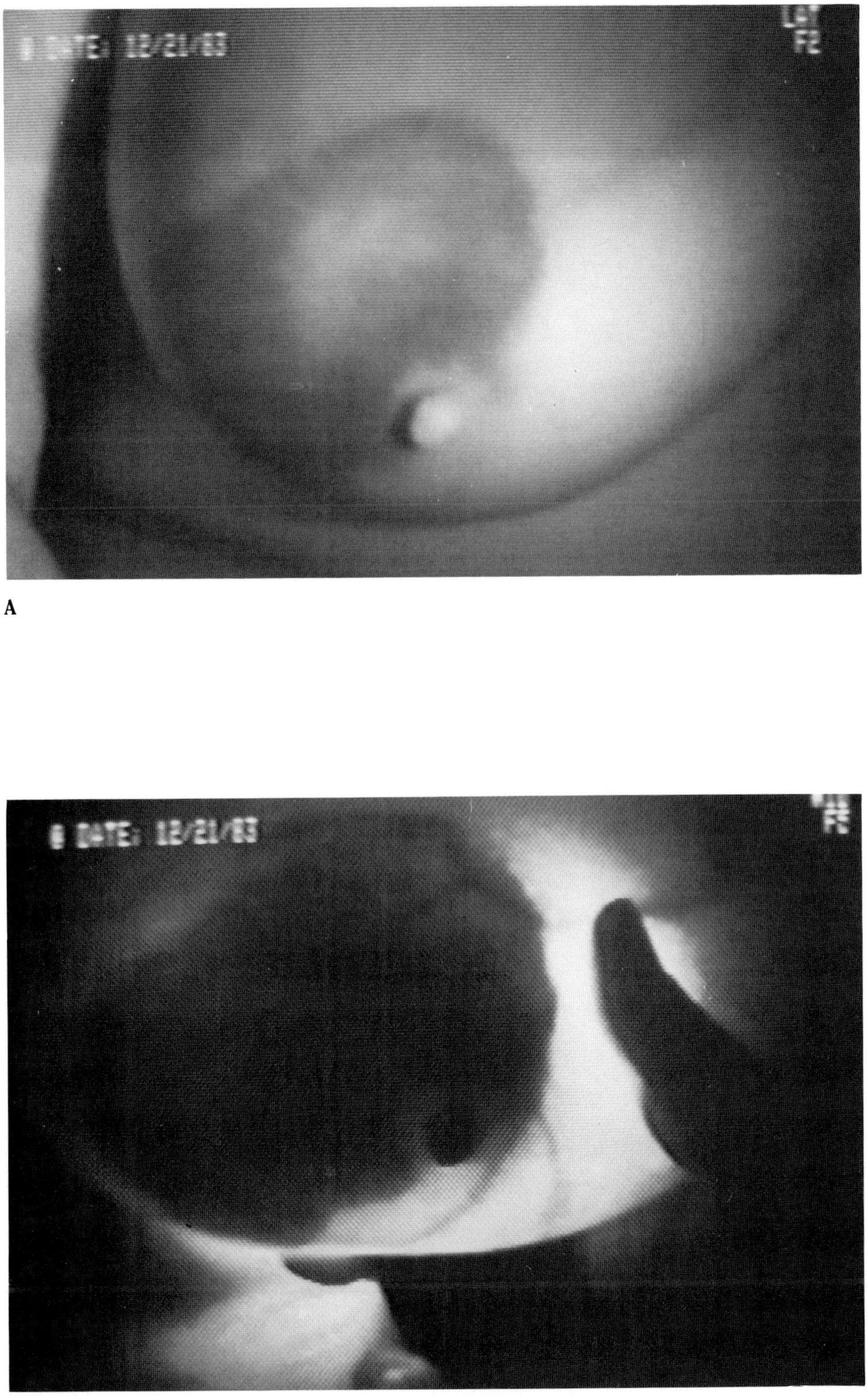

A

B

Fig. 14-1 A: Light shining on breast, utilizing an infrared television camera to show area of hemorrhage. **B:** Diaphanography. Note the marked light absorption by the hemorrhagic area. Compare with **A.** (*Figure continues.*)

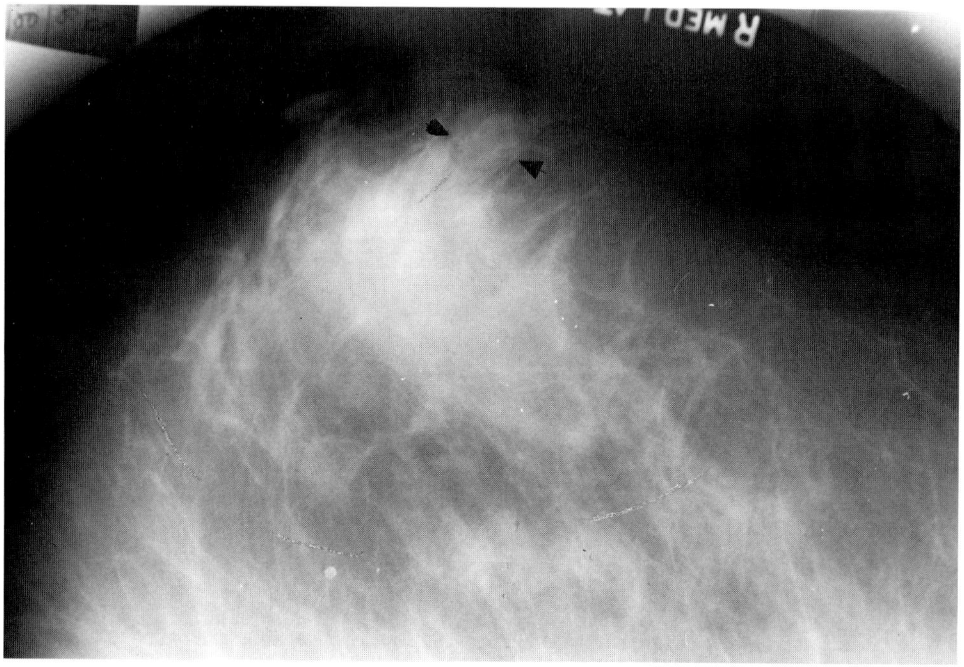

C

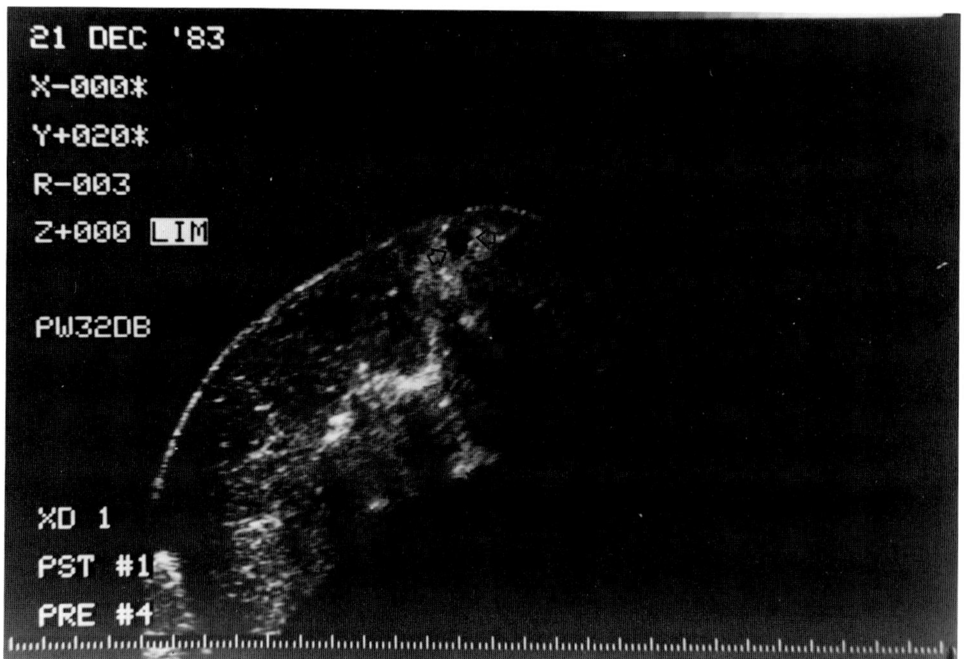

D

Fig. 14-1 **C:** Mammogram, lateral view. Note the well defined nodule. **D:** Ultrasound. Anechoic area is surrounded by an area of increased density (open arrows).

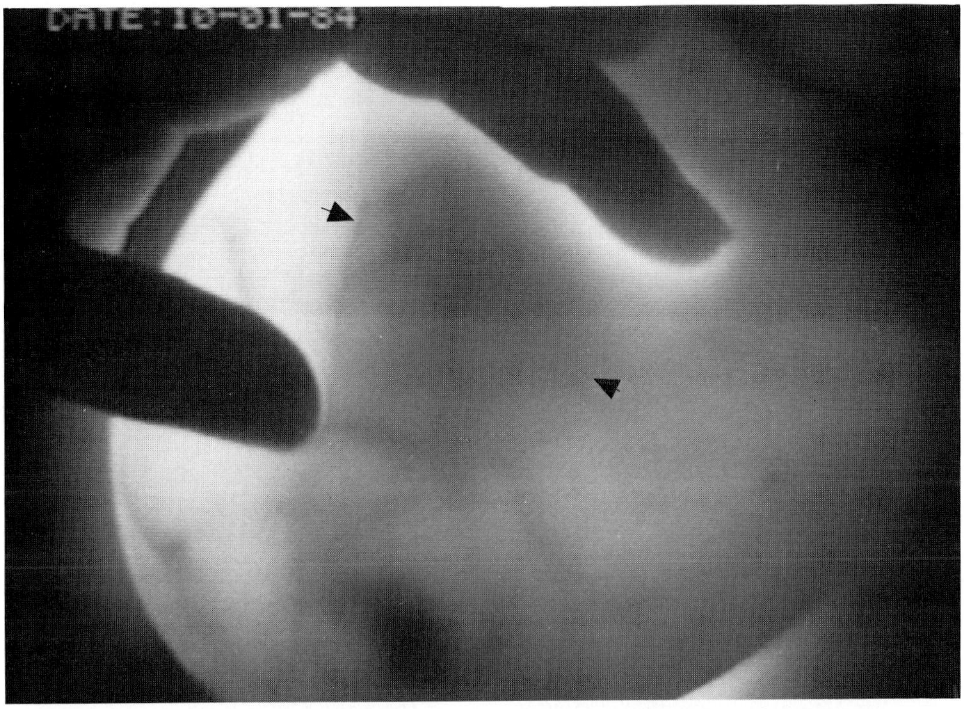

A

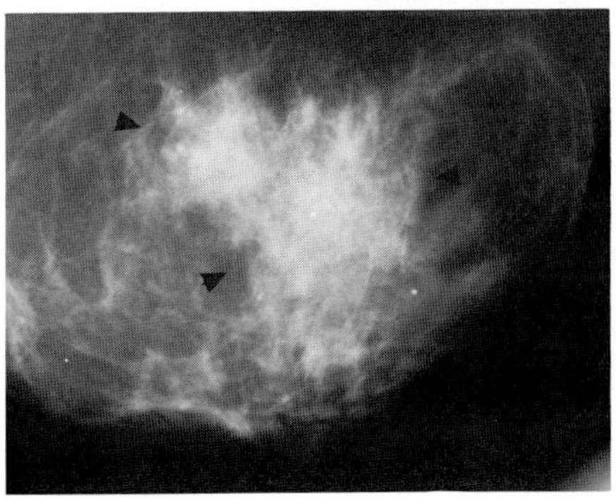

B

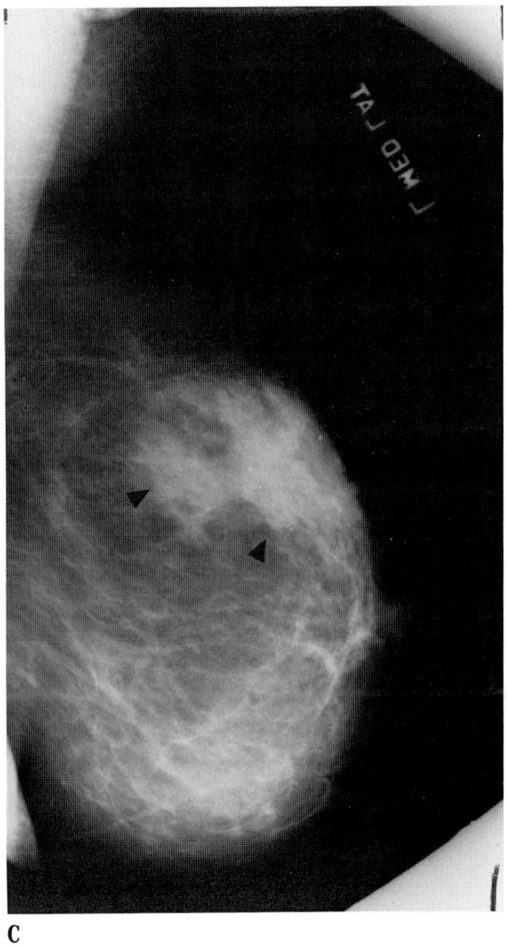

C

Figure. 14-2 A: Diaphanography. Note the marked light absorption (arrows). **B:** Mammogram, CC view. The area of increased density corresponds to the area of decreased light noted in **A** (arrowhead). **C:** Mammogram, lateral view. The area of increased density (arrowheads) seen in both mammogram views corresponds to a breast lobule. (*Figure continues.*)

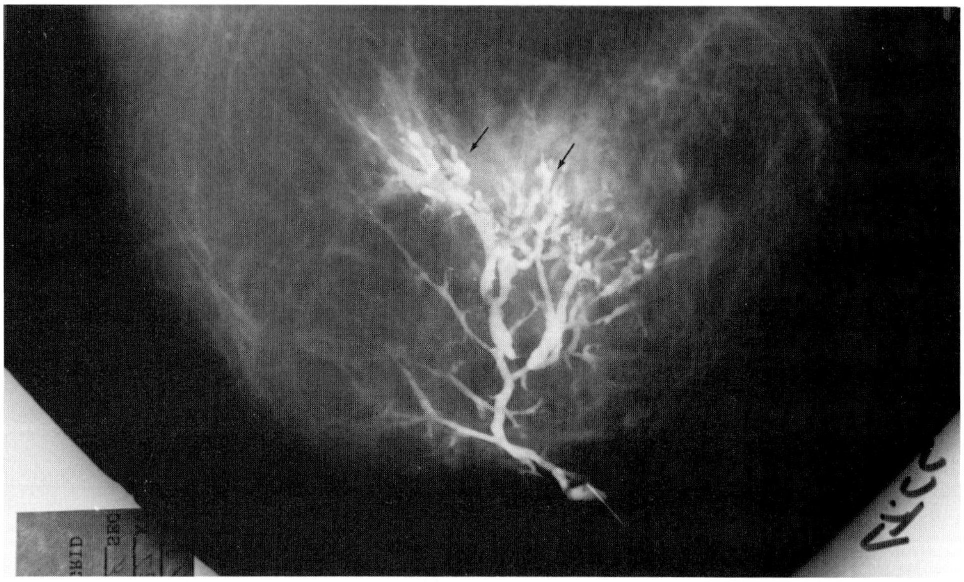

D

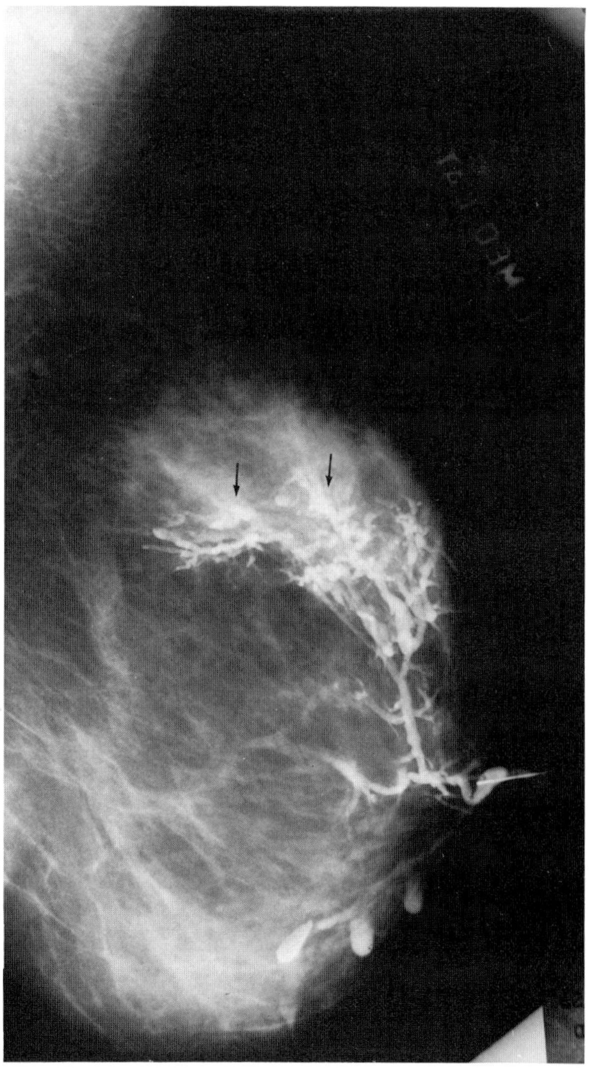

E

Fig. 14-2 D: Ductogram, CC view. **E:** Ductogram, lateral view. The ductogram outlines the lobule involved. The proximal ducts are dilated (arrows). Note that there is some layering of the dye in the dilated duct, as this view is taken across the interface of dye and duct fluid; this is not seen in the CC view.

vention to rule out malignancy. Resection of the mass revealed blood in the ducts, fibrocystic changes with hyperplasia, and florid papillomatosis. It is probable that minimal trauma caused the bleed secondary to the papillomatosis.

Case 3

A.G. is a 56-year-old woman who noted a bruise and a small mass on the lateral aspect of the right breast. On physical examination there was a large ecchymotic area measuring almost 4 cm across with a tender 1.5 cm center. Thermograms were normal. On light scanning there was marked absorption over the area of the hematoma (Fig. 14-3A). The mammograms were essentially normal with marked glandularity (P2 pattern). Ultrasound demonstrated skin thickening and a small area of increased echogenicity with shadowing (Fig. 14-3B).

The patient initially denied any trauma. On further inspection there was a bruise over the lateral right lower ribs as well. The patient then remembered walking into a door about a week before.

Discussion

It is not uncommon to find minor hemorrhages in the breast of which the patient is unaware; she may not even remember the episode of trauma, as in case 3. In the

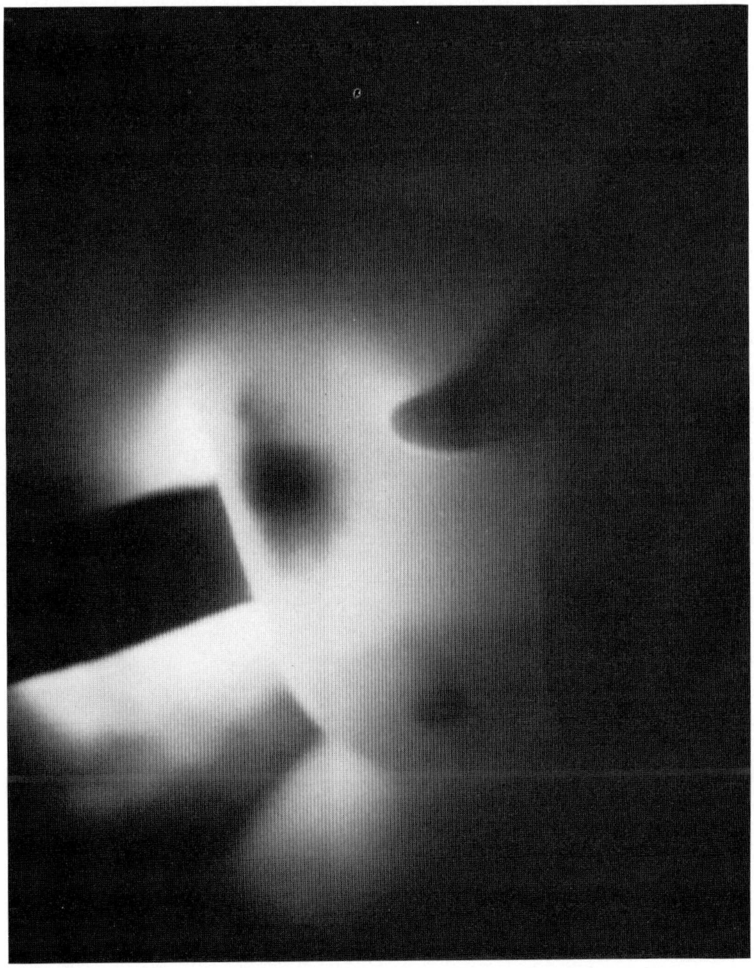

Fig. 14-3 A: Diaphanography. There is marked light absorption over the area of the hematoma.

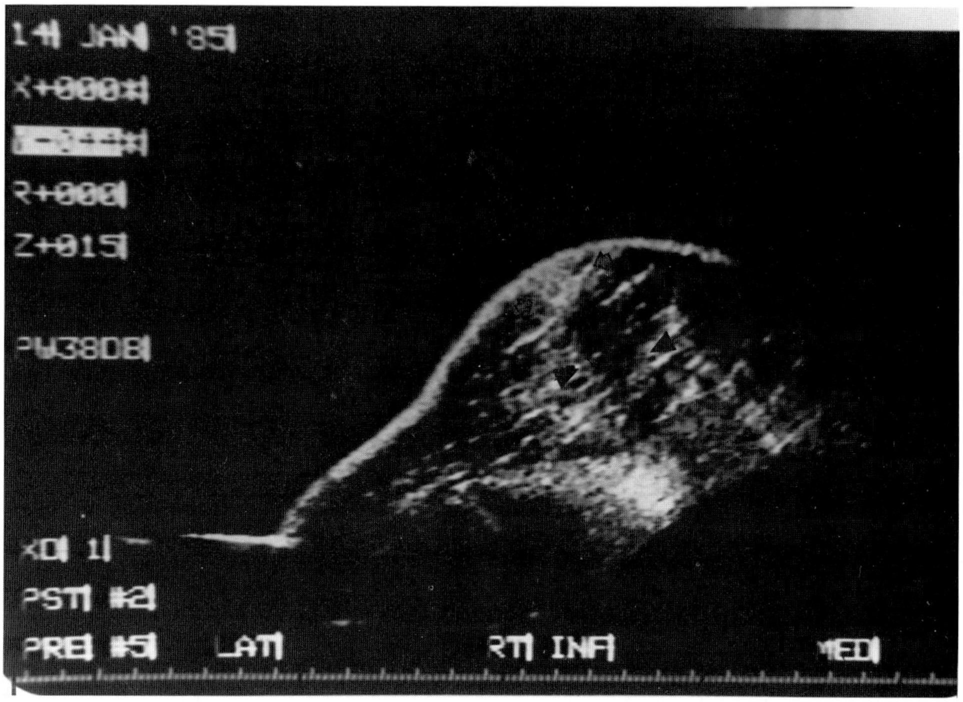

Fig. 14-3 **B:** Ultrasound. There is skin thickening and markedly increased echoes in the subcutaneous area (open arrow) with posterior shadowing (arrow).

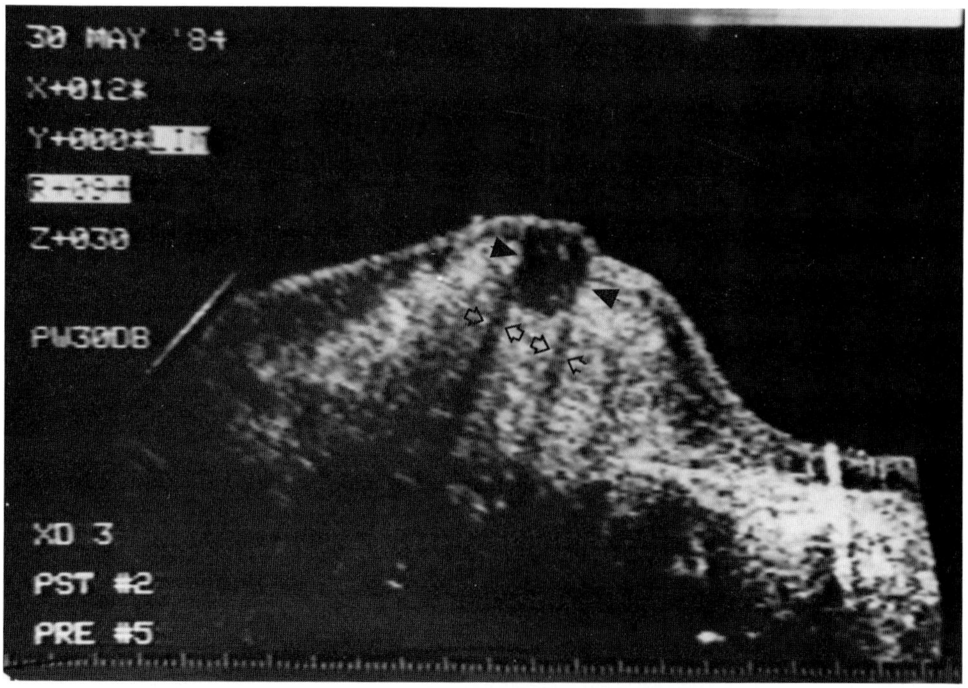

Fig. 14-4 Ultrasound. Note the large low-level echo area behind the nipple (arrowhead) with internal echoes and posterior edge shadowing (open arrows).

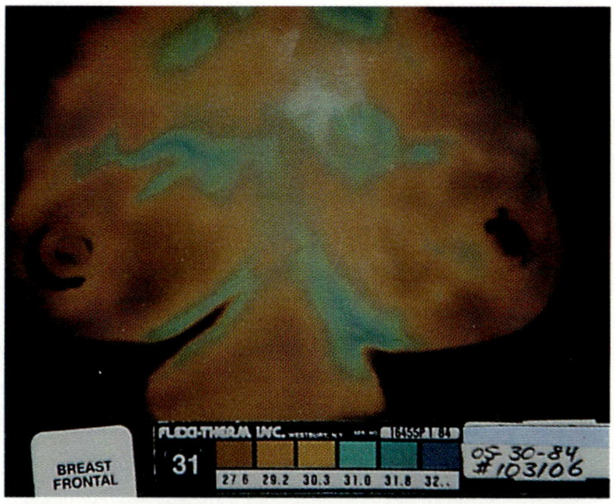

Fig. 1 Postoperative hemorrhage. Note the increased right nipple heat. The dark semicircular area beneath the nipple is the recent operative scar. (Color scales are at the bottom of the thermogram: brown = cold, blue = hot.)

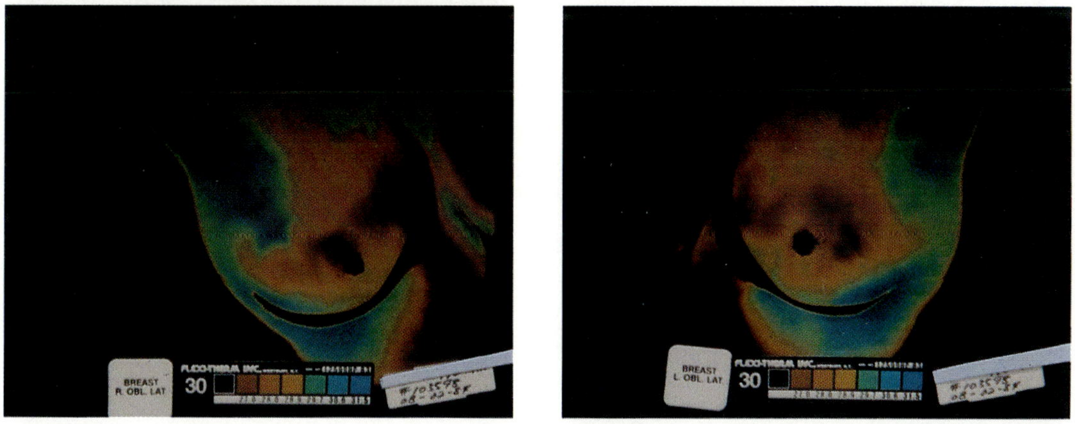

Fig. 2 Postoperative hemorrhage. Note the dark blue area on the lateral right breast extending toward the right nipple.

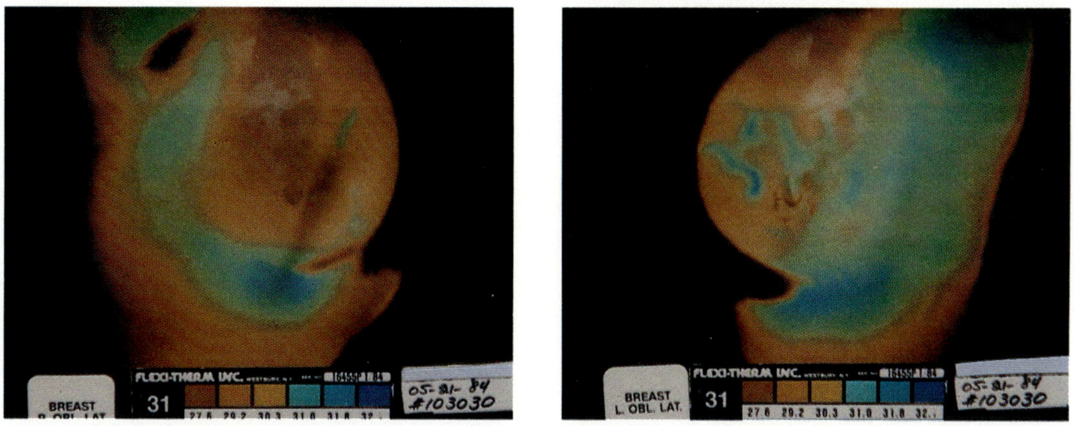

Fig. 3 Infection. Note the increased left nipple heat and adjacent vascularity (green and blue area).

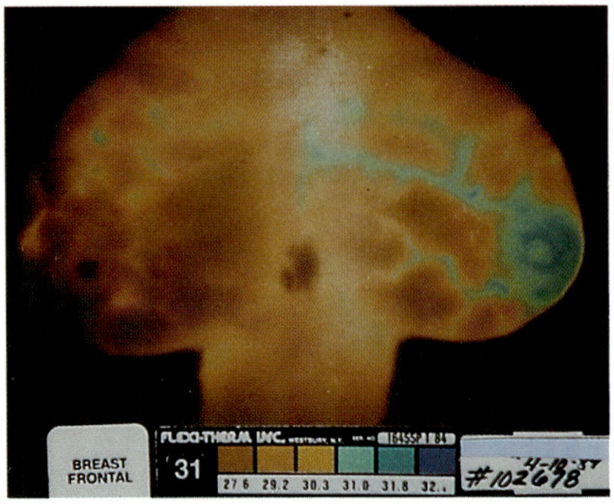

Fig. 4 Infection. Note the markedly increased left nipple heat and vascularity. (The left nipple is 4°C warmer than the right nipple.)

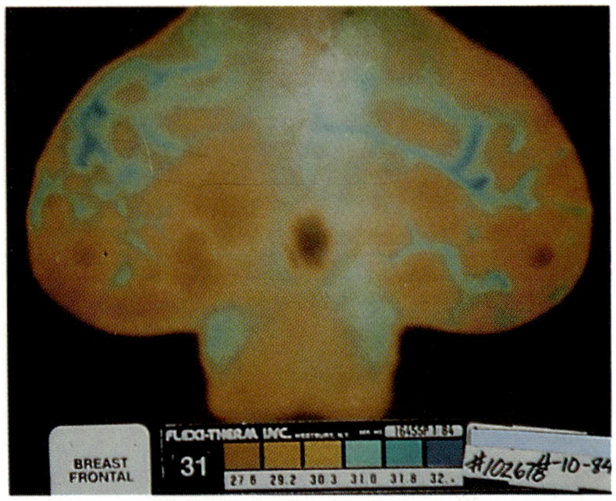

Fig. 5 Same case as in Fig. 4. This is a normal thermogram, obtained after a course of antibiotics. Note that the nipple areas show equal heat, and that the vascularity has diminished on the left.

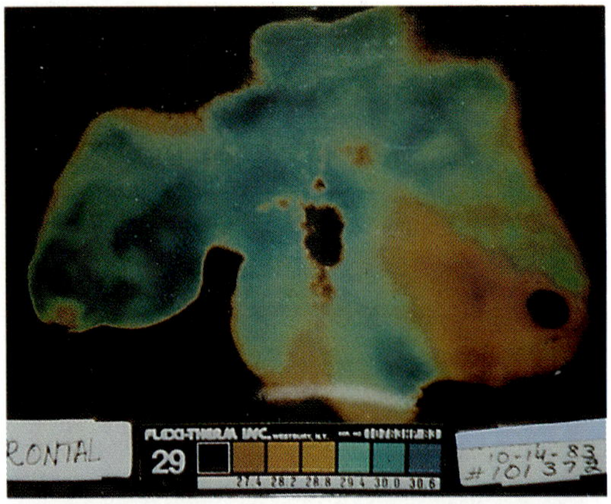

Fig. 6 Implant: global hyperthermia. Note the entire right breast (blue-green). The breast on the right seems smaller; this is due to loss of contact on the thermogram caused by contraction of the breast. Compare with Figs. 8, 24, and 33.

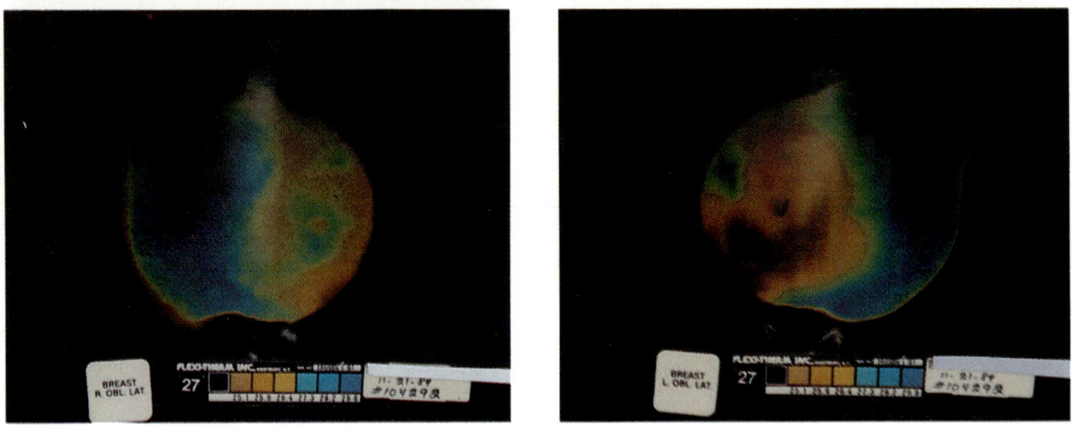

Fig. 7 Skin infection just under the right nipple. Note the increased heat of the right nipple.

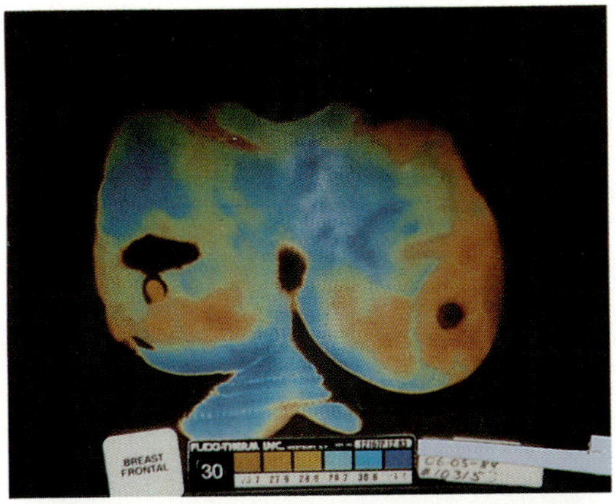

Fig. 8 Postoperative changes. Note that the right breast is smaller. The dark area above the right nipple is caused by poor contact of the thermographic plate over an area of postsurgical retraction. Note the elevated right nipple, increased right nipple heat, and increased vascularity.

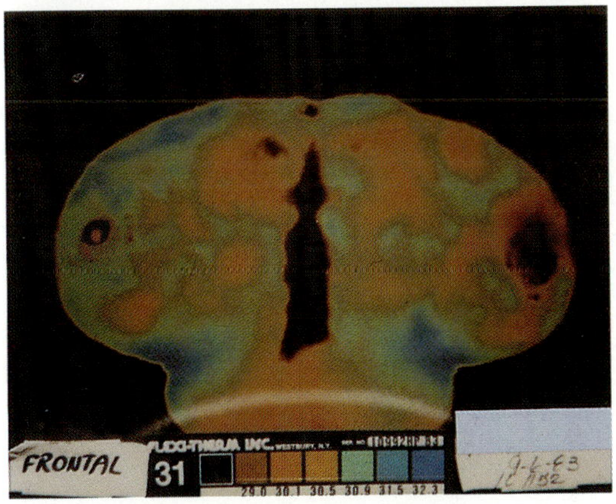

Fig. 9 Postoperative changes. Note the increased nipple heat and vascularity on the right.

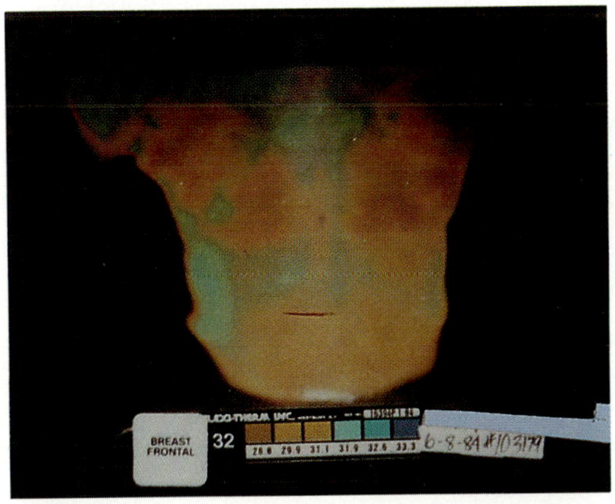

Fig. 10 Prepubescent breast. Note the green area representing increased right nipple heat.

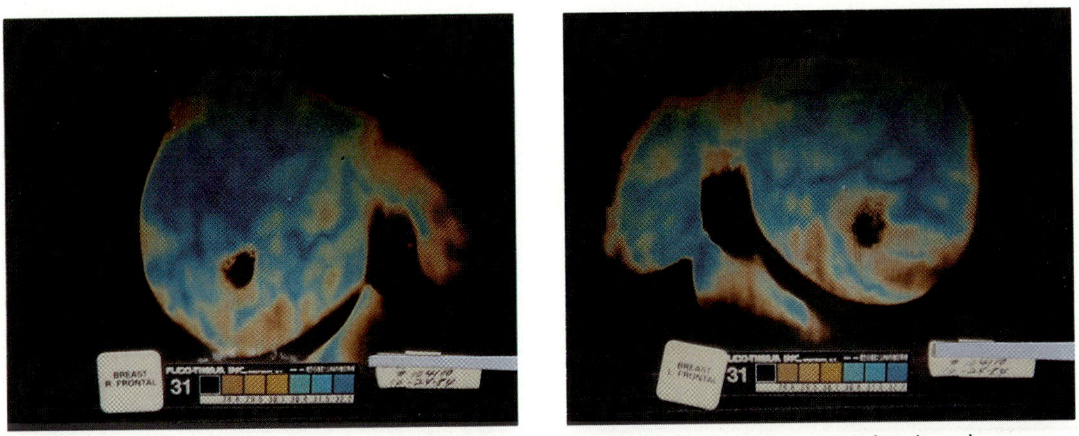

Fig. 11 Lactating woman. Note the marked bilateral vascularity. This was present despite a long cooling period.

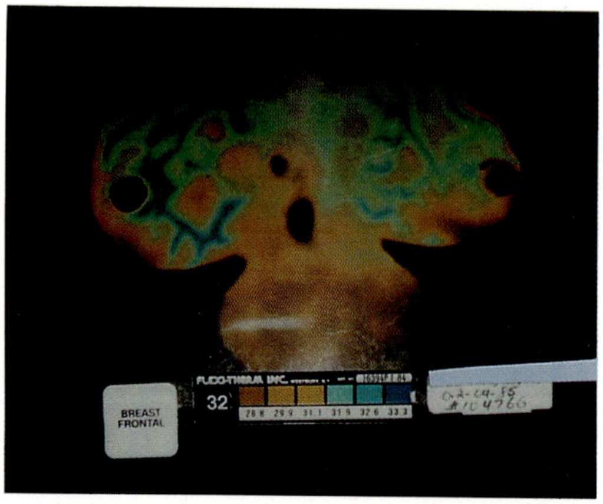

Fig. 12 Pregnant woman. Note the marked bilateral vascularity similar to that in Fig. 11.

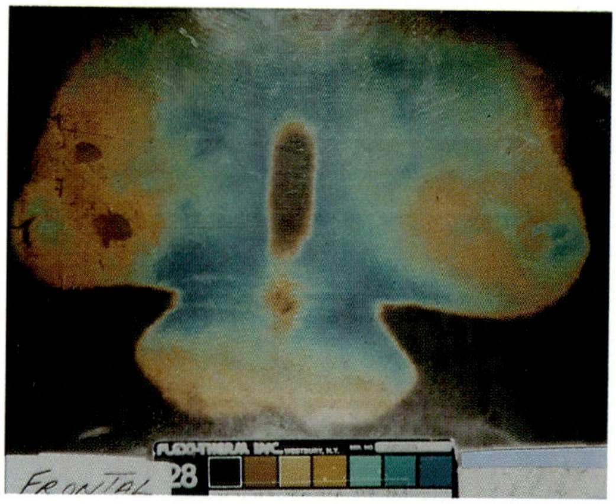

Fig. 13 Infiltrating ductal carcinoma. Note the increased left nipple heat and periareolar vascularity.

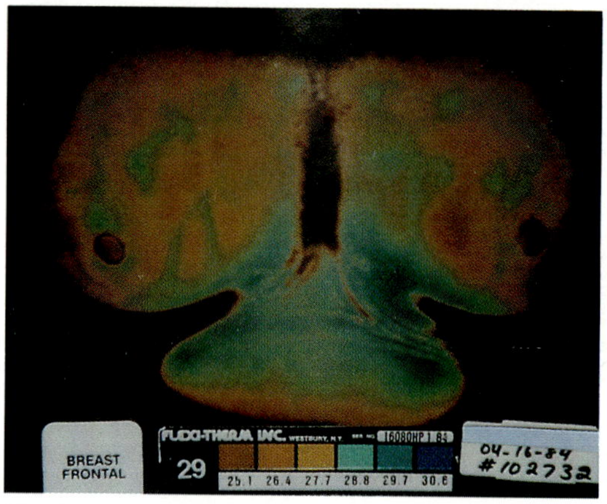

Fig. 14 Infiltrating ductal carcinoma. Note the increased right nipple heat.

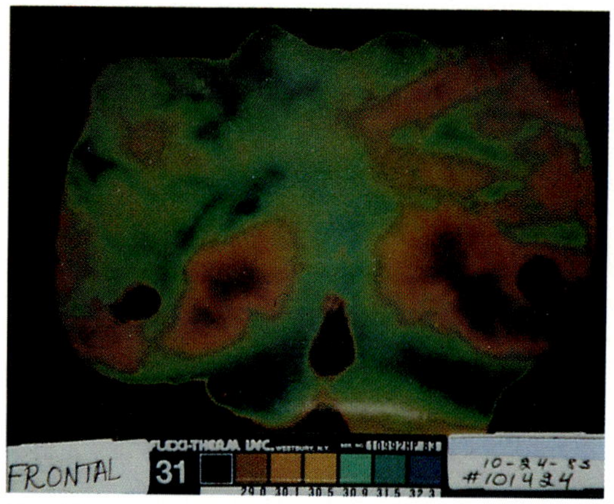

Fig. 15 Infiltrating ductal carcinoma. Note the increased vascularity and slightly increased right nipple heat. (Part of the nipple shows increased heat.)

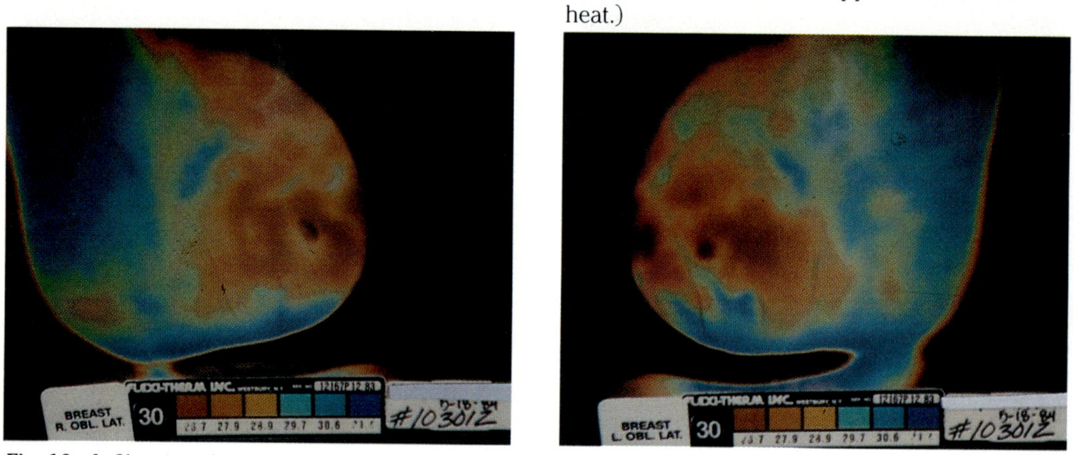

Fig. 16 Infiltrating ductal carcinoma. Oblique views. Note the draining vein (blue area) on the inferior left breast, extending towards the nipple.

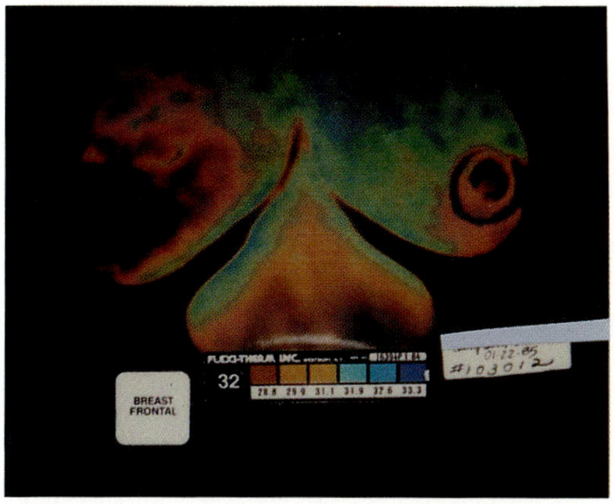

Fig. 17 Infiltrating ductal carcinoma, after irradiation. There is a marked increase in vascularity in the left breast, as well as a swollen and hot left nipple.

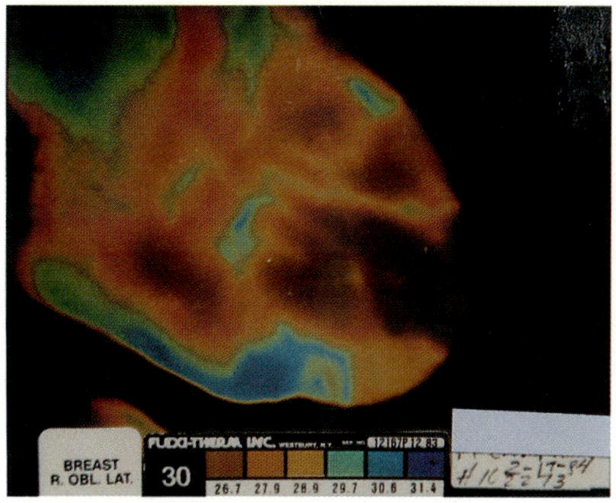

Fig. 18 Multicentric carcinoma. Note the irregular outline on the inferior portion of the breast (edge sign) and the markedly increased heat in this area.

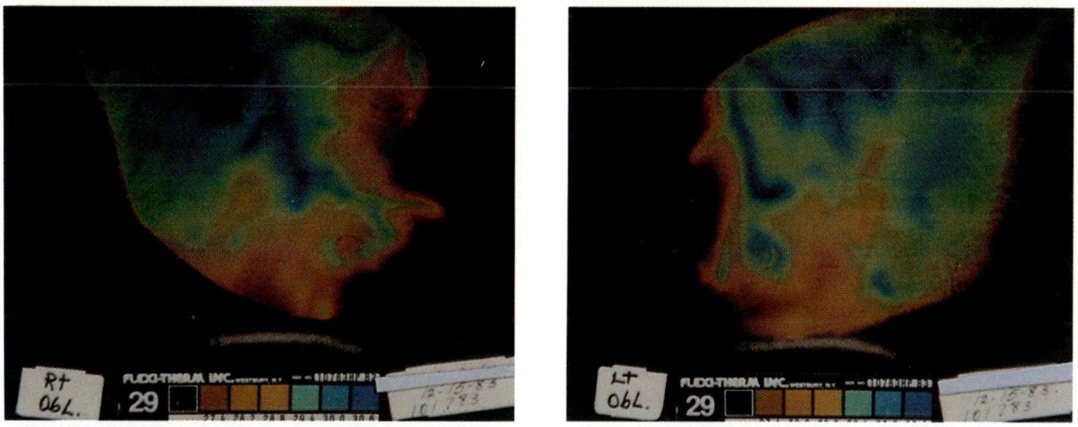

Fig. 19 Paget's disease, oblique views. Note the increased ieft nipple heat. The nipple on the left is blue (hotter) and nipple on the right is yellow (cooler).

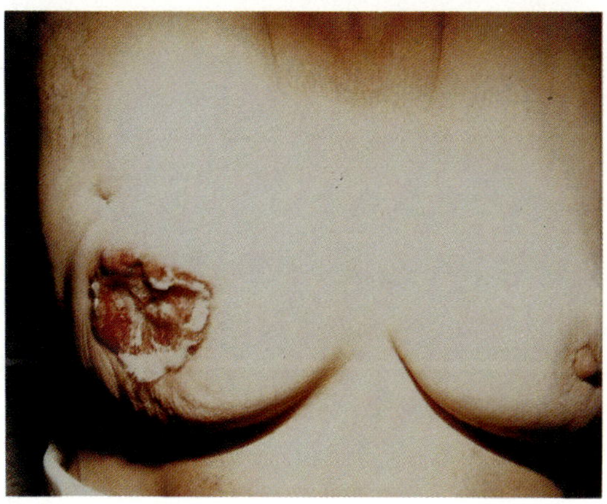

Fig. 20 Ulcerating carcinoma. There is partial autoamputation of the anterior right breast.

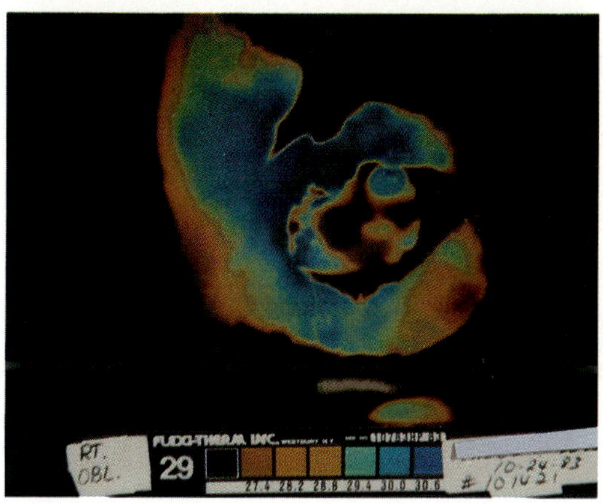

Fig. 21 Ulcerating carcinoma, same patient as in Fig. 20. There is global hyperthermia (blue color showing increased heat). The dark area in the mid-breast represents ulceration with a lack of contact to the thermographic plate.

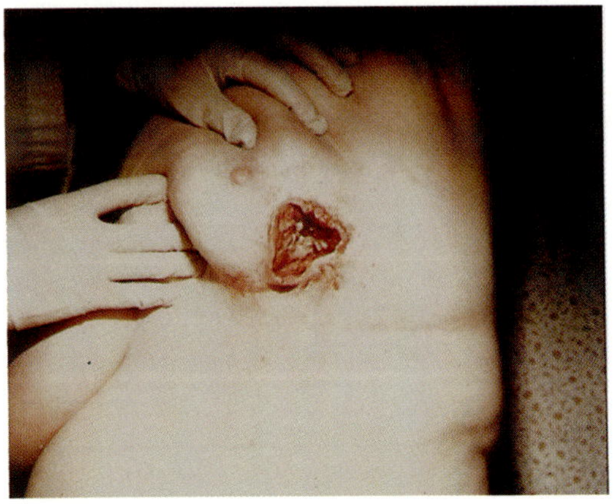

Fig. 22 Ulcerating carcinoma. Note the large cavitating carcinoma under the left breast.

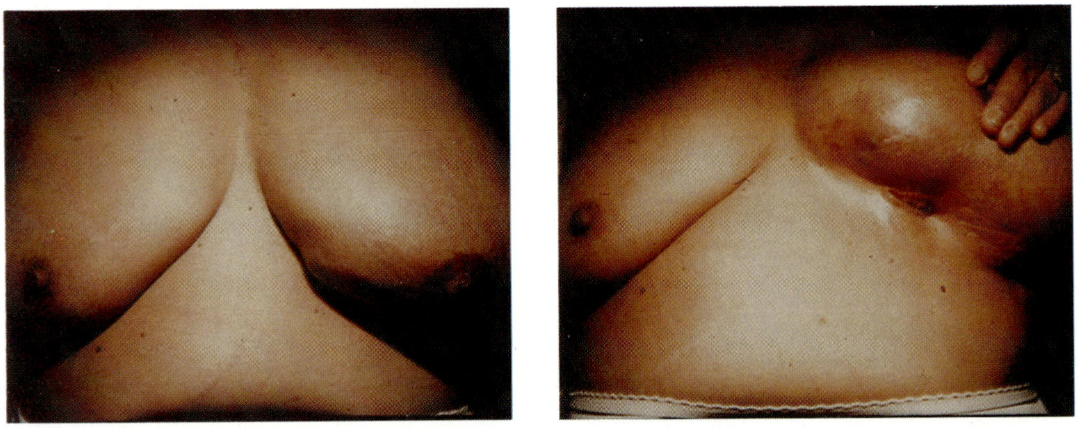

Fig. 23 Necrotic carcinoma. Note the bulging of the inner, lower aspect of the left breast in the left photograph. A small ulceration in the inframammary fold is seen in the right photograph.

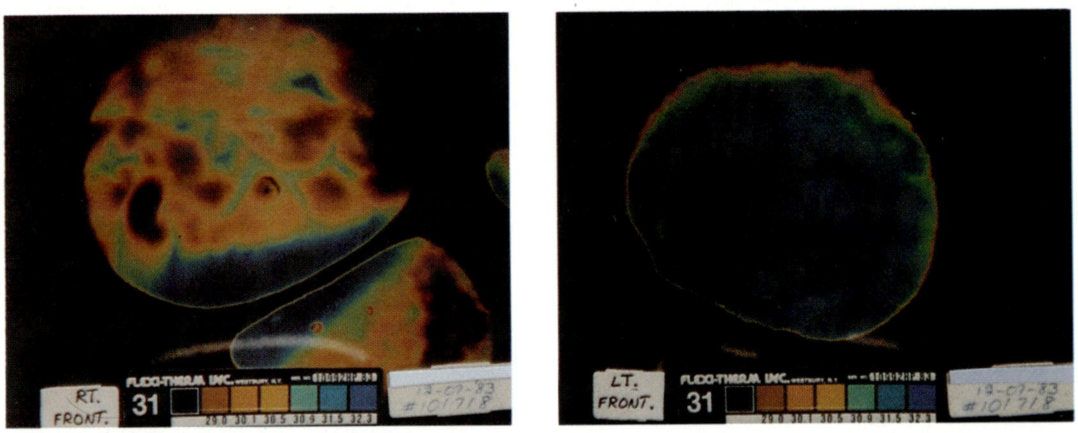

Fig. 24 Necrotic carcinoma, same patient as in Fig. 23. There is global hyperthermia of the left breast (breast is totally blue). The blue area seen in the inferior aspect of the right breast is due to incomplete cooling of a large-breasted woman, the breast resting against the obese abdomen.

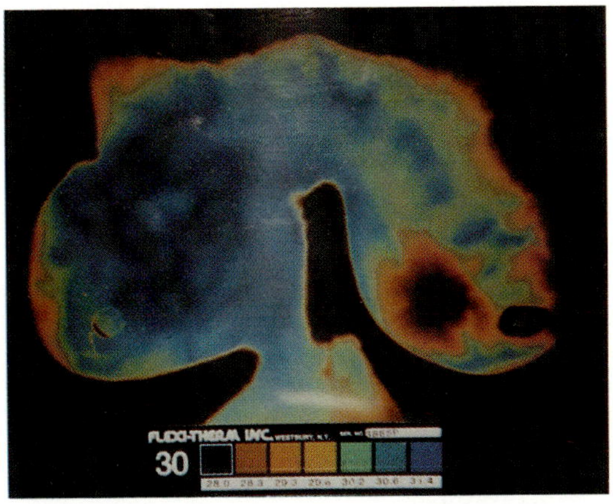

Fig. 25 Missed carcinoma. Note the global hyperthermia of the right breast (almost totally blue).

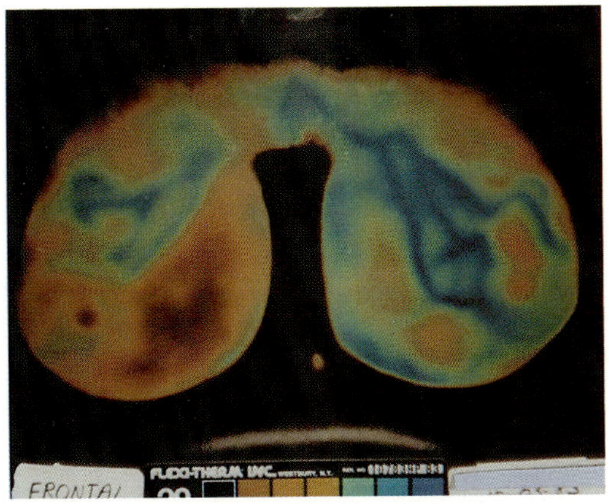

Fig. 26 Medullary carcinoma. Note the marked increase in vascularity and nipple heat in the left breast.

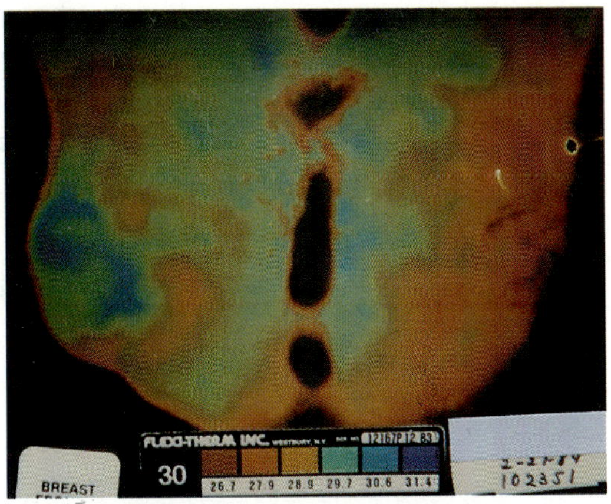

Fig. 27 Gynecomastia in a boy. Note the marked increase in vascularity and nipple heat in the right breast.

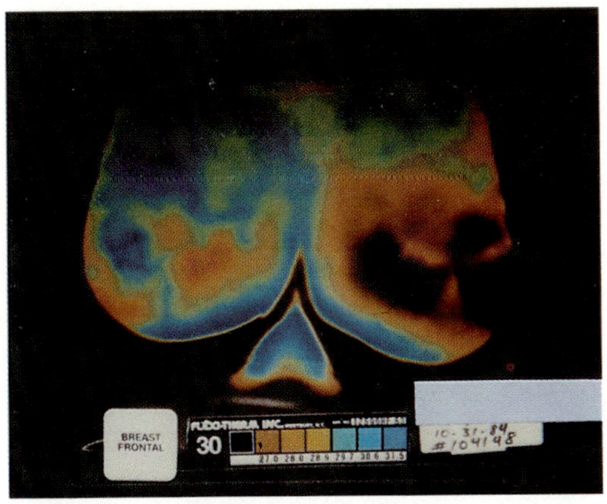

Fig. 28 Postirradiated breast. Note the marked right nipple heat and adjacent vascularity. The right breast is smaller.

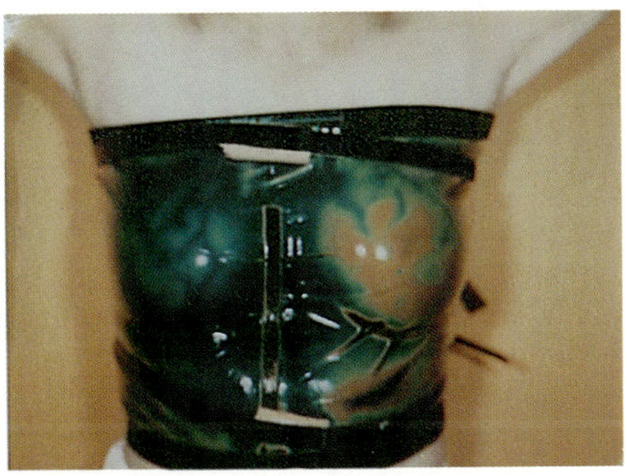

Fig. 29 Infiltrating ductal carcinoma. This thermogram was done in 1982 wth the flexi-therm wrap around thermographic sheet. Note the marked global hyperthermia of the right breast.

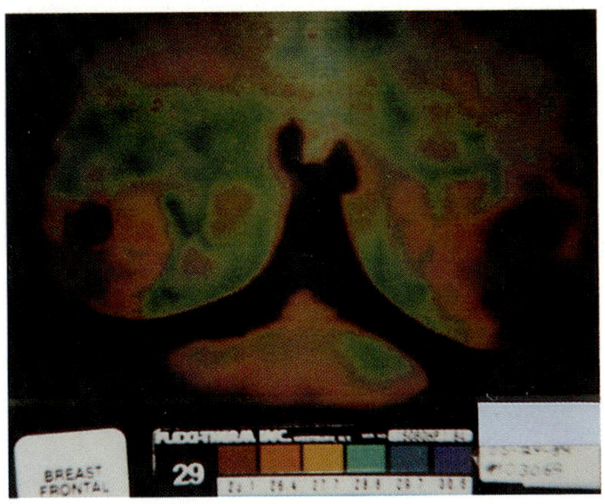

Fig. 30 Postirradiated breast. Same case as in Fig. 29, but 2 years later in 1984. Note the diffuse increased vascularity in the right breast.

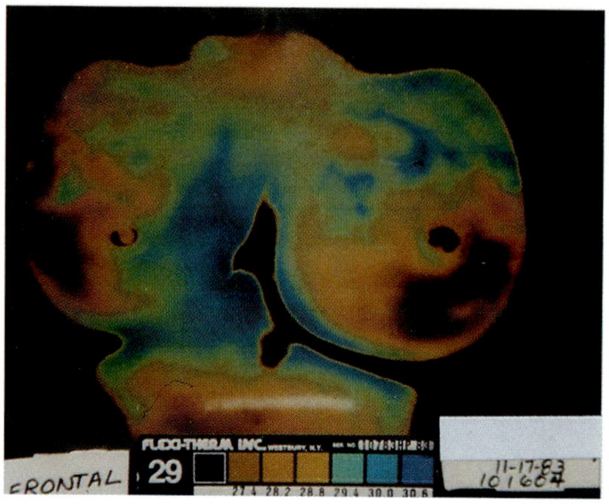

Fig. 31 Postirradiated breast, recurrent tumor. Note the increased right nipple heat and markedly increased vascularity in the inner right breast.

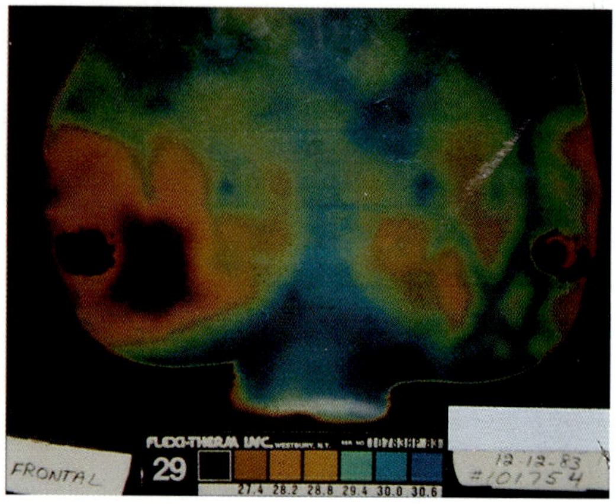

Fig. 32 Infiltrating ductal carcinoma (12/83). Note the increased left nipple heat and vascularity.

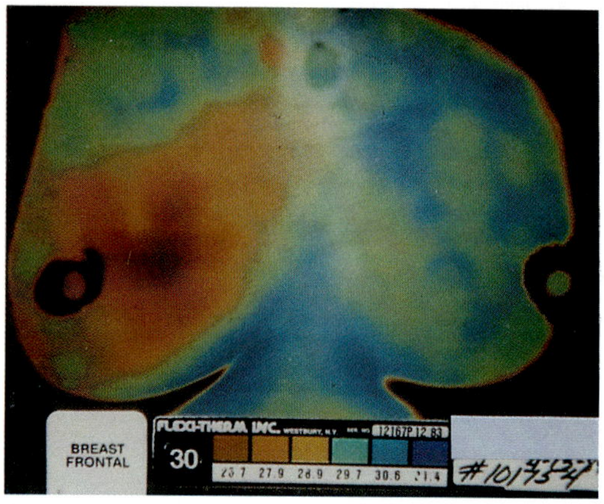

Fig. 33 Breast during radiation therapy (4/84). Note the global hyperthermia of the left breast.

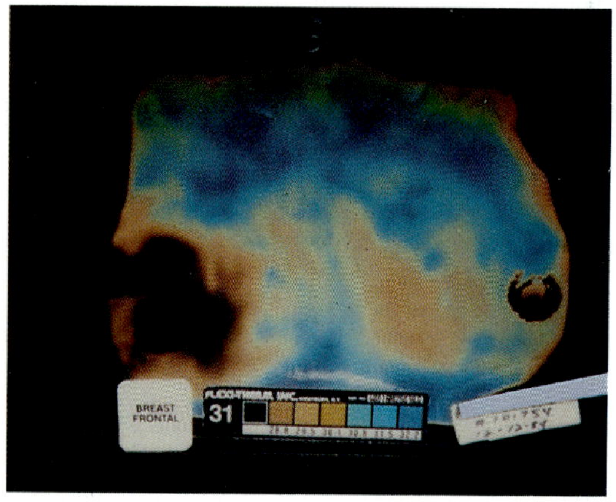

Fig. 34 Postirradiated breast (12/84). Note the increased left nipple heat and vascularity. There has been a decrease since 4/84 (Fig. 33).

*The fact that fewer thermograms than other studies are demonstrated reflects the cost of color photography; it does not mean that the author believes thermography is of less value.

cases presented, the amount of hematoma was large. Thermography is usually normal. Diaphanography is the most sensitive of the imaging procedures, being markedly absorptive of light transmission because of the hemoglobin present in the ecchymotic area. The results of mammography vary. In the first two cases there was a mass present, whereas in case 3 no mass was detected. These variations are due in part to the amount of blood present and the fact that a mass of hematoma was seen in one case but not in the others. In case 3 the ultrasound demonstrated a highly echogenic mass with shadowing, whereas in case 1 a cystic area of liquefied blood was noted, and in case 2 only diffuse shadowing was seen. In case 2 the diffuse nature of the shadowing on ultrasound was probably due to the diffuse nature of the blood collection in the lobule.

Case Studies: Postoperative Hemorrhage

Case 4

I.B. is a 39-year-old woman who on 3/26/84 had a fibroadenoma resected deep within the right breast. On two occasions blood was aspirated from the surgical area. She had pressure dressings for the first month postoperatively. The most recent needle aspiration was on 5/25/84. She presented to the Woman's Breast Center on 5/30/84 complaining that the right breast was still swollen.

On physical examination there was a firm, swollen mass 5 cm in diameter in the anterior portion of the right breast behind the right nipple and a recent scar in the inferior periareolar area. The mass was slightly tender.

Liquid crystal thermograms showed increased right nipple heat (Color Fig. 1). On diaphanography there was an inability to penetrate the mass with light. Ultrasound showed the presence of a 2 cm cystic area with some internal echoes (Fig. 14-4). On aspiration 0.5 cc of bright red blood was obtained.

Because of the depth of the lesion it was not possible to fully appose the tissues at surgery, and a hematoma filled the space. It takes a long time for this size hematoma to resolve, but it eventually will do so. Further surgical exploration raises the risk of infection and recurrent hemorrhage. Six months later there was complete resolution of the mass and only slight persistence of the tenderness.

Case 5

D.H. is a 30-year-old woman who presented with a painful breast lump of 8 months' duration. She had been told by a physician that it was a dilated milk duct.

On physical examination there was an ill-defined, tender, 2 cm area at 9 o'clock on the right breast. Thermograms showed some increase in vascularity on the right, a slightly positive thermogram (Color Fig. 2). Diaphanography was normal. Mammograms showed a poorly defined density without calcifications, thought to represent glandular tissue. Ultrasound showed glandularity without a mass.

At surgery an area of breast tissue with duct ectasia and fibrosis was found draped about a well circumscribed lipoma that had not been appreciated on the imaging studies.

The patient returned 1 week after surgery because of bleeding from the right nipple. On physical examination there was a scar in the outer aspect of the right breast with induration over the entire outer aspect of the breast. With minimal pressure to the lateral aspect of the breast there was a discharge of dark brown blood from two ducts on the lateral aspect of the nipple.

Thermograms showed increased heat and vascularity consistent with recent postoperative changes. On diaphanography there was a marked decrease in light absorption over the entire lateral inferior aspect of the breast.

The patient was reassured that this postoperative bleeding was caused by transection of the two ducts at surgery and that the hematoma would regress slowly. Two

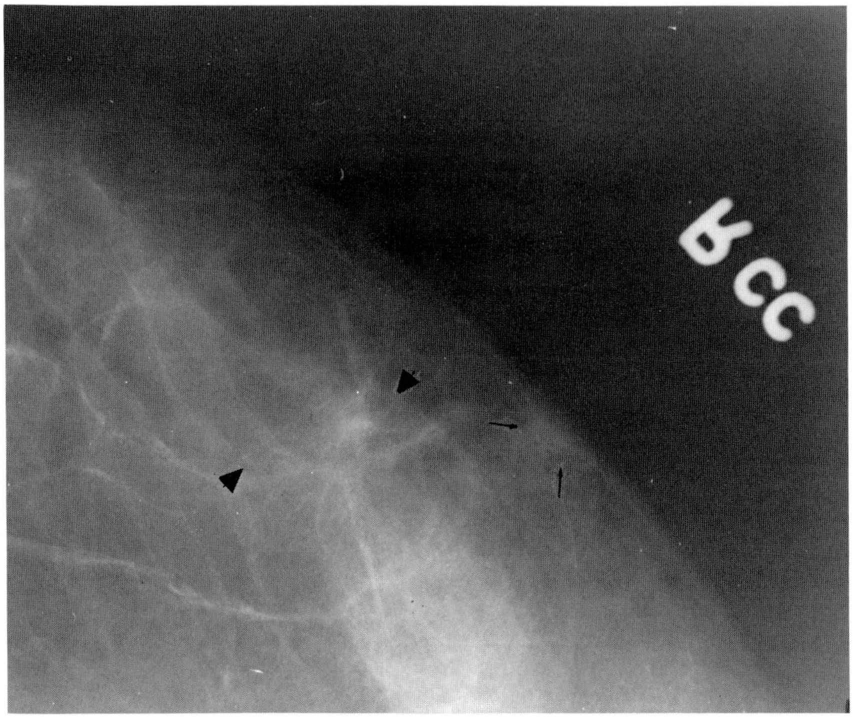

Fig. 14-5 Magnification mammogram. Note the slight skin thickening (small arrows) and slight spiculization from the area of biopsy (arrowheads).

months later on reexamination there was slight pain in the outer breast and some old clotted blood extruding from a single duct in the outer aspect of the nipple. The thermogram remained slightly positive on the right. Diaphanography showed decreased light transmission over the outer aspect of the breast, less than on the earlier examination. There was decreased light transmission throughout the ductal system lateral to the nipple. Mammograms showed duct dilatation and slight skin thickening in the area of the scar. The original density was no longer present (Fig. 14-5).

The hematoma was slowly resolving. The ducts contained old blood that could be expressed with some difficulty. It was suggested to the patient that she use warm compresses and continue to gently milk the ducts to remove the old blood. The area continued to resolve and 2 months later was clinically normal.

Discussion

Postoperative hematomas resolve slowly; the larger the hematoma, the longer is the period of recovery. This slow resolution can be very disturbing to the patient, who must be reassured. Diaphanography is the most sensitive imaging procedure to detect blood in the tissues. A good physical examination with a history of the recent surgery usually suffices to establish the diagnosis.

Bibliography

Hemorrhage

Barth V: *Atlas of Diseases of the Breast*. Stuttgart, Georg Thieme, 1979.

Egan RL, McSweeney MB: Breast sonography—interpretative criteria, in Jellins J, Kobayashi

T (eds): *Ultrasonic Examination of the Breast*. London, Wiley, 1983, pp 307–318.
Homer MJ: Mammographic appearance of the breast after needle localization biopsy. *Breast* 1985;11(2):26–31.
McCrea ES: Hemorrhage into the breast. *J Can Assoc Radiol* 1981;32:62–63.
Porrath S, Sandhu R, McNeil J: Thermography and benign breast disease. Proceedings American Academy of Thermology, Los Angeles, 1984 (in press).
Sickles EA, Klein DL: Effects of needle aspiration on the mamographic appearance of the br ast: A guide to the proper timing of the mammography examination. *Radiology* 1982; 145:44.
Sonnenfeld M, D'Orsi CJ, Sadowsky NL, et al: Mammographic patterns of unusual breast lesions. *JCE Radiol* 1979;1(4/5):13–30.
Tabár L, Dean PB: *Teaching Atlas of Mammography*. New York, Thieme-Stratton, 1983.

Postoperative Hemorrhage

Homer MJ: Mammographic appearance of the breast after needle localization biopsy. *Breast* 1985;11(2):26–31.
Sickles EA, Klein DL: Effects of needle aspiration on the mammographic appearance of the breast: A guide to the proper timing of the mammography examination. *Radiology* 1982;145:44.

15

Infections

Saar Porrath

There are many locations in the breast that can become infected: the nipples, the ducts, Montgomery's glands, the skin, glandular tissue, lesions such as cysts and hematomas, and lymph nodes. The clinical presentation varies depending on the location; however, there are a few basic underlying signs. The onset is usually fairly precipitous, with a rapid presentation of clinical signs from the first symptom. The skin overlying the area may become red and thick. There is on occasion localized lymphedema and rarely red streaking from lymphatics. The area is usually tender to touch, may be painful, and shows increased heat. A palpable mass may be present.

These symptoms and signs are usually localized to the breast. Occasionally, however, the pain radiates to the axilla or shoulder. No matter how noxious the breast infection the patient almost never responds with temperature or malaise.

When the nipple or areolar area is the site of inflammation, it becomes red and tender. Nipple discharge is rare unless the adjacent ducts are infected. There is usually some pain. A mass is seldom present unless the infection goes untreated. The nipple may become enlarged.

Mammography may show some skin thickening. It may be otherwise unhelpful except to rule out the presence of a mass. Thermography is exquisitely sensitive to any inflammatory reaction and shows a positivity out of proportion to the physical findings. The entire anterior portion of the breast may demonstrate a marked increase in heat of 3° to 5°C more than the normal opposite side. There is also an increase in vascularity. Diaphanography shows decreased light transmission with any skin thickening. The infected area shows as a "blackened area," with marked light absorption due to the increased blood. The involved area of infection is smaller on light scan than the area seen on thermography. Ultrasound may show the skin thickening. There may be increased echoes in the subcutaneous tissues and some increase in the shadowing from the nipple and periareolar area. Treatment with antibiotics and the applications of warm compresses are usually all that is necessary (see Chapter 19).

Montgomery's glands are blind-ending sebaceous glands. They surround the nipple and are located on the edge and within the areola. They serve as a source of lubrication. When infection occurs in one of these blind ducts an abscess may quickly develop. A tender mass is present clinically, usually at the edge of the areola. It may be small or up to a few centimeters in size.

The thermogram is very positive in the entire anterior portion of the breast. Diaphanography shows a generalized marked decrease in light transmission in the surrounding area with a clear delineation of the "infected mass." Ultrasound shows the mass to be semisolid with thickened walls and internal echoes in the "fluid area." Mammography may demonstrate the mass if attention is paid to soft tissue detail.

Warm compresses and antibiotic therapy usually suffice, although in some cases surgery is necessary as the infection sometimes smolders and recurs if not completely abated (see Montgomery's gland abscess case report, below).

Duct infections may be accompanied by a nipple discharge of either serous fluid, which will show inflammatory cells, or frank pus, depending on the location of the duct. If the infection is deep or the infected portion is blocked from egress to the nipple, no discharge may be present. There may be itching or a sensation of pulling in the nipple. Unless an abscess develops, the mammogram and ultrasound may be normal, although a slightly dilated duct may be seen on ultrasound. The light scan may show an area of decreased light transmission. Thermography is very positive. Again, as with superficial infections, antibiotics and warm compresses are usually sufficient unless an abscess develops.

With mastitis, an inflammation of the glandular tissue, the signs depend on the location of the infection. There may be localized redness or increased redness of a large segment of the breast, with associated pain and tenderness. The light scan and thermography reflect the process, showing a generalized decrease in light transmission in the involved area and a generalized increase in heat and vascularity on the thermogram. Mammography is usually negative except for skin thickening and an increase in the subcutaneous lymphatics. There may be a poorly defined area of increased density seen in the glandular tissue, but it is variable. Ultrasound reflects these changes as well. A focal mass is seldom present.

The treatment is again antibiotics and warm compresses. The mastitis tends to recur if incompletely resolved. Not infrequently, mastitis recurs in the same site, even when treated adequately, although the recurrence may be months or years later.

When a focal abscess develops, the clinical signs and diagnostic tests reflect it. If the abscess is deep, the findings are less distinct than if the location is more superficial. The clarity of findings also depends on the size of the abscess. The larger the abscess the more generalized the symptoms and the more distinct the resultant signs.

Diaphanography is more positive if the lesion is more superficial or large, or if the breast is small in relation to the size of the abscess. The light scan in infections, especially when localized, is the most positive of the entities (along with hematomas) seen on diaphanography. There is almost total absorption of the light. Thermography is almost always positive, irrespective of the location unless the abscess has been treated with antibiotics and is sterile. With a sterile abscess the other tests may remain positive, whereas the thermogram reflects the decrease in the inflammation and is normal. In the dense glandular breast (Wolfe P2, DY) an abscess may be ill-defined on mammography or even lost in the adjacent tissue. If the abscess is small and deep and the adjacent inflammation localized, mammography may be inconclusive or negative. There may be a well defined mass seen. Ultrasound shows the abscess with relative clarity as a thick-walled density with a "fluid center" containing some internal echoes.

Although antibiotics may suffice, surgical intervention in the form of incision and drainage or removal of the abscess, is more common than in the infections described above. (The reader is referred to case studies under Infections in Adults and Infections in Teenagers, below.)

Infectious swelling of the axillary lymphatics does not imply a breast etiology. Although it can occur with almost any of the infectious processes mentioned above, it may also be due to infections in the upper extremity. It may also occur because of a generalized condition such as tuberculosis (see the case study, below).

In the United States tuberculosis, syphilis, and fungal disease (except superficially on the skin) of the breast are rarely seen. When they do occur, they can appear as either a diffuse but localized area or an abscess.

Postoperative inflammation is not a true infectious process but may mimic one. The breast may present with skin thickening and even a peau d'orange appearance (skin changes resembling an orange peel). The breast is tender and firm owing to the recent incision. The thermogram is positive because of the inflammatory response. Diaphanography shows a generalized decrease in light transmission, especially when there is skin involvement and hematoma. Ultrasound may show skin thickening and an increase in the subcutaneous echoes, and there is shadowing from the recent incision. There may be fluid in the tissues. Mammography shows a diffuse increase in density with thickening of Cooper's ligaments from lymphatic engorgement. The findings described are related to the amount of surgery. If there has been a simple biopsy, the findings may be localized to the area. If there has been a larger surgical procedure in which more of the breast was involved, the findings are more generalized. The abnormalities tend to resolve within a few weeks to months depending on the amount of surgery. Most radiologists are unfamiliar with this process as they seldom see the immediate postoperative breast. If there has been extensive hemorrhage into the breast, the findings take longer to resolve, diaphanography remains positive longer, and ultrasound shows more tissue disruption.

Inflammatory carcinoma of the breast is not a true infection but a blockage of the lymphatics by tumor cells with an intense skin reaction. (This subject is discussed further in Chapter 21.)

Case Studies: Breast Abscesses and Infections in Adults

Case 1

E.O. is a 39-year-old woman who came self-referred because of a lump of 4 weeks' duration. On physical examination a small-breasted woman was seen with a 3 cm well defined soft nodule in the upper outer aspect of the right breast. Small lymph nodes were felt in the right axilla. The mass was neither tender or painful.

Thermography showed increased heat in the upper right breast and nipple area when compared to the left. On diaphanography there was marked light absorption through the mass (Fig. 15-1A). Mammography showed marked glandularity to the breasts, a Wolfe DY pattern. There was an indistinct bulge in the upper outer right breast without calcifications (Fig. 15-1B). Ultrasound showed a well defined nodule with diffuse internal echoes, the central portion being almost echo-free. There was shadowing from the edge of the nodule (Fig. 15-1C). Pus was obtained on needle aspiration, and *Staphyloccoccus aureus* grew out on culture. The patient was referred to a surgeon who incised and drained the abscess. The patient recovered completely following antibiotic therapy.

Case 2

S.Q. is a 41-year-old woman who in May 1983 had had a cyst adjacent to the right nipple that was aspirated by a surgeon with fluid obtained. She had had chronic drainage from the area since that time. She was treated on one occasion with antibiotics. She came to the Woman's Breast Center on 2/16/84 because of pain in the area.

On physical examination there was a hard 2 cm area just medial and superior to the right nipple. In the center of the nodule was a small area containing pus. The pus was removed and sent for culture, growing out diphtheroids. Thermography was positive in the right nipple and periareolar area. Diaphanography showed a marked light decrease with a lucent center where the pus had been removed (Fig. 15-2). Mammograms showed marked glandularity (P2 pattern), without a mass. Ultrasound demonstrated a small echo-free area extending into the base of the nipple.

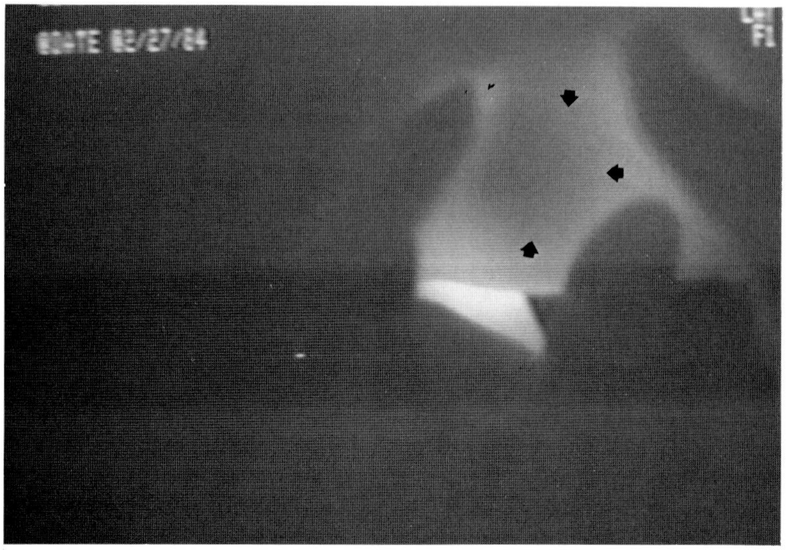

A

Fig. 15-1 **A:** Diaphanography. Note the decreased light transmission through the mass (arrows). Compare with cysts (Fig. 10-1) showing increased small Light Transmission, and with fibroadenomas (Figs. 12-2A and 15-5A) demonstrating another cause of decreased light transmission. Note that the decreased light transmission is less than with hemorrhage (Fig. 14-3A). **B:** Mammogram, lateral view. There is a slight bulge in the glandularity (open arrows) but no well defined mass. **C:** Ultrasound. There is a mass with diffuse internal echoes (arrowheads). Compare with the echo patterns of giant fibroadenomas (Figs. 12-4B and 12-5B) and an infected cyst (Fig. 10-5C); note the difference, with only a few internal echoes and a thick wall noted in the infected cyst.

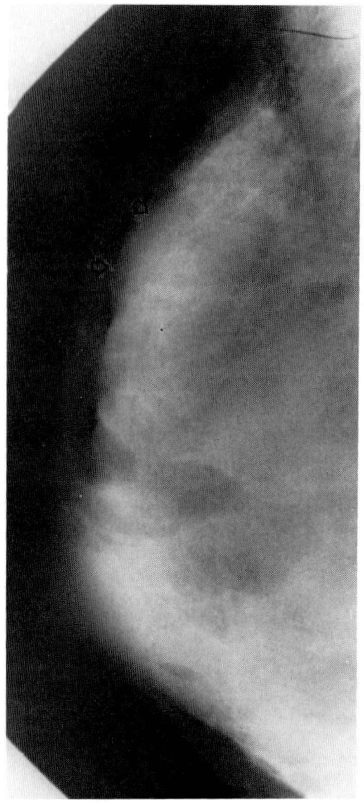

B

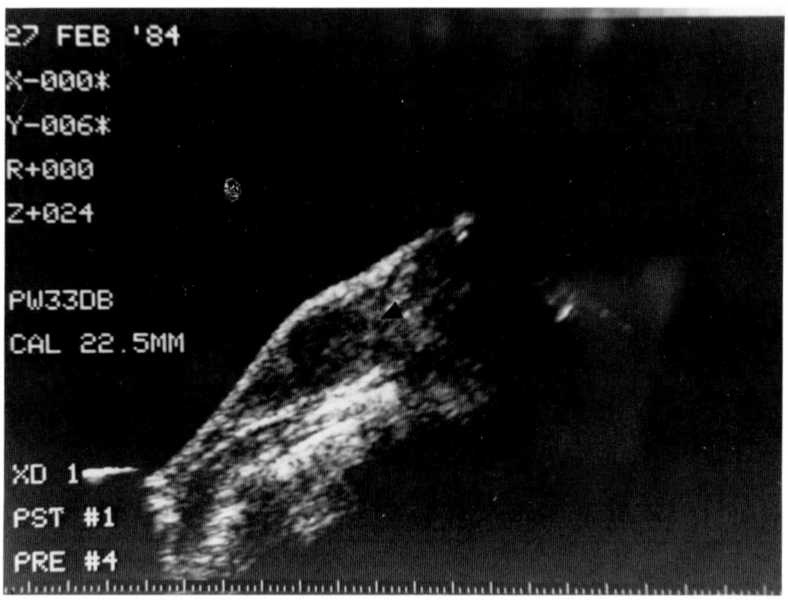

C

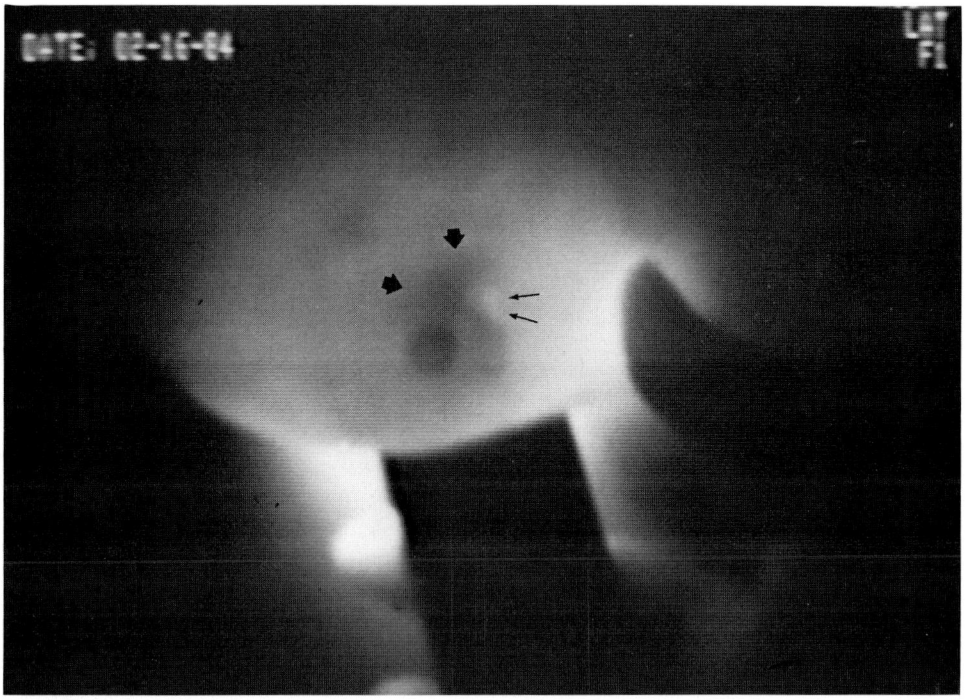

Fig. 15-2 Diaphanography. Note the area of decreased light transmission (thick arrows) and the lucent area (thin arrows) where pus had been removed.

The patient was referred to a surgeon for removal of the chronically draining area, which was acting as a nidus of infection. At surgery cystic hyperplasia with focal chronic inflammation was found. The patient had been symptom-free since the surgery.

Case 3

J.W. is a 43-year-old woman referred because of a painful left breast lump of 1 week's duration. On physical examination there was a 4 cm firm, indurated area extending laterally from the nipple and involving the outer aspect of the nipple. There was no nipple discharge.

Thermograms and diaphanography were both very positive in the area of the induration and lump (Fig. 15-3A). Mammography showed thickening behind the nipple area without a discrete mass. Ultrasound demonstrated a 1.5 cm echo-free area (Fig. 15-3B). On needle aspiration 0.5 cc of pus was obtained, which grew out *Escherichia coli.*

The patient underwent incision and drainage on two occasions, as well as an extended course of antibiotics. The infection cleared.

Case 4

M.T. is a 27-year-old woman who presented with a 4-day history of a very painful, swollen right nipple. On physical examination the right nipple was swollen with a reddened bubblelike area that involved about one-third of the nipple, measuring 5 by 8 mm. Thermograms were very positive in the nipple and periareolar area. The bubblelike area showed markedly diminished light transmission on diaphanography.

The area was punctured with a needle, and a small amount of whitish, puslike material was obtained. The patient was told to use warm compresses. On follow-up examination 2 weeks later the area was clinically normal, as was the repeat thermography.

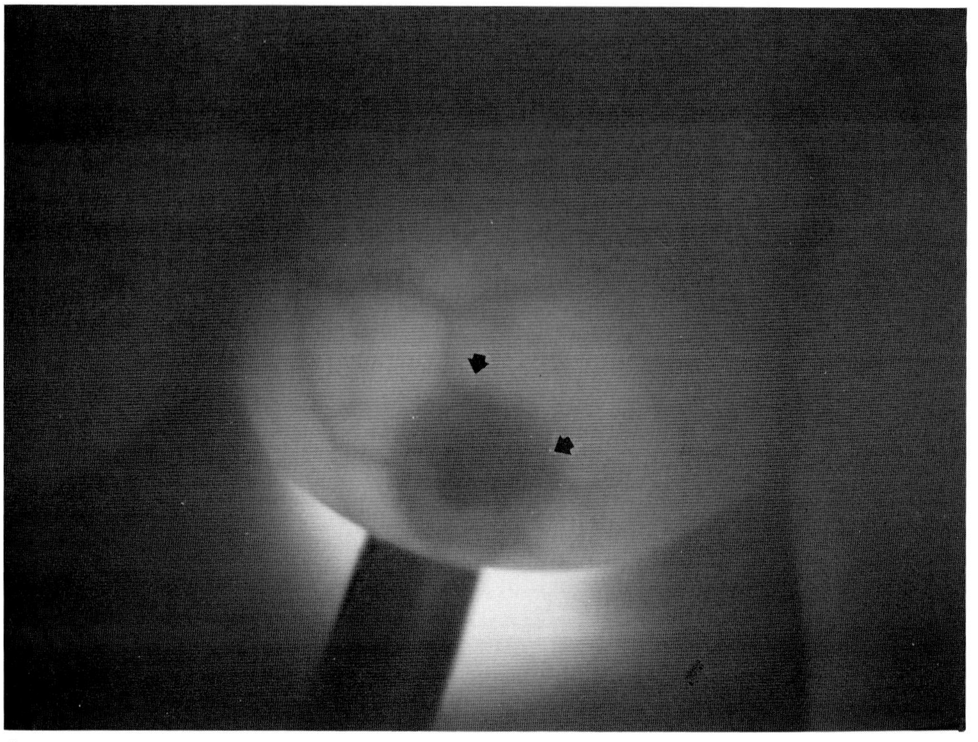

A

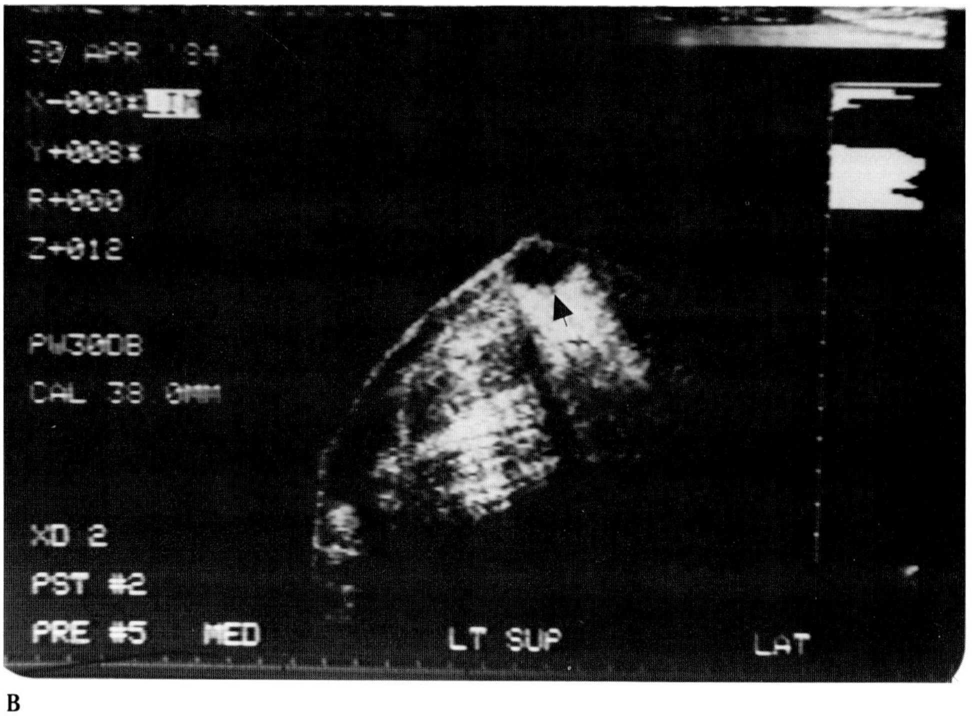

B

Fig. 15-3 A: Diaphanography. There is markedly decreased light transmission above and lateral to the left nipple (arrows). **B:** Ultrasound. There is an echo-free area behind the nipple with increased sound transmission (arrow). Compare with another abscess (Fig. 15-1C), showing diffuse internal echoes, and cysts (Fig. 10-2A). Note that abscesses can have a varied pattern and may appear like simple cysts, as did this one, or like a solid tumor (Fig. 15-1C).

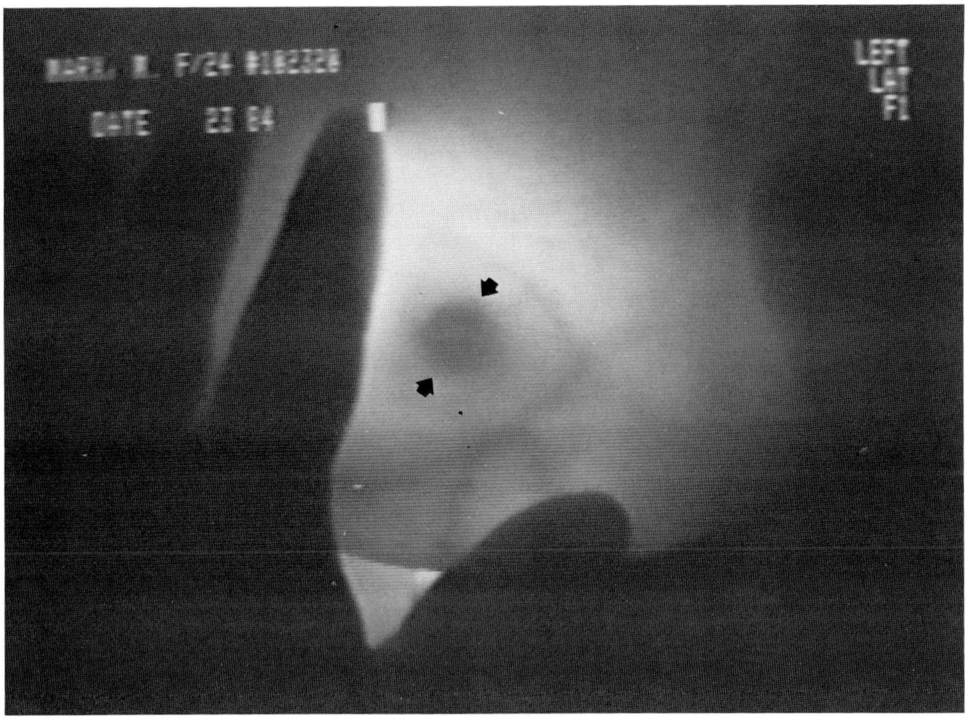

Fig. 15-4 Diaphanography. Note the swollen, poorly defined left nipple (arrows). Compare with a nipple shadow with hemorrhage (Fig. 14-1B) and a hematoma (Fig. 14-3A). The nipple is usually well demarcated and very light-absorptive; if it is not, swelling should be considered.

Case 5

M.M. is a 24-year-old woman who was referred because of a painful left breast mass. Physical examination was extremely difficult because of the patient's anxiety and the marked tenderness. The left nipple was swollen to twice the size of the right and was reddened, but no mass was present. Thermography was very positive in the left nipple area. Diaphanography demonstrated the swollen nipple (Fig. 15-4).

She was placed on antibiotics and warm packs. On reexamination 2 weeks later the thermogram was normal, and the size of the left nipple had reduced to equal that of the right nipple. The redness was gone, as was the tenderness. The patient had been having multiple infected hair follicles surrounding the areola, and it was thought that this problem may have led to the nipple infection.

Six weeks later the patient returned with a tender left nipple and a firm 1 cm mass directly behind the nipple. The thermogram was again markedly positive in the area of the nipple. Ultrasound demonstrated a poorly defined density with diminished echoes behind the nipple. She was treated with antibiotics, with no resolution of the mass. She remained on periodic antibiotics for 2 months, finally consenting to surgery. The surgery demonstrated chronic periductal inflammation and an area of acute and and chronic inflammation with foreign body giant cells consistent with an abscess. She remained symptom-free for about 4 months after surgery, then again developed another abscess in the left nipple area.

Discussion

Staphylococcus aureus is an unusual bacterium in breast abscesses and infections; more commonly a gram-negative bacterium is cultured. The source of entry is not known, but with *S. aureus* being cultured as in case 1, it may be that a hair follicle became infected and developed an abscess.

Although it is very unusual for a cyst that has been aspirated to become infected, it can obviously occur, as in case 2. In case 4 there was a localized infection of a distal portion of a duct, or a blind duct, in the nipple. Because it was well localized it was necessary only to lance the area and apply warm compresses. This case of treatment is in contradistinction to case 5, where there were multiple recurrences of a nipple inflammation. It is probable that there was a low-grade infection of the ducts in this case that "seeded" the nipple area.

Thermography is extremely sensitive to active infections but is nonspecific. On diaphanography the greatest degree of light absorption occurs with hemorrhage and localized infections such as abscesses. (The reader is referred to the case report section of Montgomery's gland abscesses, below.)

Case Study: Montgomery's Gland Abscess

Case 6

M.P. is a 58-year-old woman whose family history included a mother who developed unilateral breast cancer at age 85. The patient presented with an extremely tender 3 cm mass behind the right nipple of 2 days' duration, with increasing tenderness. Because of the marked tenderness it was difficult to determine the boundaries of the mass. There was bulging of the areola but no nipple discharge.

The thermogram was acutely positive with the right nipple exhibiting a 5°C difference from the left. There was an increased temperature in the surrounding tissue as well. On diaphanography there was a marked decrease in light transmission through the mass (Fig. 15-5A).

Mammography demonstrated increased tissue density on the right, adjacent to the nipple, but no defined mass (Fig. 15-5B). Automated breast ultrasound showed the presence of a poorly defined 2 cm cystic area with some internal echoes. There was dilatation of the adjacent ducts (Fig. 15-5C).

Needle aspiration produced 0.5 cc of reddish brown fluid. There were many inflammatory cells and no bacterial growth at 48 hours.

The patient was started on cephalexin (Keflex) and warm compresses. When rechecked 3 days later there was less tenderness. The thermographic difference of the nipples had decreased to 3°C. The light scan showed a diminished size to the mass. The cephalexin and warm compresses were continued.

When seen 3 weeks later there was minimal induration behind the right nipple, with no true mass identified. The thermogram showed a minimal increase in temperature, and diaphanography showed the presence of a 1 cm darkly light absorptive mass just lateral to the nipple within the areola. The findings continued to resolve slowly. At 3 months all studies were normal.

Discussion

Montgomery's glands are blind-ending ducts of sebaceous cysts that surround the nipple and serve as a source of lubrication. When infected they may be difficult to treat with antibiotics only, and surgery may be necessary.

When an infection occurs in the area of the areola it may not be possible to discern at the initial examination the location of the nidus of infection. The thermogram is very sensitive to any infection but not specific to location. The thermogram is the most sensitive test for residual infection. Diaphanography and ultrasound tend to be more definitive regarding location. The mammogram may not be specific.

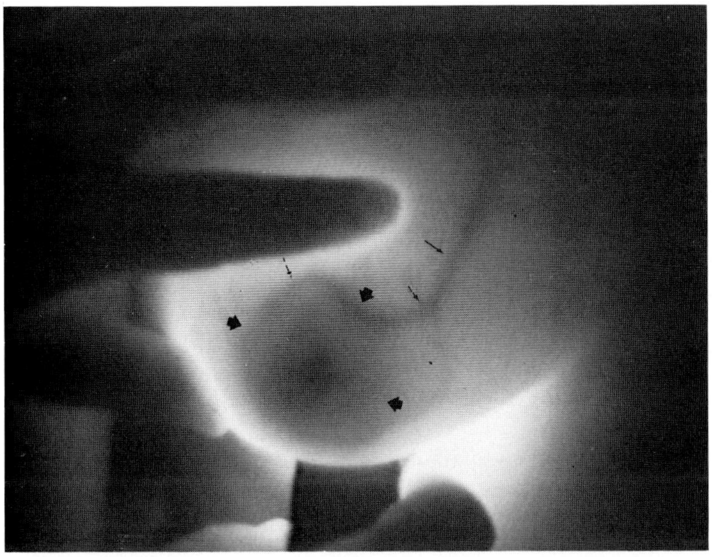

A

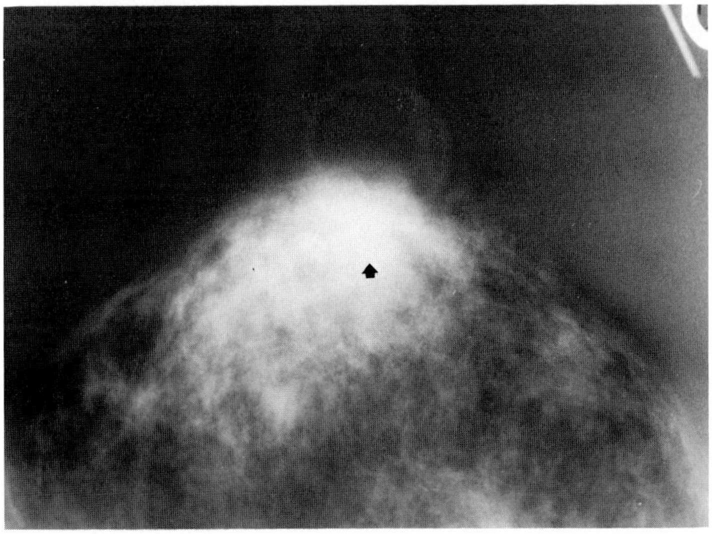

B

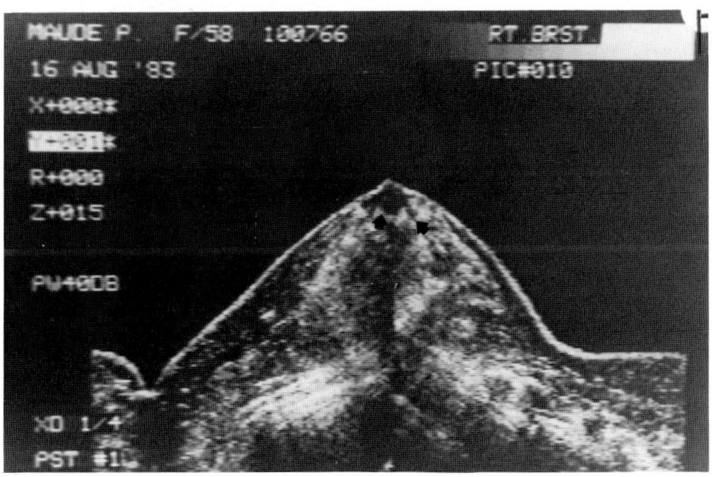

C

Fig. 15-5 **A:** Diaphanography. There is decreased light transmission in the nipple area (thick arrows). Note the prominent superficial vein to the infected area (thin arrows). **B:** Mammogram, CC view. Note the area of increased density; no mass (arrow) is present. **C:** Ultrasound. There is an echo-free area behind the nipple without increased through transmission or shadowing (arrows).

Case Studies: Infections in Teenagers

Case 7

A.D. is a 14-year-old girl who 2 months earlier was treated by her pediatrician with antibiotics for a left breast infection, with resolution. Two days prior to being seen this time she developed tenderness, pain, and swelling in the left breast in the same area as the previous infection. Physical examination revealed erythema of the anterior portion of the breast and a 1 cm firm area just lateral to the left nipple, at the edge of the areola.

Liquid crystal thermograms showed increased heat over the entire anterior left breast (Color Fig. 3). Diaphanography showed markedly decreased light transmission over the mass (Fig. 15-6A). A 2 by 8 mm fluid area was seen on ultrasound just beneath the skin, with increased attenuation of sound waves (shadowing) adjacent to this area (Fig. 15-6B).

This case was presumed to represent a recurrent infection with a small abscess. The patient was restarted on antibiotics and warm compresses. It is probable that the original infection was incompletely treated, and a nidus of infection remained that flared up at a later date. There was complete resolution within a week.

Case 8

R.C. is a 15-year-old girl who was seen by a surgeon on 5/7/84 with a 1-day history of severe breast pain. The left breast was erythematous with a slightly inverted nipple and a minimal peau d'orange appearance. There was fullness without a mass. Aspiration revealed some watery purulence but no pus. There was no growth at 48 hours. The patient was started on antibiotics. When seen at follow-up on 5/11/84 the erythema was gone, the tenderness was less, but induration and a mass effect were present. She was referred to us for further evaluation.

On 5/21/84 she had minimal erythema anteriorly, and a tender density about 2 cm in size adjacent to the nipple. Liquid crystal thermograms showed a diffuse area of increased heat over the nipple and periareolar region on the left. Diaphanography showed a marked decrease in light transmission in the same area (Fig. 15-7). Ultrasound showed a 2 mm fluid area and marked shadowing. The patient was restarted on antibiotics and warm compresses. There was complete resolution of the infection without recurrence.

Case 9

N.L. is a 13-year-old girl who presented with a 2-day history of a painful left breast lump. Physical examination showed diffuse redness in the periareolar area just lateral to the left nipple. There was marked firmness of the area, with a 2.5 cm mass present.

Thermograms showed marked left nipple and periareolar heat, with a 5°C difference from the right side (Color Fig. 4). Diaphanography demonstrated diminished light transmission in the area. Ultrasound revealed a 1 cm area of relatively few echoes, with a marked increase in echogenicity in the area (Fig. 15-8).

Needle aspiration obtained 0.5 cc of pus, which grew out gram-negative cocci. The patient was treated with antibiotics and warm compresses. On a return visit 2 weeks later the area was normal on physical examination, and the thermogram had also reverted to normal (Color Fig. 5).

Discussion

Infections of the breast in teenagers occur more commonly than is realized, especially because the imager seldom has the opportunity to consult on these cases. It is not infrequent to obtain no growth on the aspirated fluid or pus. The source of the infection is probably hematogenous, with no good explanation as to why the breast becomes infected. It is not dissimilar to what occurs in the older patient.

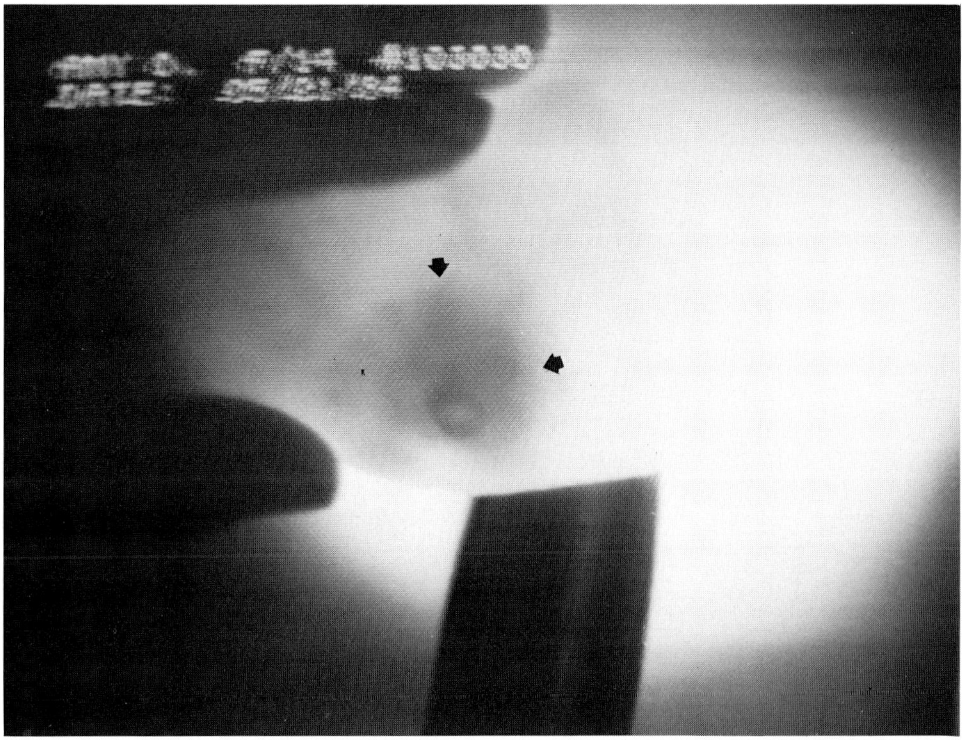

A

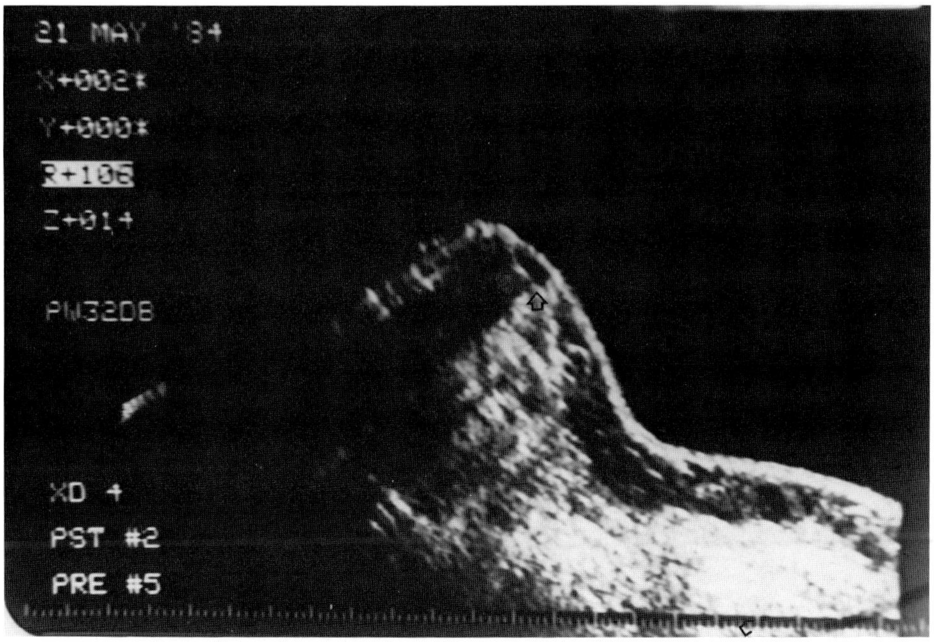

B

Fig. 15-6 **A:** Diaphanography. Light transmission is decreased adjacent to the nipple (arrows). **B:** Ultrasound, single transducer. There is an echo-free area with no increased through transmission (open arrows). Compare with other abscesses (Figs. 15-1C and 15-3B).

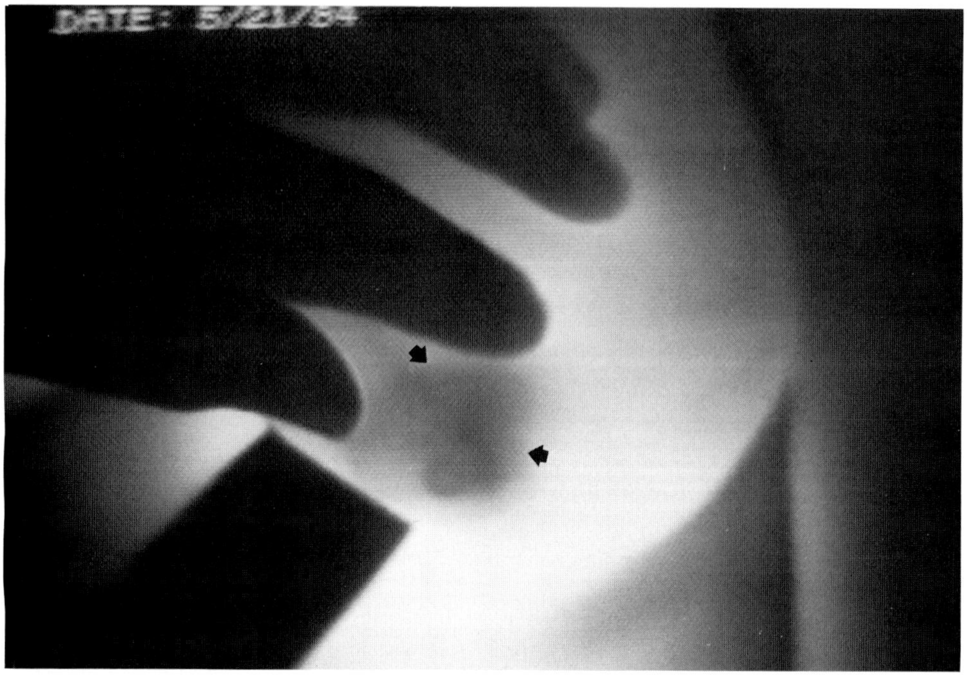

Fig. 15-7 Diaphanography. Note the decreased light transmission adjacent to the nipple (arrows).

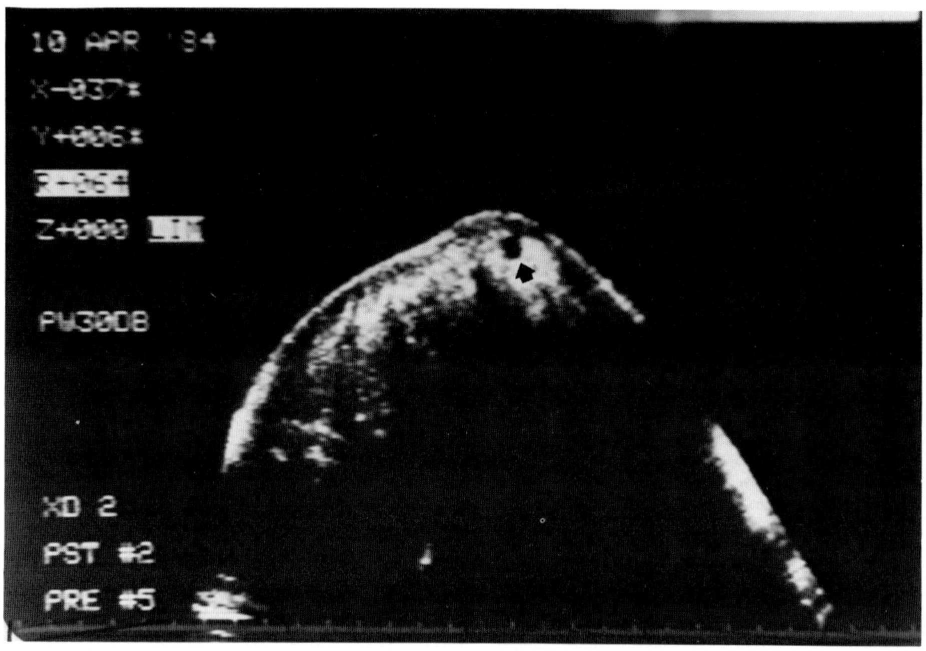

Fig. 15-8 Ultrasound. Note the echo-free area (arrow).

It is interesting to note how quickly a very positive thermogram, as in case 3, reverts to normal. This result reflects the value of thermography for assessing and following infectious processes.

In case 3 the area of abscess was smaller than the surrounding area of tissue reaction. This surrounding area was demonstrated on thermography, diaphanography, and ultrasound. The use of mammography in a patient of this age is not advocated unless there is no resolution of the problem, and even then it is best to do a biopsy without mammography. When evaluating a teenager under these circumstances, if the imager has only mammography available the patient should be referred elsewhere or treated clinically, rather than undergoing mammography.

Case Study: Tuberculous Adenitis and Lymphedema of the Breast

Case 10

M.A. is a 74-year-old woman who was diagnosed as having polyarteritis nodosa 15 years earlier. She had been on intermittent steroid treatment during that time. In January 1984 she presented with increasing weakness and masses in the right supraclavicular and lower left axillary areas. Excisional biopsies of these lymph node masses revealed caseating and noncaseating granulomas containing acid-fast bacilli consistent with tuberculosis. She was placed on antituberculous therapy. The patient was seen in June 1984 because of enlargement of the left breast and a peau d'orange appearance.

On physical examination there was a scar in the lower left axilla. The left breast was twice the size of the right breast and was firm without a discrete mass. There was skin thickening and a moderate peau d'orange appearance on the left breast.

Liquid crystal thermography showed global hyperthermia on the left of 2.7°C as well as increased nipple heat. Diaphanography showed a generalized decrease in light transmission on the left. Mammography revealed moderate glandularity bilaterally consistent with a Wolfe P2 classification. There was enlargement on the left breast with skin thickening and changes consistent with lymphedema. No mass or calcifications were identified (Fig. 15-9A).

The findings were consistent with lymphedema of the left breast secondary to lymphatic blockage, partially due to the removal of a portion of the lower axillary chain, and in part due to involvement of other left axillary nodes with tuberculous changes. The patient was informed there there would be slight resolution of the changes but not complete regression. By February 1985 there was a marked decrease in lymphedema of the left breast. The thermogram, although still positive on the left side, had cooled down. Diaphanography was normal. On mammography there was a marked diminution in the subcutaneous changes and skin thickening (Fig. 15-9B).

Discussion

It is important to remember that all breasts that present with a peau d'orange appearance do not contain inflammatory carcinoma, although this diagnosis must be ruled out. Other causes include infection (as in this case), postsurgical dissection of the axilla, postirradiation effects, and marked congestive heart failure. The findings on thermography, diaphanography, and mammography in this case are nonspecific and simply reflect the skin and lymphatic changes. Ultrasound, not done on this patient, would reflect the same changes.

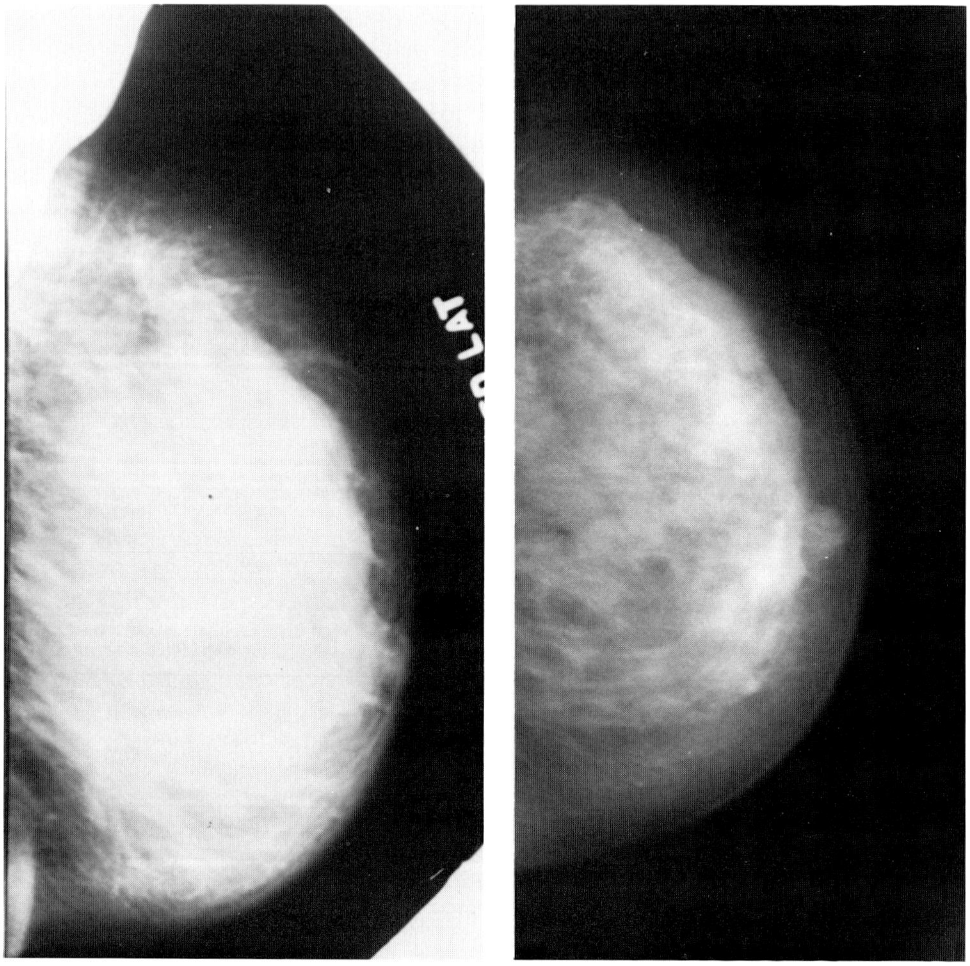

A B

Fig. 15-9 Left (**A**) and (**B**) lateral mammograms obtained in June 1984 and February 1985, respectively. Compare the mammograms. Note the marked skin thickening, especially inferiorly, the increased subcutaneous markings, and the increased density of the glandularity in the first film. These abnormalities are resolved in the second film.

Bibliography

Breast Abscesses and Infections in Adults

Barth V: *Atlas of Diseases of the Breast.* Stuttgart, Georg Thieme, 1979.

DiMaggio C, Muzzio P, DiBello A, et al: Transillumination of the breast. *la Radiol (Torino)* 1976; 62(6):401–413.

Hobbins WB: Thermography of the breast—a skin organ, in Gautherie M, Albert E, Keigh L (eds): *Thermal Assessment of Breast Health.* Lancaster, MTP Press, 1984, pp 37–48.

Kopans DB, Meyer JE, Proppe KH: The double line of skin thickening on sonograms of the breast. *Radiology* 1981; 141:485–587.

Schwartz GF: Benign neoplasms and "inflammations" of the breast. *Clin Obstet Gynecol* 1982; 25(2):373–385.

Tabar L, Dean PB: *Teaching Atlas of Mammography.* New York, Thieme-Stratton, 1983.

Montgomery's Gland Abscess

DiMaggio C, Muzzio P, DiBello A, et al: Transillumination of the breast. *Radiol Med (Torino)* 1976; 62(6):401–413.
Hobbins WB: Thermography of the breast—a skin organ, in Gautherie M, Albert E, Keith L (eds): *Thermal Assessment of Breast Health.* Lancaster, MTP Press, 1984, pp 37–48.
Schwartz GF: Benign neoplasms and "inflammations" of the breast. *Clin Obstet Gynecol* 1982; 25(2):373–385.

Infections in Teenagers

Hobbins WB: Thermography of the breast—a skin organ, in Gautherie M, Albert E, Keigh L (eds): *Thermal Assessment of Breast Health.* Lancaster, MTP Press, 1984, pp. 37–48.
Kopans DB, Meyer JE, Proppe KH: The double line of skin thickening on sonograms of the breast. *Radiology* 1981; 141:485–487.
Martin JE: *Atlas of Mammography.* Baltimore, Williams & Wilkins, 1982.
Sandison AT, Walker JC: Diseases of the adolescent female breast. *Br J Surg* 1968; 55(6):443–448.
Schwartz GF: Benign neoplasms and "inflammations" of the breast. *Clin Obstet Gynecol* 1982; 25(2):373–385.

Tuberculous Adenitis and Lymphedema of the Breast

Grausman RI, Goldman JL: Tuberculosis of the breast: Report of nine cases including two cases of co-existing carcinoma and tuberculosis. *Am J Surg* 1945; 67:48–56.
Hobbins WB: Thermography of the breast—a skin organ, in Gautherie M, Albert E, Keith L (eds): *Thermal Assessment of the Breast Health.* Lancaster, MTP Press, 1984, pp 37–48.
Homer MJ: Cardiopulmonary pathology masquerading as primary breast disease. *Breast* 1984; 10(2):6–9.
Kopans DB, Meyer JE, Proppe KH: The double line of skin thickening on sonograms of the breast. *Radiology* 1981; 141:485–587.
Martin JE: *Atlas of Mammography.* Baltimore, Williams & Wilkins, 1982.
Sandison AT, Walker JC: Diseases of the adolescent female breast. *Br J Surg* 1968; 55(6):443–448.
Schwartz GF: Benign neoplasms and "inflammations' of the breast. *Clin Obstet Gynecol* 1982; 25(2):373–385.
Tabar L, Dean PB: *Teaching Atlas of Mammography.* New York, Thieme-Stratton, 1983.
Tabar L, Kett K, Nemeth A: Tuberculosis of the breast. *Radiology* 1976; 118:587–589.

16

Mondor's Disease

Saar Porrath

The breast has an extensive vascular supply, both venous and arterial. These vessels are subject to the same diseases that occur elsewhere in the body. Arteriosclerosis with calcification of the arteries is commonplace in any mammography practice that includes older patients.

Thrombosis and thrombophlebitis of veins can occur in the breast. The occurrence of thrombophlebitis of the lateral thoracoepigastric vein with retraction of the overlying skin is known as Mondor's disease, named for the physician who first described it. The thrombophlebitis of the vein may set up an inflammatory reaction in the adjacent tissues. As this reaction subsides, the tissues retract, causing retraction of the overlying skin, which stimulates the skin reaction seen with cancer. The underlying vein may be tender, and there may be pain in the initial stages. The vein feels ropelike.

Although originally reported in the lateral aspect of the breast, affecting the branches of the thoracoepigastric vein, in reality thrombophlebitis can occur anywhere in the breast. Not uncommonly it occurs after surgery in the inferior aspect of the breast and usually goes unrecognized.

The thrombosis and thrombophlebitis are self-limited and most often do not cause skin retraction. The patient may have pain and tenderness, but not always. The vein almost always feels firm and ropey.

Martin demonstrated a vein on mammography that is listed as the vein of Mondor's disease. It appears similar to other prominent veins. Clinical correlation is usually necessary to establish the diagnosis. Thermography, if done in the acute stages, may show increased heat, but by the time the patient is usually seen the process is old and the thermogram normal. Ultrasound is noncontributory. Diaphanography may show the vein, which can be correlated clinically as it can be seen to "roll" under the light.

Treatment is symptomatic; hot compresses may help. The disorder is almost always self-limited, with the patient being given reassurance.

Case Studies

Case 1

P.D. is a 28-year-old woman who presented with a very tender ropelike area in the tail of the left breast. It measured just under 1 cm in width by 4 cm in length. The pain and palpable density appeared shortly after an exercise session, about 3 weeks prior to being seen.

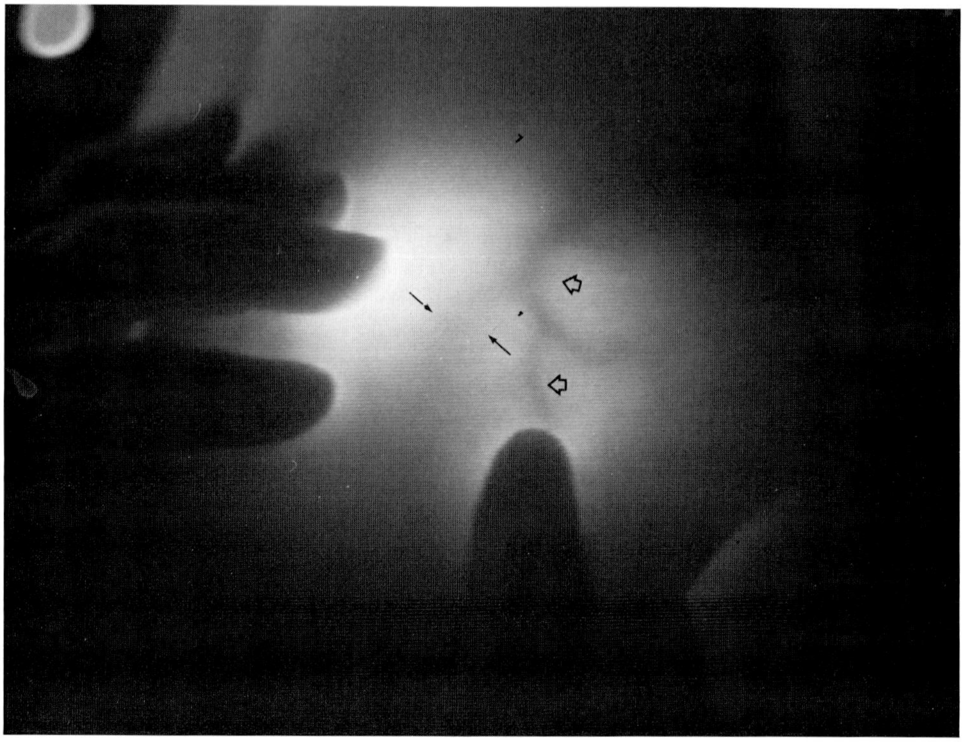

Fig. 16-1 Diaphanography. The deep vein shows as a widened area of slightly decreased light transmission (thin arrows). It could be rolled between the fingers causing pain. Note the better definition of the superficial veins (open arrows).

Thermography and diaphanography were normal. A single-view mammogram showed marked glandularity (Wolfe DY pattern) but no lesion. Ultrasound showed a similar picture.

The patient was reassured and told to apply warm compresses to the area. A month later the lesion and tenderness were gone.

Case 2

Y.B. is a 32-year-old woman who presented with a tender, ropelike area of sudden onset in the upper outer area of the left breast. It was painful and had been present for the 2 weeks prior to being seen. No event was linked to the onset.

The density measured 1 by 6 cm. It was possible to roll the area between the fingers and isolate it from the underlying glandular tissue. The thermogram showed slightly increased heat in the area, but it was within normal limits. The mammogram and ultrasound were noncontributory. On diaphanography the ropelike structure showed decreased light transmission and could be seen when rolled between the fingers (Fig. 16-1).

The patient was treated with reassurance and warm compresses. The pain and tenderness resolved in 3 weeks, but the ropelike area persisted for 6 months.

Discussion

Although both of these cases presented in the classic location described by Mondor—the distribution of the lateral thoracoepigastric vein—this site is by no means the only location within the breast that the disorder can occur. It also appears in almost all age groups. The skin retraction which is described as accompanying this entity was not seen in either of these patients and may indeed be more unusual than suspected.

Bibliography

Haagensen CD, Bodian C, Haagensen DE: *Breast Carcinoma.* Philadelphia, Saunders, 1981, p 431.

Martin JE: *Atlas of Mammography.* Baltimore, Williams & Wilkins, 1982, p 285.

17

Papillomatous Lesions

Saar Porrath

Papillomatous lesions are papillary growths arising from the epithelial lining of the ducts. They include papillomatosis; solitary papillomas; nipple papillomas, a variety of solitary intraductal papillomas; multiple papillomas; papillary cystadenomas, a variety of solitary or multiple papillomas; and papillary carcinomas.

Papillomatosis is an overgrowth of the lining of a single or multiple ducts. It is spread along the duct surface and does not exhibit a stalk as do the other varieties of papillomatous lesions. The duct may be partially or completely filled. It can be limited to a single area or, not uncommonly, is seen in multiple locations in one or both breasts.

It is usually a microscopic finding and seldom presents either as a mass or with distinct physical findings. Haagensen et al. thought that because it does not form a palpable mass it is not a clinical entity, and therefore the main differential is to exclude carcinoma.

Although usually asymptomatic, on rare occasions it presents as a nipple discharge; clear and serous or even bloody. Smears of the fluid are usually normal and acellular, although rarely clusters of papillary cells are seen.

The mammography may be normal or show an area of ill-defined increased density. Occasionally there are small calcifications, punctate or blunted. Sometimes a single or a group of prominent ducts are seen. A ductogram may show slight irregularities of the duct wall, appearing in a sawtooth fashion. There is rarely a blocked duct. More often there is a slightly dilated but empty duct, signifying that the papillomatosis has resolved or sloughed, leaving behind only the residue of the dilated duct.

The value of ultrasound in the diagnosis is that the slightly dilated ducts may be visualized, or it may show that a mass is not evident. Thermography is normal unless the condition is florid and very active metabolically, a rare circumstance. Light scanning may be normal unless there is blood in the duct, and then the duct may show as a darkened area extending from the nipple. On occasion the ill-defined area seen on mammography is evident as an area of diminished light transmission.

Because it is usually an incidental finding, the excisional biopsy is often enough. In those cases where the presentation is a group of calcifications, prebiopsy localization with mammography followed by excision may be necessary to rule out cancer.

Single or solitary papillomas can be found in any duct. They are a localized proliferation of ductal epithelium forming a polypoid mass, usually with a stalk. They may measure from a few millimeters to many centimeters. The more common presentation is the small papilloma of less than 1 cm, which has few symptoms and signs. When the papilloma is larger, up to a few centimeters, and surrounded by a duct so that it appears as if it were a growth within a cyst, it has been incorrectly termed a papillary cystadenoma, incorrect because it is neither a true adenoma or within a cyst.

Papillomas are almost always benign, although on rare occasions there can be malignant degeneration. Because of the increased area of ductal surface there may be an increase in secretion. The secretion may cause some degree of duct dilatation, seen both proximal and distal to the papilloma. The secretion may present as a nipple discharge. It comes from a single duct orifice and is usually clear or serous. Because of the friability of the tissue of the papilloma, even minimal trauma may cause slight sloughs of tissue, which may present as clumps of papillomatous cells on a smear. This same friability may lead to bleeding and a bloody or rust-colored discharge. Papillomas are the commonest cause of a bloody nipple discharge (see Chapter 6). Not infrequently the area of bleeding or slough scleroses or scars, the bleeding and discharge of abnormal cells then ceasing. On occasion the entire papilloma sloughs, leaving behind an area of scarring at its base in the duct wall and an otherwise empty but slightly dilated duct.

If the papilloma grows large enough, usually 1 cm or more, there may be a mass felt on physical examination. Milking the area of the mass toward the nipple may produce an exuberant discharge, often bloody. If no mass is present, the milking usually identifies the approximate location of the lesion.

Mammography, especially in the glandular breast, may show nothing. The mass, if present, is usually poorly defined from the surrounding glandularity; however, if the mass is large enough, it may be well defined. The dilated duct may be apparent. Calcifications may occur in the areas of sclerosis or throughout the papilloma but are not common. The calcifications may be single or multiple, small and benign in appearance, or punctate.

Diaphanography has been shown to be extremely valuable in the diagnosis; the accuracy rate on light scanning may approach 80 percent, depending on the size of the lesion, whereas plain mammography is less than 50 percent accurate at best. The papilloma on light examination shows as an intense area of diminished light depending on its depth from the surface. The closer to the surface it is, the darker and more defined is the area. This is especially true if the lesion is blood-filled. In those cases the duct which contains blood also shows as a darkened area. If the papilloma is small or deep in the breast, it may not show at all.

Thermography is normal in most circumstances. If the papilloma is large or superficial, there may be an area of increased heat or vascularity. Ultrasound may show the dilated duct and even, on occasion, the papilloma within the duct. If the lesion is large enough and the duct markedly dilated, it may appear as a filling defect within the duct. The papilloma seldom obstructs the duct so that by properly aligning the transducers the duct surrounding the mass can be seen on three sides of the mass, giving the appearance of a cyst adenoma. In cases of a sloughed papilloma only the empty duct is seen.

Ductography can be a valuable adjunct. A single duct with a rust, clear, or bloody discharge should always be cannulized and dye-injected. The purpose is to identify a defect, if any exists, and to rule out another cause such as cystic hyperplasia or possibly malignancy. Although the picture of a lobulated defect within a dilated duct is extremely suggestive of a benign papilloma, removal of the lesion is suggested, as accurate differentiation from an intraductal papillary carcinoma is not possible on the basis of a ductogram alone. Extravasation of dye is an indication of a cancer, as the integrity of the duct is seldom compromised by papillomas.

Ductography is also done to demonstrate the presence of any other filling defects in the same ductal system, a not uncommon occurrence. Ductography is not 100 percent accurate in the diagnosis of papillomas. Although many lesions are seen only on ductography, it may not be possible to delineate the lesion or even to fill the duct or the section of the duct containing the papilloma. It has been said by surgeons that once a solitary nipple discharge with papillomatous cells is found there is no place for ductography or further work-up, as the surgeon will explore the duct. This author believes that if preoperatively we can map out the duct and show that there is more than one lesion in the duct there is less likelihood of the second lesion being overlooked at surgery; moreover, the surgery is simpler if the rest of the duct is clear. In addition, if the duct is clear of a lesion, many surgeons watch the breast, without performing surgery. Preoperative localization with methylene blue filling the duct makes delineation of the involved duct easier at surgery.

Haagensen et al. defined an additional entity, the nipple papilloma. It is in essence a solitary papilloma in the distal aspect of the duct, adjacent to the nipple. It is an uncommon lesion. It may present as a mass extruding from the nipple or, as with other papillomas, with a discharge. It may be incompletely removed at surgery as the surgeon using a periareolar incision clears the proximal portion of the duct but may neglect to clear the portion of the duct distally, leaving a portion of the papilloma, which may regrow. With the exception of the external presentation, the findings may be similar to those discussed under other solitary papillomas (see case 1, below).

Multiple papillomas are more than just many solitary papillomas. According to the extensive and excellent long-term studies done by Haagensen et al., the multiple variety carries the onus of a more serious, possibly premalignant condition. In an excellent article by DuPont and Page, papillomas are noted to be proliferative lesions with an increased associated incidence of cancer. DuPont and Page did not differentiate between solitary and multiple papillomas.

The same diagnostic characteristics are present for single or multiple papillomas. When a solitary papilloma is found by the radiologist, additional papillomas should be sought so as to rule out missed lesions. Multiple papillomas tend to appear at a younger age than the solitary variety. They are more commonly bilateral and present as a mass more often than do solitary papillomas. In addition, they less often show a nipple discharge possibly because they are usually located more peripherally, whereas solitary papillomas are more common in the periareolar area.

Treatment for both solitary and multiple papillomas is simple excision, being sure that the duct that is involved does not contain additional lesions. Multiple papillomas tend to recur more often, possibly because of incomplete excision of all the lesions.

Papillary carcinoma is an unusual lesion that usually cannot be differentiated clinically from benign papillomas. It may have the same presentation and findings as the benign lesion except when it is invasive and large enough to distort normal findings. There may be extravasation on ductography. It is for that reason that intraductal growths seen on ductography or ultrasound should be explored. The differentiation lies in the hands of the pathologist.

Case Studies: Papillomas

Case 1

P.E. is a 30-year-old woman who presented because of a bloody right nipple discharge. Two years earlier she had ductal surgery on the right side for a ductal papilloma. A year later she had a recurrence of the papilloma with a second surgery. On physical examination there were bilateral implants, with scars present in the inferior aspect of the breasts. There were two scars in the right periareolar area. The nipple on the right was slightly smaller than on the left, and there was a slit across the front of the nipple

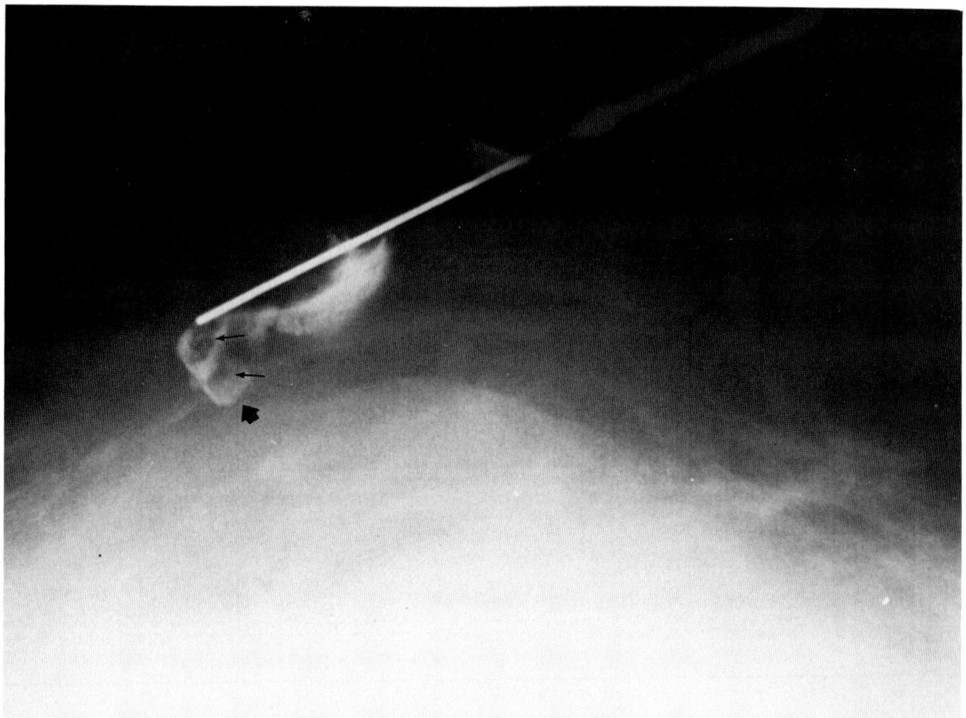

Fig. 17-1 Ductogram, magnified. The filling defects (thin arrows) represent intraductal papillomas. The blunt end (thick arrow) of the duct is from previous surgical transection.

from the previous surgeries. A small drop of blood could be extruded from the mid-portion of the nipple slit. No masses were felt.

Liquid crystal thermograms showed increased nipple heat and vascularity on the left (Th III thermogram). This picture has remained unchanged at 1 year and is thought possibly to be due to hormonal changes and the previous nipple surgery on the right. Diaphanography was normal. Mammograms demonstrated bilateral silicone gel implants and marked glandular tissue. Ultrasound showed slightly dilated ducts bilaterally.

A ductogram was performed by probing the nipple slit on the right. A single duct was encountered that extended medially. Dye injected into this duct demonstrated a slightly dilated duct measuring less than 2 cm in length; multiple filling defects were seen within it (Fig. 17-1).

It was thought that this lesion represented a duct that had been excised twice previously, which would account for its shortness. The filling defects were thought to be due to a papilloma. Preoperatively the duct was outlined with methylene blue. At surgery a duct extending into the nipple area filled with a papilloma was found.

Case 2

C.S. is a 54-year-old woman who was referred because of a left breast mass of 1 year's duration and a persistent yellowish left nipple discharge. On physical examination there was a firm, somewhat poorly defined 2 cm mass in the upper outer aspect of the left breast and a profuse yellowish discharge from the left nipple. There was a transverse scar through the right nipple and surgical changes to the right nipple.

Thermograms showed increased nipple heat and increased vascularity on the left (Th III thermogram). There was a slight decrease in light transmission over the left mass. Mammograms demonstrated a poorly defined area with questionable spiculization containing some benign-appearing calcifications (Fig. 17-2A.) Prominent ducts

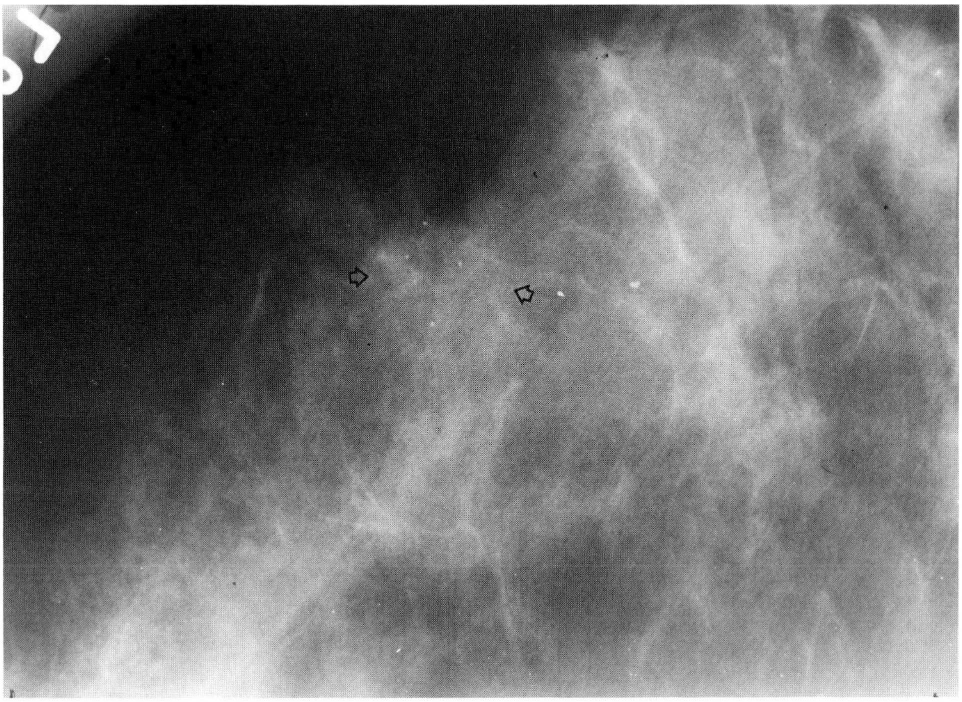

A

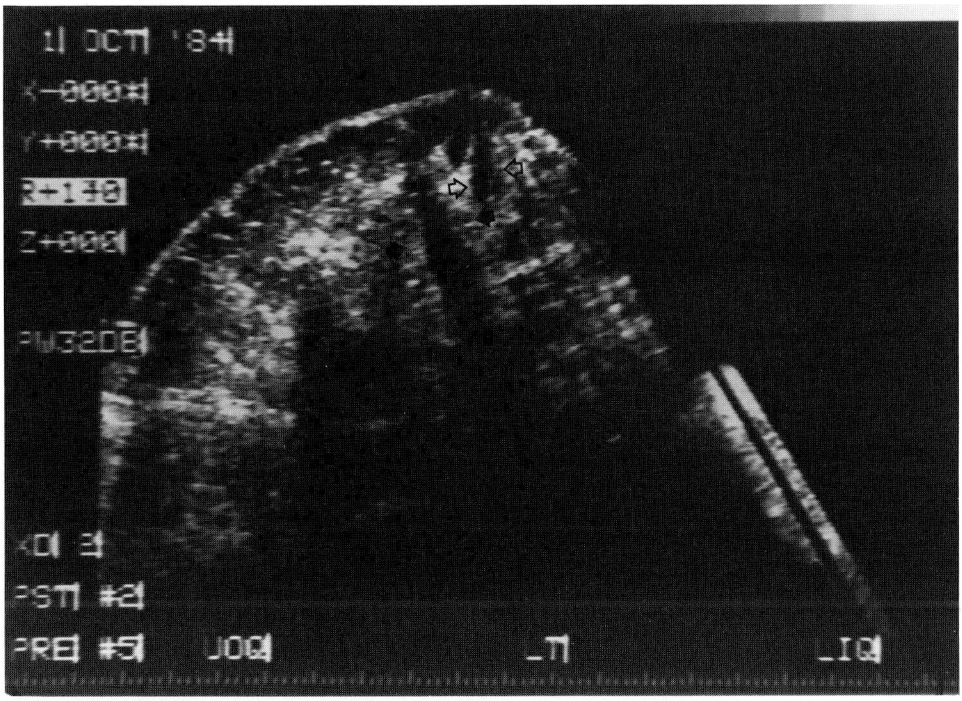

B

Fig. 17-2 A: Mammogram magnified, CC view. Note the poorly defined area (open arrows) with a suggestion of spiculization and benign-appearing calcifications. **B:** Ultrasound, rotary, around nipple. Note the area of marked shadowing (arrows) and the dilated ducts (open arrows).

were also seen on the left. Ultrasound showed the markedly dilated ducts on the left and persistent shadowing in the upper outer left breast (Fig. 17-2B). An attempt was made to cannulize the duct with the discharge, but it could not be done. Smears of the nipple discharge demonstrated epithelial cells suggestive of papillary hyperplasia. A papilloma was found at surgery.

Case 3

C.S. is a 49-year-old woman referred because of a left breast nodule. On physical examination there was a firm 1 cm nodule just medial to the left nipple. There was no nipple discharge.

Liquid crystal thermograms demonstrated increased left nipple heat (Th III thermogram). On diaphanography there was some decrease in light transmission over the nodule. There was mild glandularity seen on mammography (P1 pattern), with a well defined nodule of tissue density noted; no calcifications were seen (Fig. 17-3A). On ultrasound there was an area of almost cystic density with some internal echoes and no increased through transmission. There were some small ducts seen entering this area (Fig. 17-3B).

At surgery there was a well differentiated cyst containing an intraductal papilloma. Fibrocystic changes and chronic nonspecific mastitis were also found.

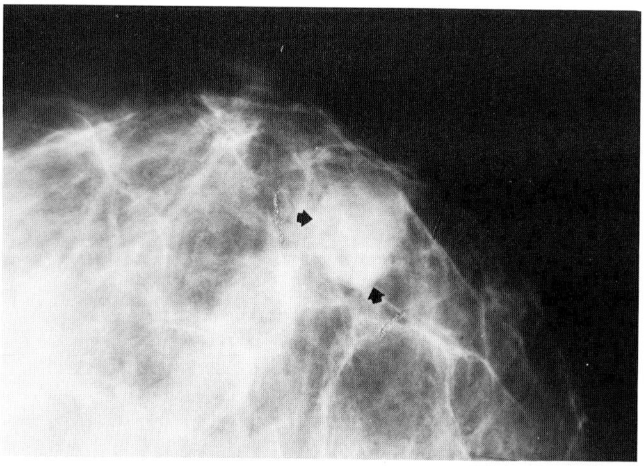

A

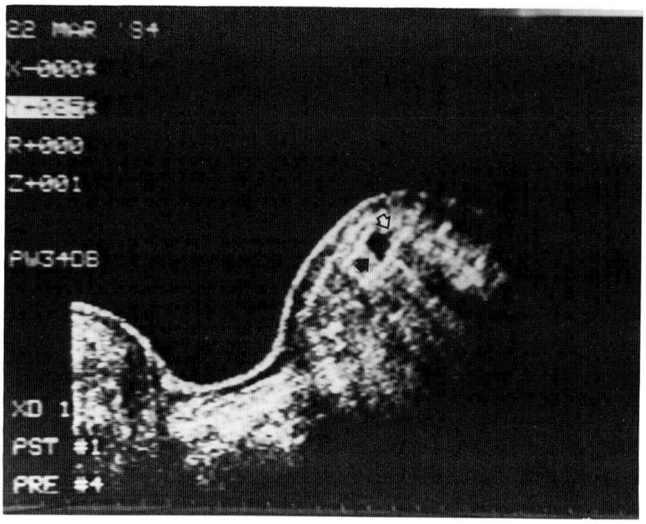

B

Fig. 17-3 **A:** Mammogram, CC view. Note the well defined nodule (arrows). **B:** Ultrasound. Note the irregularly shaped echo-free area. There is no increased through transmission (arrow). Note also the duct entering the area (open arrow). Compare with a cyst (Fig. 10-2B), which shows an echo-free area with increased transmission; fibrocystic disease (Fig. 13-3C); hemorrhage (Fig. 14-1D); postoperative change (Fig. 20-1); and teenage infection (Fig. 15-1B). Note that all except cysts are echo-free areas with no increased through transmission.

Case 4

D.B. is a 30-year-old woman who presented with a bloody right nipple discharge. The discharge was from a single duct in the center of the nipple. No masses were felt.

Liquid crystal thermograms demonstrated increased nipple heat and vascularity on the right (Th III thermogram). On diaphanography there was a marked decrease in light transmission in the medial superior portion of the right areola, with extension toward the nipple (Fig. 17-4A). There was marked glandularity (DY pattern) on mammography, without a lesion identified. Ultrasound demonstrated glandular tissue but no mass.

A ductogram showed a dilated duct with a large filling defect, 9 mm in width by more than 3 cm in length (Fig. 17-4B). At surgery a large intraductal papilloma with areas of fibrosis and collagenous hyalinization was found. Adjacent to the duct were areas of ductal ectasia with sclerosing adenosis and chronic inflammation.

Case 5

A.P. is a 65-year-old woman who presented with a profuse yellowish discharge from a single duct in the mid-portion of the left nipple. No masses were felt.

Liquid crystal thermograms demonstrated increased left nipple heat (Th III thermogram). Diaphanography was normal. There was marked glandularity (P2 pattern) on mammography with scattered benign calcifications; no mass was seen. Ultrasound demonstrated a slightly dilated duct on the left. Ductography demonstrated a slightly dilated duct with at least two filling defects measuring about 3 mm in size (Fig. 17-5). At surgery intraductal papillomas were found.

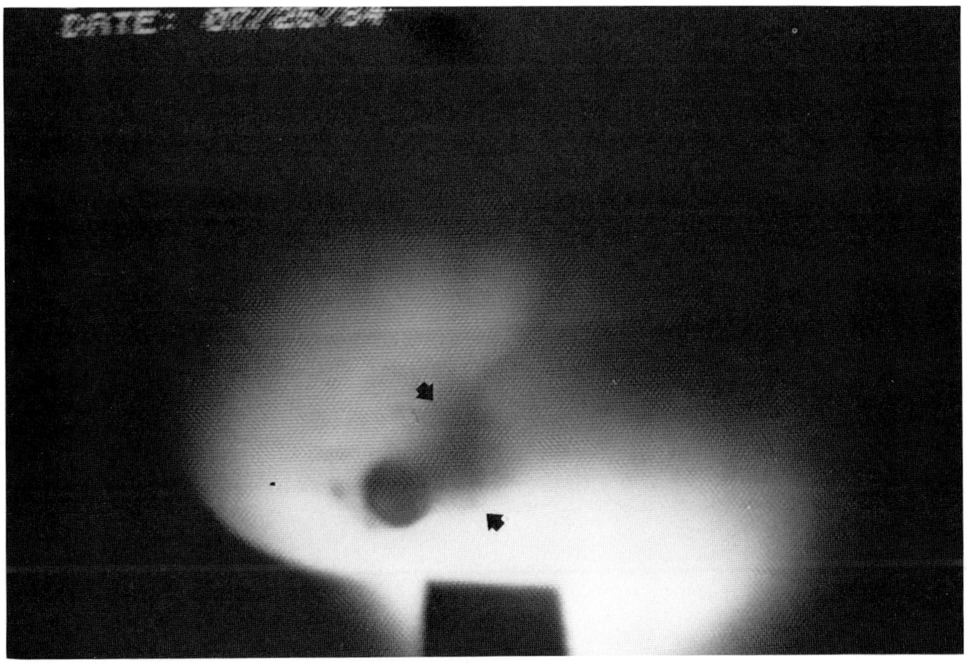

A

Fig. 17-4 A: Diaphanography. Note the marked decrease in light transmission (arrows). Compare with diaphanography of fibroadenomas (Figs. 12-2A and 12-5A) and infection Figs. 15-1A and 15-3A). These are less distinct, whereas this diaphanography is more similar to that seen with hemorrhage (Fig. 14-3A).

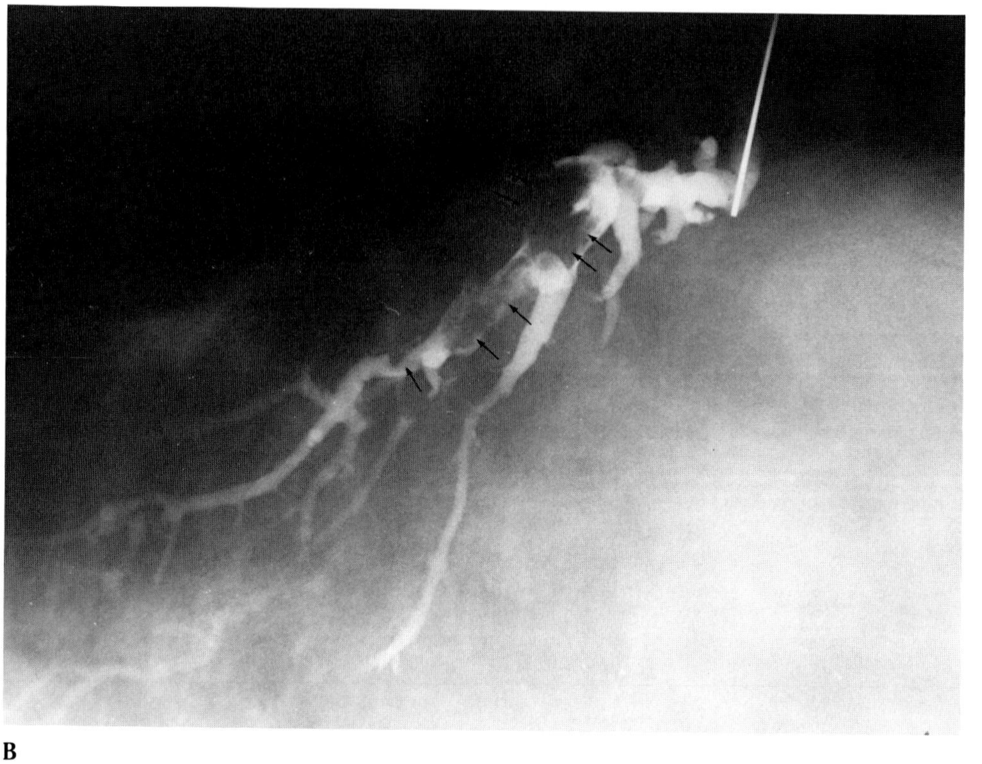

B

Fig. 17-4 B: Magnified ductogram. Arrows define the multiple filling defects, which are intraductal papillomas.

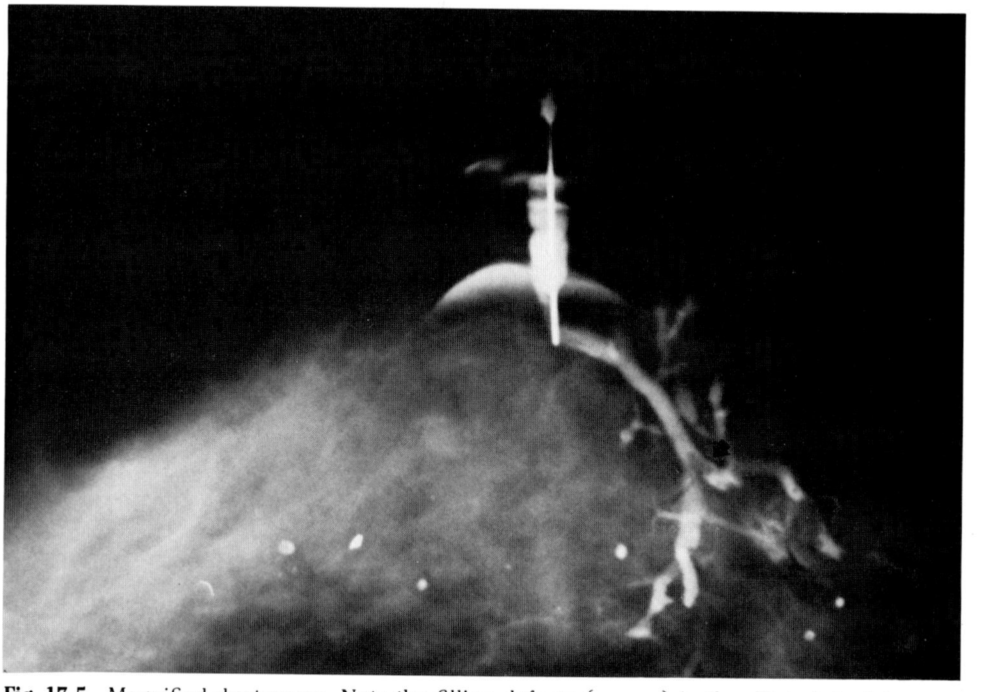

Fig. 17-5 Magnified ductogram. Note the filling defects (arrows) in the dilated ductal system.

Discussion

Case 1 demonstrates a nipple papilloma. At the previous two surgeries the incision had been a periareolar approach, and the duct had been cleared out from the level of the incision into the breast. The duct extending into the nipple area had not been removed. It was in this portion of the duct that the papilloma continued to grow. This case is an example of incomplete removal of the nipple papilloma, not a recurrence. Without the methylene blue dye localization outlining the duct, the surgeon would have been unable to identify the duct because of the scarring from the two previous surgeries.

The nipple discharge from a papilloma is more often serous or yellowish than it is bloody, although both types of discharge are demonstrated in the above cases (see Chapter 6).

Diaphanography often demonstrates the lesion or the duct, as in case 4. Ductography on many occasions demonstrates the defects. Unless the duct or portion of the duct can be filled, the papilloma may not be demonstrated.

Although most papillomas do not present as a palpable mass, they do on occasion. The size of papillomas can vary greatly, as can be seen in the above cases.

Case 3 is unusual in that it was a papilloma within a cyst. It can be speculated that this case represented cystic dilatation of a duct due to obstruction; however, there was a well defined cyst wall found at pathologic examination.

Case Studies: Papillomatosis

Case 6

K.D. is a 36-year-old woman who was referred because of a mass present at 10 o'clock in the left breast. On physical examination there was an ovoid 1 by 2 cm firm density in the inner aspect of the left breast. The patient related that it had been present and had not changed in 10 years.

Thermography and diaphanography were normal. Mammography revealed marked glandularity (DY pattern) with a semicircular, slightly irregular group of calcifications and the impression of a very faint density associated with the calcifications (Fig. 17-6). To be sure that these corresponded to the mass felt clinically, a needle was inserted into the mass, and on repeat mammography the calcifications were indeed seen to correspond to the mass. Ultrasound showed some shadowing in the area but no mass.

Mammograms from 10 years earlier were not available, but the report on them did not mention calcifications. Biopsy was recommended. Preoperative mammographic localization was done. At surgery apocrine adenosis, diffuse papillomatosis, and microcalcifications were found.

Case 7

R.P. is a 75-year-old woman self-referred for screening mammography. Twelve years previously she had had a papilloma removed from the right breast. The physical examination at this time was negative except for a right superior periareolar scar. Thermography and diaphanography were normal. Mammograms showed a 10 by 12 mm somewhat poorly defined density in the inner lower aspect of the right breast (Fig. 17-7). On the left there were two groups of calcification without masses, thought to be benign. Old mammograms were not available.

Preoperative mammographic localization was done. At surgery a firm mass was found that was thought clinically to represent carcinoma. Pathologic evaluation demonstrated sclerosing intraductal papillomatosis.

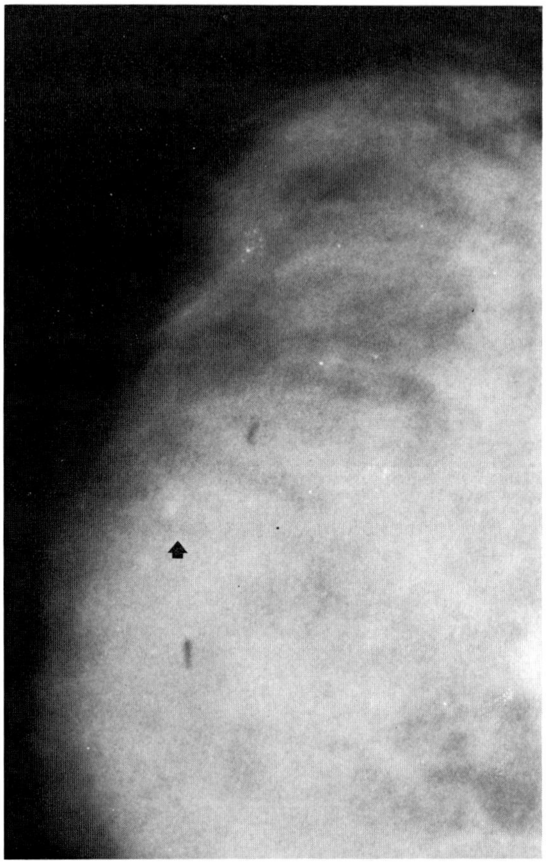

Fig. 17-6 Mammogram, magnified. Amorphous calcifications (arrow) are present without a mass.

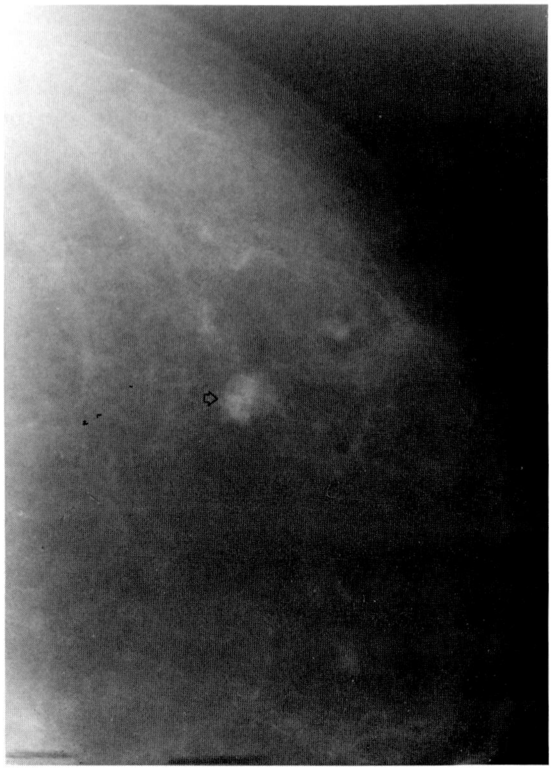

Fig. 17-7 Mammogram, magnified. Note the irregular mass without calcifications (open arrow) in this fatty breast.

Discussion

Papillomatosis is usually an incidental finding at surgery; however, these two cases were presented to demonstrate that this is not always the case. It is not known if in case 1 the calcifications were caused by apocrine adenosis, diffuse papillomatosis, or a combination of the two. It is interesting to note that the patient in case 2 had a previous papilloma removed from the same breast. It is possible that the benign calcifications on the left, not biopsied, could also represent papillomatosis. For additional cases involving papillomatosis the reader is referred to the case studies on fibrocystic disease in Chapter 13 and case 2 in Chapter 14.)

Case Study: Papillary Carcinoma

Case 8

H.H. is a 57-year-old woman whose sister had a mastectomy at age 40 for breast cancer. The patient was referred because of a reddish stain on her nightgown.

Physical examination showed mild glandularity of the breast, and there was a minimal bloody discharge from a single duct of the left nipple. Thermograms and diaphanography were normal. Mammography showed mild glandularity (P1 pattern), and no mass or malignant calcification was seen. A ductogram showed slight duct

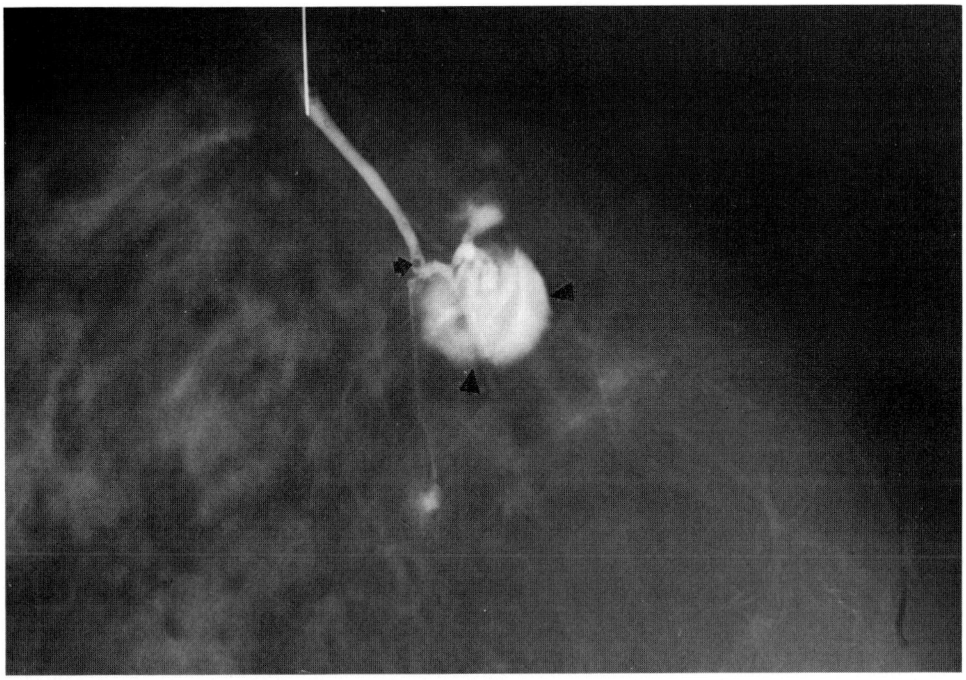

Fig. 17-8 Ductogram. The distal duct is slightly dilated. There are air bubbles adjacent to the needle filling a defect in the mid-duct (arrow) that is very similar to an air bubble. The extravasation (arrowheads) from the duct is highly suggestive of malignancy with disruption of the duct wall integrity.

dilatation, and a filling defect within the duct. There was extravasation of contrast material from the duct (Fig. 17-8). The probability of malignancy was raised.

A preoperative ductogram was done using methylene blue, as the nipple discharge was not spontaneous and the surgeon was not sure he could localize the duct. At surgery an intraductal papillary carcinoma with foci of infiltration was found. There were adjacent areas of intraductal papillomatosis and fibrocystic disease. The patient underwent an axillary node dissection and a course of radiation therapy.

Discussion

Although the vast majority of intraductal filling defects found at ductography are benign, the diagnosis cannot be made preoperatively with any assurance. Extravasation of dye, suggesting loss of normal continuity of the duct wall, raises the possibility of a malignancy. Preoperative localization with a methylene blue ductogram can be very helpful in cases where the discharge is not adequate to be seen at surgery. This procedure also allows for less tissue to be removed at surgery.

Bibliography

Papillomas

Barth V: *Atlas of Diseases of the Breast.* Stuttgart, Georg Thieme, 1979.

Carter D: *Interpretation of Breast Biopsies: Biopsy Interpretation Series.* New York, Raven Press, 1984.

DiMaggio C, Muzzio P, DiBello A, et al: Transillumination of the breast. *Radiol Med (Torino)* 1976; 62(6):401–413.
Dupont WD, Page DL: Risk factors for breast cancer in women with proliferative breast disease. *N Engl J Med* 1985; 312:146–151.
Egan RL, McSweeney MB: Breast sonography—interpretative criteria, in Jellins J, Kobayashi T (eds): *Ultrasonic Examination of the Breast.* London, Wiley, 1983, pp 307–318.
Haagensen CD, Bodian C, Haagensen D E: *Breast Carcinoma: Risk and Detection.* Philadelphia, Saunders 1981.
Kasumi F, Tanaka H: Diagnosis of intracystic tumors by ultrasound, in Jellins J, Kobayashi T (eds): *Ultrasonic Examination of the Breast.* London, Wiley, 1983, pp 283–291.
Sandison AT, Walker JC: Diseases of the adolescent female breast. *Br J Surg* 1968; 55(6):443–448.
Schwartz GF: Benign neoplasms and "inflammations" of the breast. *Clin Obstet Gynecol* 1982; 25(2):373–385.
Tabár L, Dean PB: *Teaching Atlas of Mammography.* New York, Thieme-Stratton, 1983.
Tabár L, Dean PB, Pentek Z: Galactography: The diagnostic procedure of choice for nipple discharge. *Radiology* 1983; 149:31–38.

Papillomatosis

Carter D: *Interpretation of Breast Biopsies: Biopsy Interpretation Series.* New York, Raven Press, 1984.
DiMaggio C, Muzzio P, DiBello A, et al: Transillumination of the breast. *Radiol Med (Torino)* 1976; 62(6):401–413.
Dupont WD, Page DL: Risk factors for breast cancer in women with proliferative breast disease. *N Engl J Med* 1985; 312:146–151.
Haagensen CD, Bodian C, Haagensen DE: *Breast Carcinoma; Risk and Detection.* Philadelphia, Saunders, 1981.
Morris DM, Gonzalez EG, Gelder FB, et al: Elevated hormone receptors in a patient with breast papillomatosis. *Breast* 1984; 10(1):16–17.
Tabár L, Dean PB: *Teaching Atlas of Mammography.* New York, Thieme-Stratton, 1983.
Tabár L, Dean PB, Pentek Z: Galactography: The diagnostic procedure of choice for nipple discharge. *Radiology* 1983; 149:31–38.

Papillary Carcinoma

Carter D: *Interpretation of Breast Biopsies: Biopsy Interpretation Series.* New York, Raven Press, 1984.
Haagensen CD, Bodian C, Haagensen DE: *Breast Carcinoma: Risk and Detection.* Philadelphia, Saunders, 1981.
Tabár L, Dean PB, Pentek Z: Galactography: The diagnostic procedures of choice for nipple discharge. *Radiology* 1983; 149:31–38.

18

Plastic Surgery and Complications

Saar Porrath

Case Studies: Augmented Breast

Case 1

G.W is a 40-year-old woman who was referred because of skin redness of the right breast. She had had saline implants inserted 2 years earlier. Apparently she had had a viral infection such as the flu during the previous week. When seen there was hardening of the right implant, diffuse redness of the skin overlying the implant on the right, and some slight retraction of the skin in the inner right breast.

Liquid crystal thermograms demonstrated a marked increase in heat over the entire right breast area of almost 3°C greater than the left (Th V thermogram) (Color Fig. 6). Diaphanography was normal, with increased light transmission through the implants (Fig. 18-1A). On mammography and ultrasound the saline bag implants were seen as well as a moderate amount of glandular tissue. No fluid collection or other abnormality was noted (Fig. 18-1B).

The patient, given warm packs and antibiotics, was well within 2 weeks. In the occasional patient with implants who has an infection, there may be a reaction around one or both of the implants that appears like a rejection phenomenon. In the rare patient this reaction leads to real rejection, necessitating removal of the implant.

Case 2

S.Z. is a 45-year-old woman referred for an evaluation. She had had silicone gel implants inserted in 1980. There were multiple closed capsulotomies during the next 3 years because of hardening of the implants. On the final attempt at closed capsulotomy there was a rupture of both implants. A mammogram was reported in February 1983 as no change to the implants. At surgery that same month a bilateral rupture of the silicone implants was encountered, with subsequent removal of the implants. The patient did not want new implants. She was seen by us in July 1983. Physical examination revealed scars from implantations and subsequent removal. No masses were present.

Liquid crystal thermograms demonstrated increased periareolar heat and vascularity on the left (Th III thermogram). Diaphanography was normal. On mammography there was moderate glandularity (P2 pattern). There was a 1 by 6 cm fragment of silicone in the upper portion of the right breast (Fig. 18-2A), and two smaller fragments of silicone on the left. Silicone outlined the ductal system on the left, adjacent to the nipple (Fig. 18-2B,C). The larger pieces of silicone were evident on ultrasound (Fig. 18-2D).

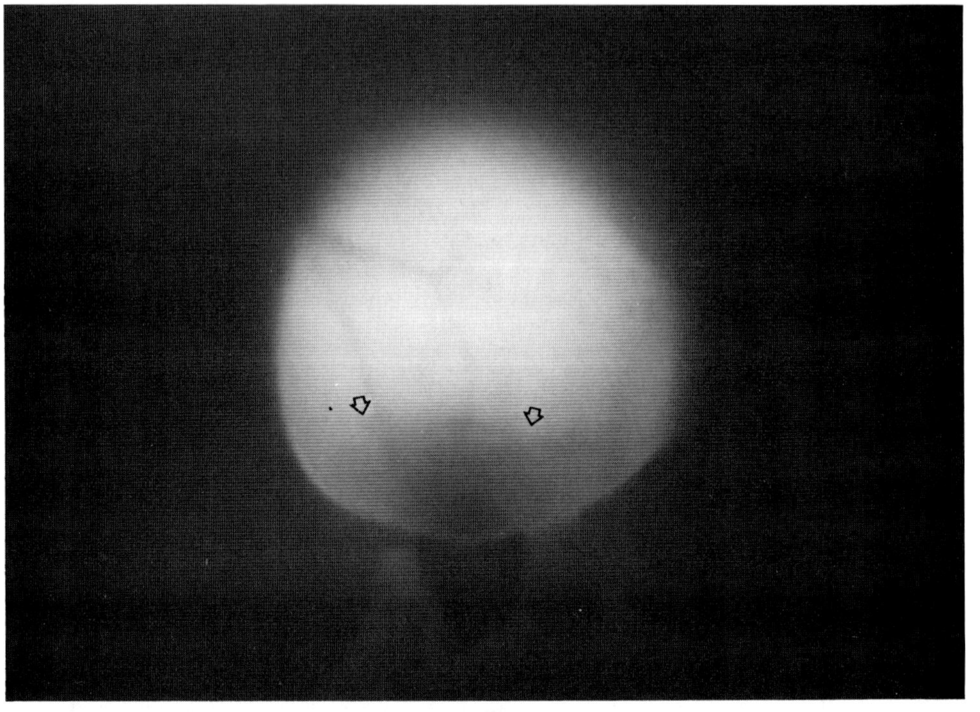

A

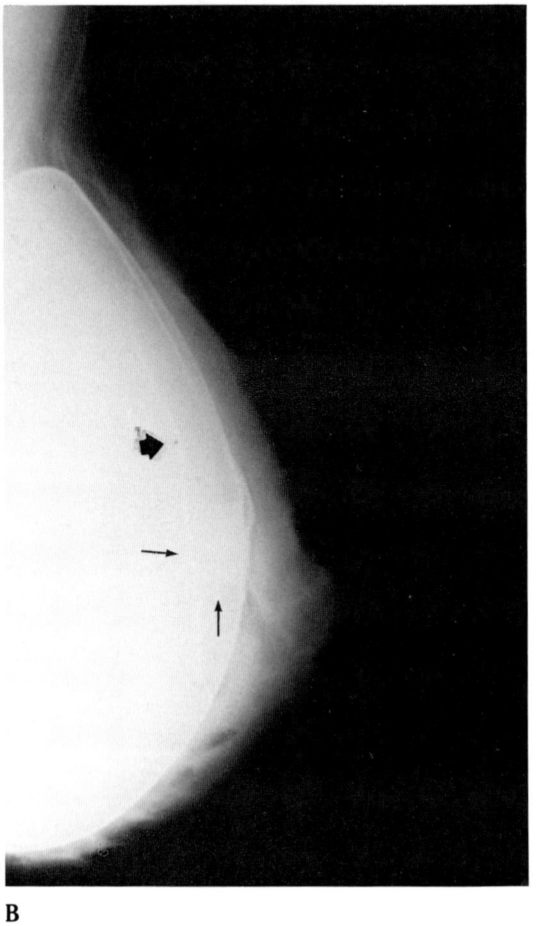

B

Fig. 18-1 **A:** Diaphanography. There is increased light transmission in the upper portion of the breast through the implant and decreased light transmission through the glandular tissue anterior to and behind the nipple (open arrows). **B:** Mammogram, lateral view: saline bag implant. Note the valve (thin arrows) and slight wrinkles (thick arrow) in the saline implant caused by minimal contraction of the capsule.

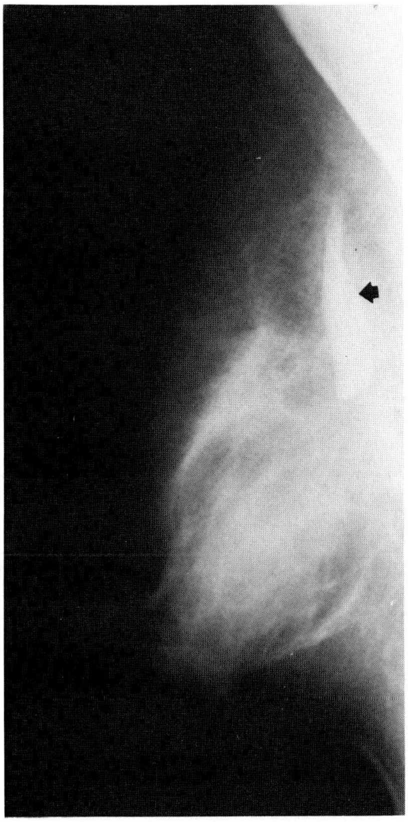

A

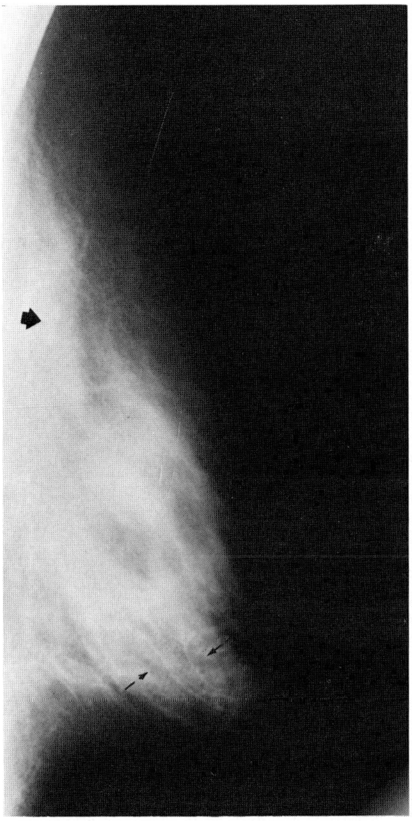

B

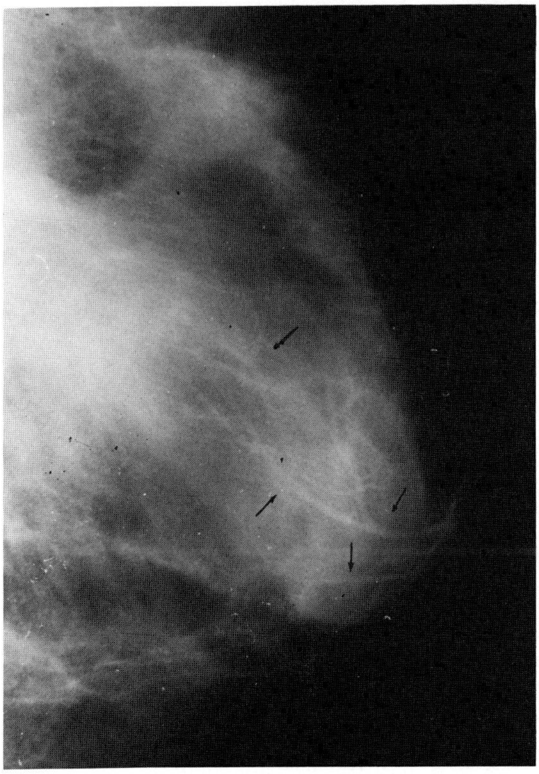

C

Fig. 18-2 A: Mamogram, right lateral view. There is a large piece of silicone from a silicone gel implant remaining in the breast (arrow). **B:** Mammogram, left lateral view. Small pieces (thick arrow) of silicone remain in the breast. Silicone is seen in the ducts (thin arrows) (see **C**). **C:** Higher magnification of **B.** Note silicon in the ducts, outlining the ducts similar to a ductogram (thin arrows). **D:** Ultrasound, longitudinal reverse image of the right breast. The echo-free areas just anterior to the pectoralis muscle corresponds to a large particle of silicone (arrow) seen on the mammogram (**A**).

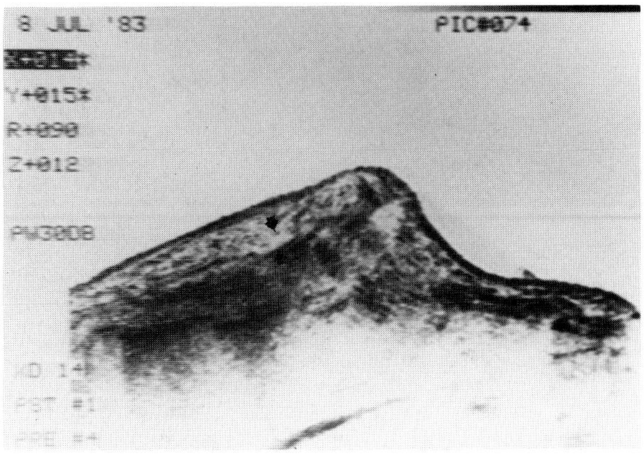

D

Silicone particles left behind in the breast following rupture of a silicone gel implant are occasionally seen. The occurrence of a silicone ductogram is extremely rare. The presence of the silicone within the duct is probably not responsible for the positive thermogram.

Case 3

V.W. is a 59-year-old woman who was referred because of breast pain. She had had previous implants that ruptured. Following removal of the ruptured implant the breast became infected. When the breast healed, silicone gel implants were inserted. On physical examination there was moderate deformity of the breasts with multiple scars. There were also marked hardening of the left implant and redness in the inner aspect of the left breast.

Liquid crystal thermograms were positive on the left owing to an edge sign, probably secondary to incomplete contact with the thermographic plate because of slight deformity on the left. There was a marked decrease in light transmission through the inner aspect of the left breast in the area of the hardness (Fig. 18-3A). Mammograms demonstrated bilateral silicone gel implants behind the muscles, as well as some calcifications surrounding the bag on the left. Silicone was noted within the tissues in the inner aspects of both breasts, with a marked tissue reaction in the inner aspect of the left breast (Figs. 18-3B,C,D). The silicone was also demonstrated on ultrasound (Fig. 18-3E).

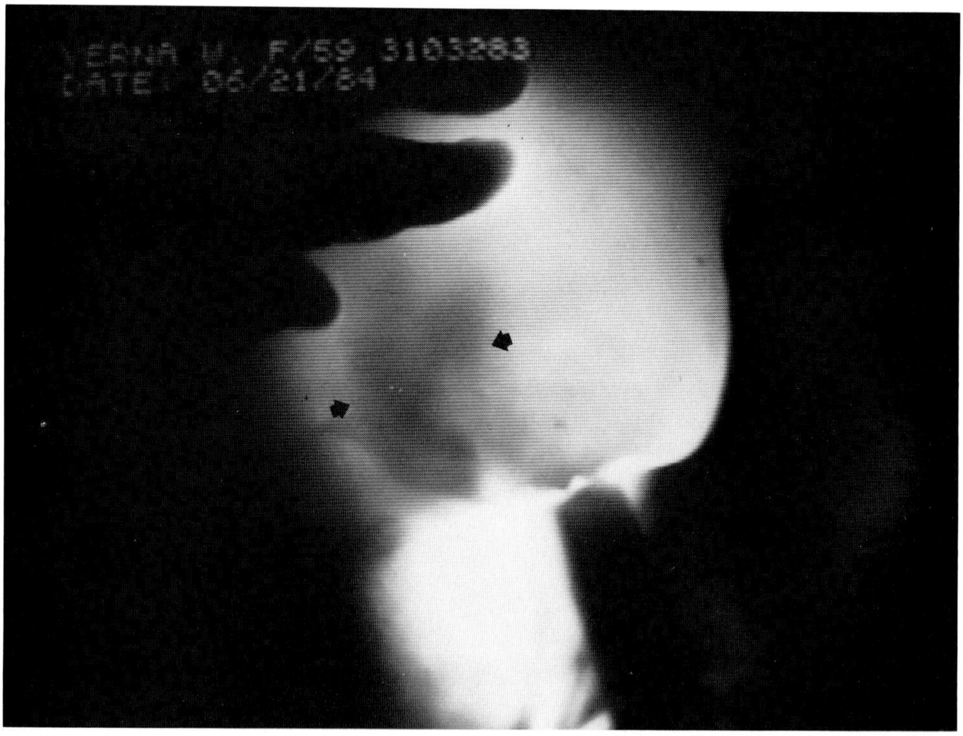

A

Fig. 18-3 A: Diaphanography. There is a marked decrease in light transmission over the inner lower aspect of the left breast (arrows).

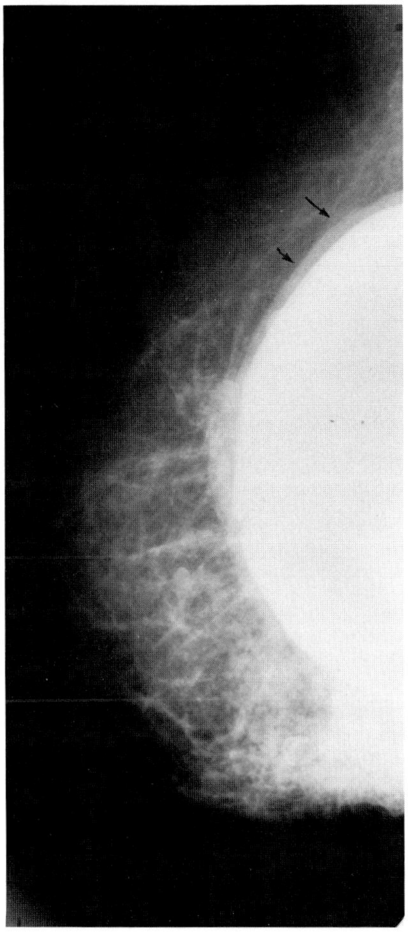

B

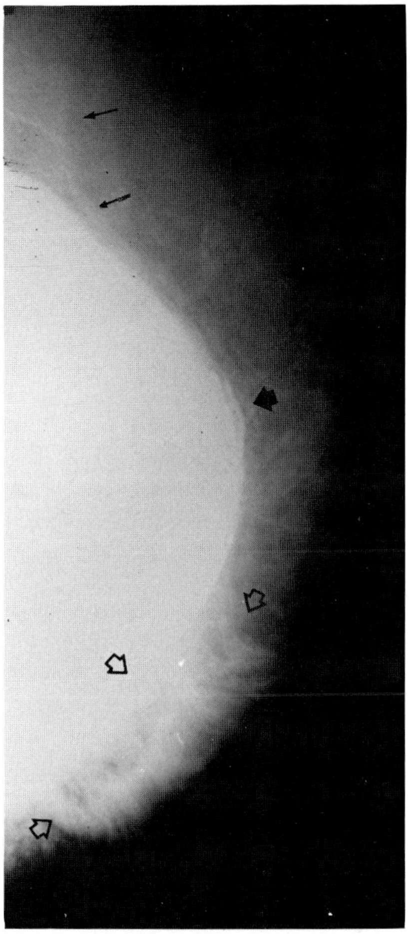

C

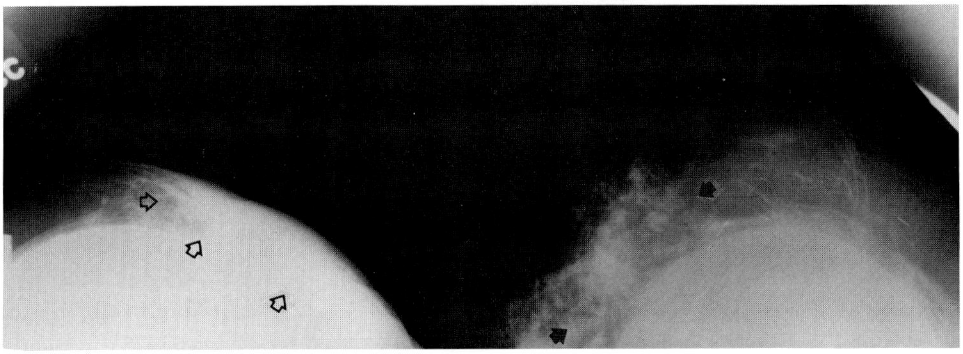

D

Fig. 18-3 **B:** Mammogram, right lateral view. The silicone gel implant behind the pectoralis muscle (thin arrows) outlines the tissue density overlying the implant. Note silicone particles in the inferior aspect of the breast. **C:** Mammogram, left lateral view. There is a silicone gel implant behind the pectoralis muscle (thin arrows). Note the small amount of calcification adjacent to the pectoralis muscle from a previous capsular contraction (arrow). There is a marked skin and tissue reaction and silicone in the inferior breast (open arrow). **D:** Mammogram, CC view of both breasts. Note the silicone and tissue reaction with obliteration of the skin line on the inner left breast (open arrows) and diffuse silicone particles on the inner right breast (arrows).

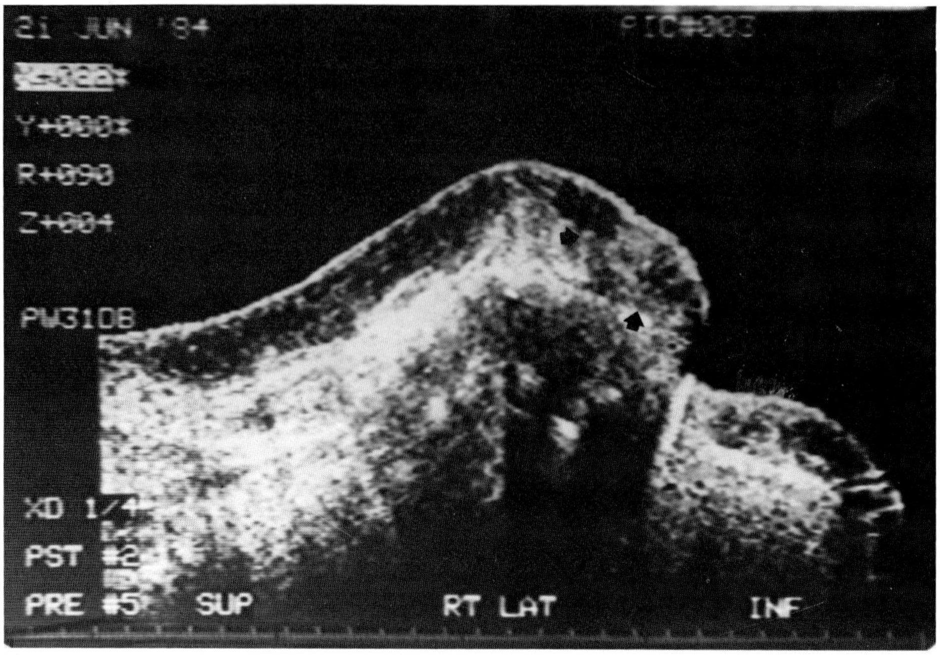

E

Fig. 18-3 E: Ultrasound, lateral view, right breast. There are slight skin retraction and increased echoes in the subcutaneous tissues from the free silicone (arrows).

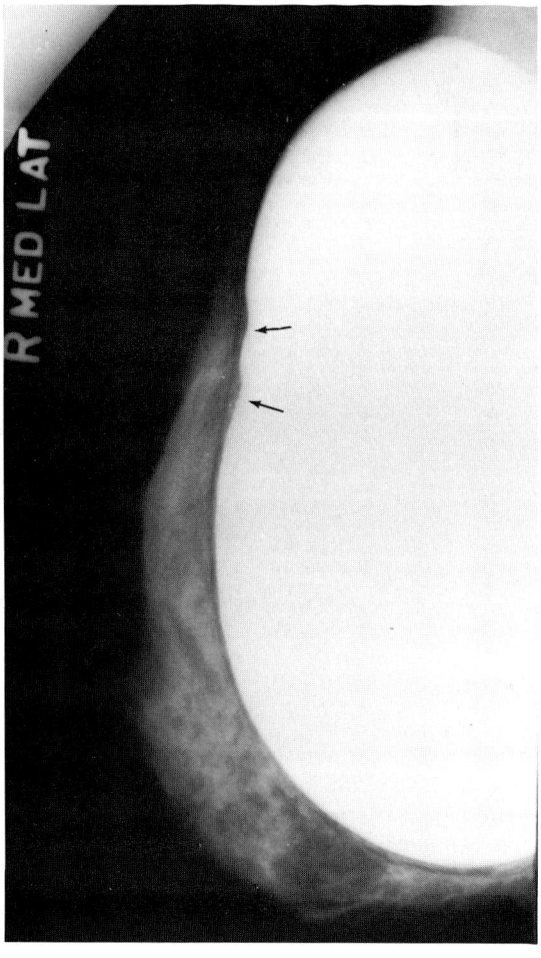

Fig. 18-4 Mammogram, lateral view. The slight irregularities of the silicone gel bag implant are due to capsular contractions (arrows).

Case 4

T.D. is a 44-year-old woman who was referred because of a change in the configuration of her breast implants. On physical examination the right implant was much firmer than the left, and the left implant was lower and more lateral in position.

Thermograms were normal. Diaphanography demonstrated increased light transmission through the implants. On mammograms there were slight irregularities of the outline of the silicone gel implants (Fig. 18-4). Ultrasound showed that the implant on the left was lower and more lateral than the right.

The changes on the mammogram were thought to be due to a capsular contraction with indentation of the implant. The patient subsequently underwent a closed capsulotomy with a decreased firmness of the right implant. The slight positional change of the left implant was due to minimal slippage of the implant within the pouch formed at surgery.

Case 5

L.H. is a 24-year-old woman referred because of a change in her breast implant. On physical examination there was a slight flattening of the inner aspect of the left breast.

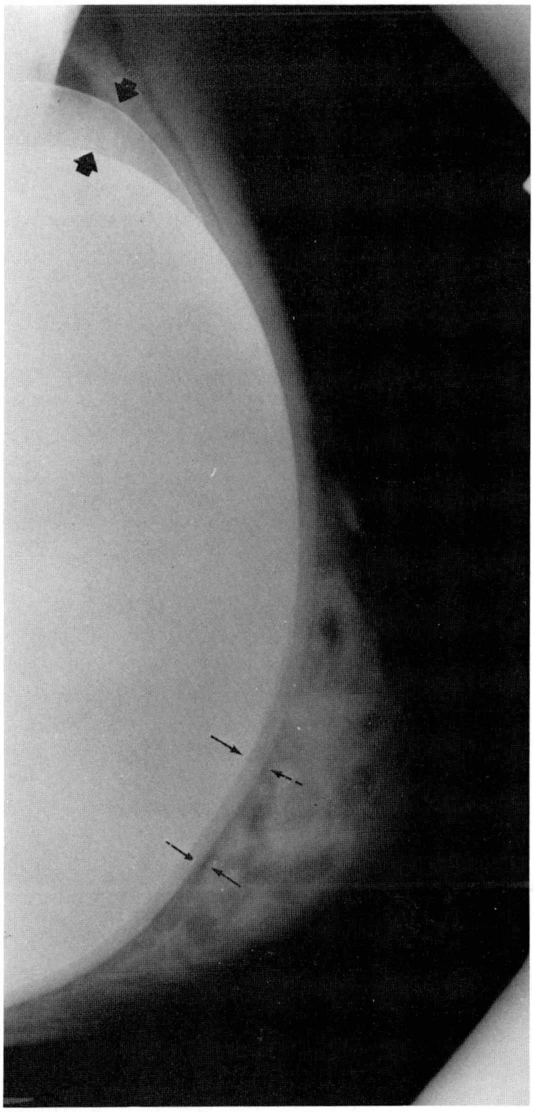

A

Fig. 18-5 A: Mammogram, lateral view: subpectoralis, double-bag implant. The inner portion is silicone, and the outer saline bag is seen predominantly in the superior area (thick arrows). The overlying pectoralis muscle is well defined (thin arrows).

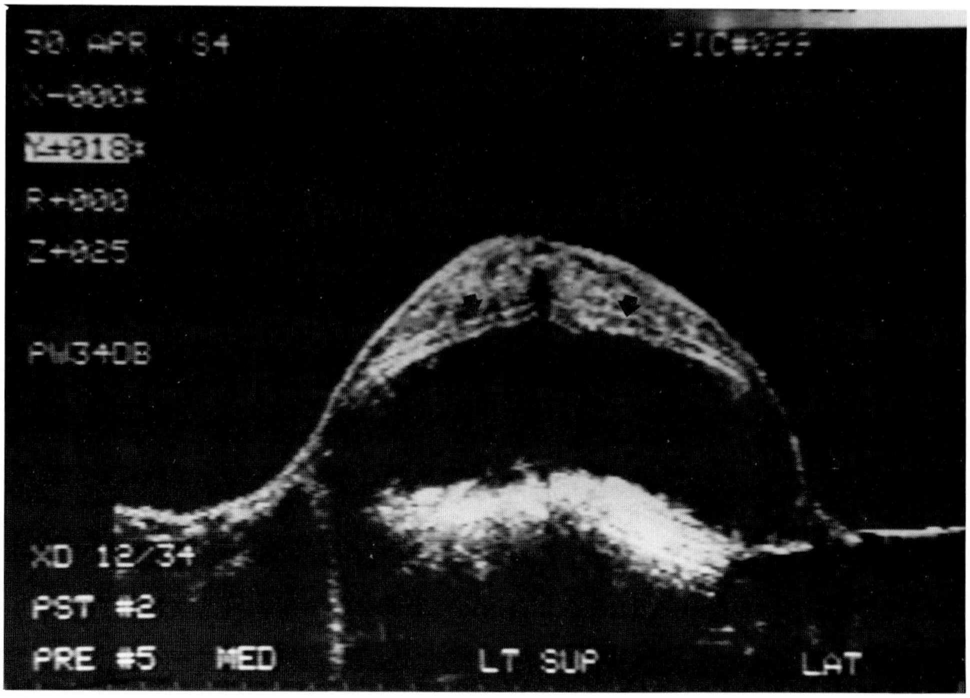

B

Fig. 18-5 B: Ultrasound, transverse view. The echo-free implant is well defined. Overlying the implant is a thin structure, the pectoralis muscle (arrows). The glandular tissue is in the anterior portion of the breast. Note that the implant appears more posterior than the adjacent chest wall owing to the increased speed of sound in fluid.

Thermograms and diaphanography were normal. Mammograms demonstrated the double-bag implants behind the pectoralis muscle (Fig. 18-5A). There was a slight difference in the distribution of the saline in the outer portion of the bag, with more saline inferiorly on the right and superiorly on the left. This finding was not thought to be significant. On ultrasound there was noted to be a slight decrease in the volume of the left implant compared to the right (Fig. 18-5B).

No cause could be identified for the slight changes present on the physical examination, and it was thought that the changes were probably secondary to a somewhat tighter pectoralis muscle overlying the left implant than on the right.

Case 6

S.S. is a 60-year-old woman who in 1969 after multiple biopsies for fibrocystic disease underwent bilateral subcutaneous mastectomies and the insertion of silicone gel implants. During the next few years she underwent numerous closed capsulotomies. In addition, she had staged reconstruction surgeries following some extrusion of gel from the capsules. In 1981 she was noted to have a lump in her right breast. It measured 2 by 3 cm on mammograms and was shown to represent a knuckle of the silicone gel implant. When she was seen in June 1983 there was a soft 5-cm nodule in the upper

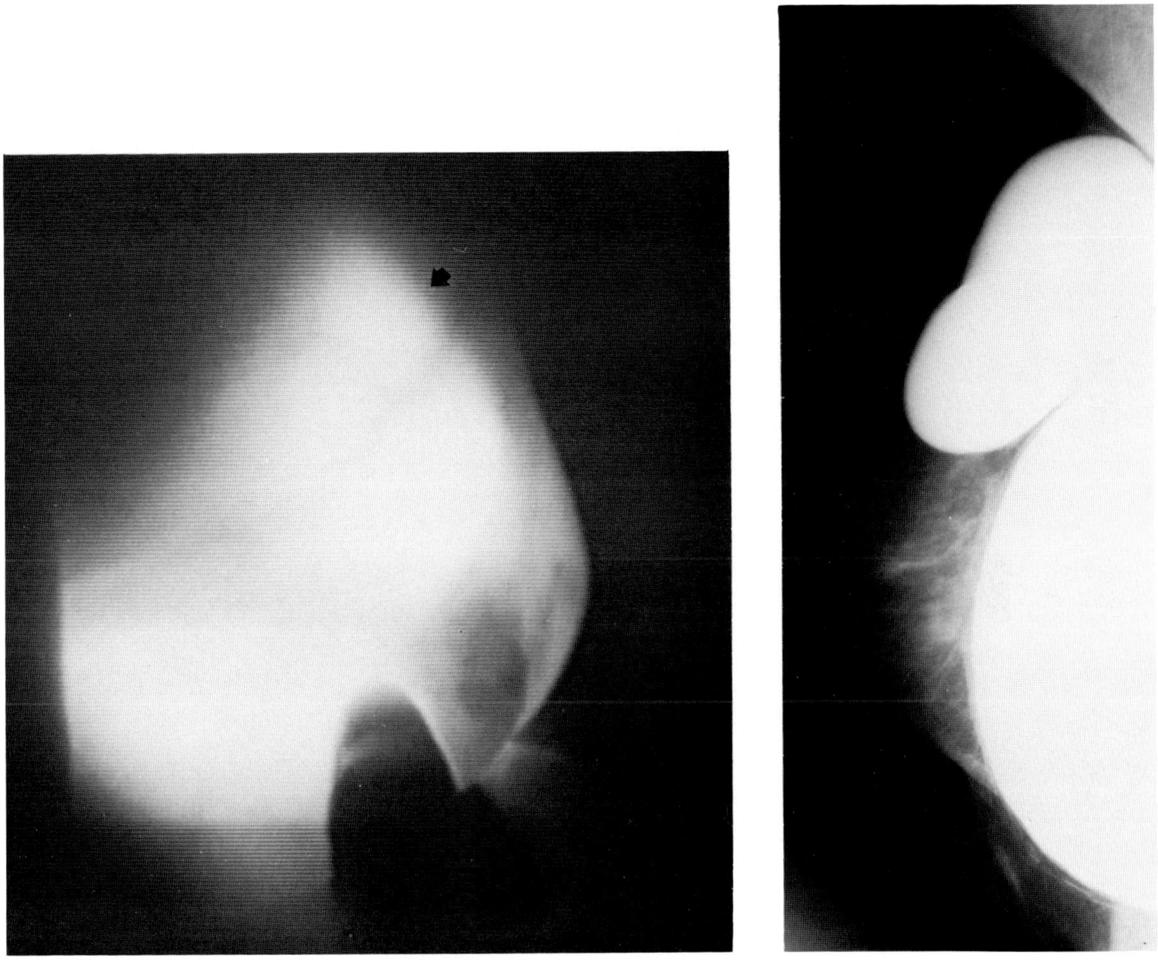

A B

Fig. 18-6 A: Diaphanography. There is increased light through the implant and the nodule. **B:** Mammogram, right lateral view. There is a large bulge of the silicone gel implant.

outer aspect of the right breast which could almost, but not entirely, be separated from the implant itself.

Thermograms were normal. On diaphanography there was increased light transmission through the implants and through the nodule itself (Fig. 18-6A). Mammography demonstrated a large silicone deposit in a globular configuration outside the major portion of the implant (Fig. 18-6B). Ultrasound showed the presence of the silicone globule adjacent to the implant.

Case 7

F.G. is a 52-year-old woman who fell on her left breast about a week prior to being seen. Eleven years earlier she had had saline bag implants inserted bilaterally. On physical examination the left breast was noted to be slightly smaller than the right, with the right implant much firmer than that on the left.

Thermograms and diaphanography were normal. On mammography a partially collapsed left implant was noted that was about 25 percent smaller than that on the right. It was also seen on ultrasound (Fig. 18-7).

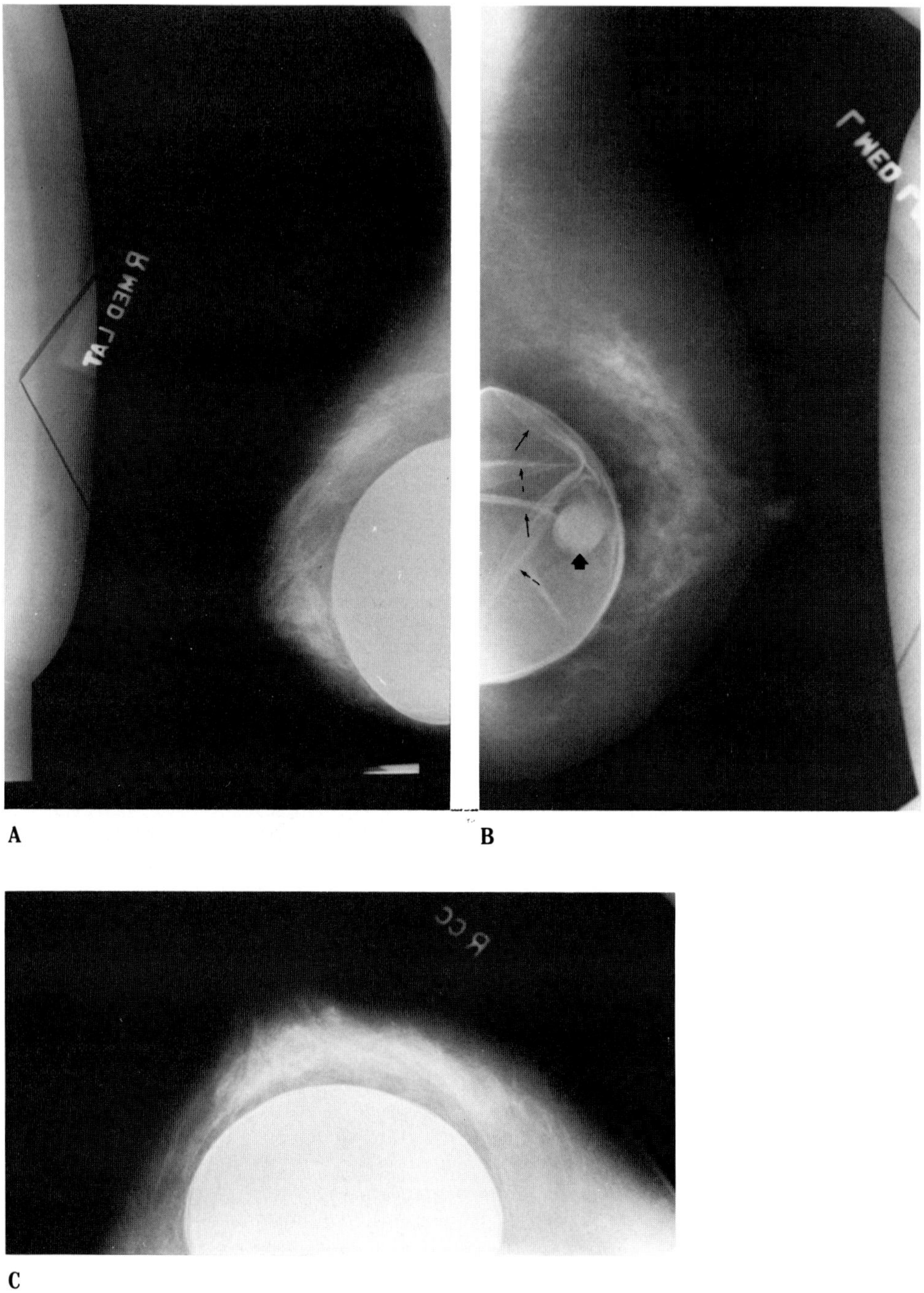

Fig. 18-7 **A:** Mammogram, right lateral view. This is the normal side with a saline bag implant. **B:** Mammogram, left lateral view: partially collapsed implant. Note the lines across the implant (thin arrows) indicating folds from loss of volume (thick arrow points to valve). **C:** Mammogram, right CC view. Normal saline implant.

Fig. 18-7 **D:** Mammogram, left CC view. Partially collapsed saline implant. **E:** Ultrasound, right transverse view. Normal saline implant (open arrows). Compare with Fig. 18-5B. This implant is smaller in comparison to the breast size. Note that the implant is not subpectoral, so no rim of tissue is present anterior to the implant. Internal echoes, especially anteriorly in the implant, are the more normal findings. **F:** Ultrasound, left transverse view. Note the small size of the implant (arrows) compared to a similar view of the right breast (**E**).

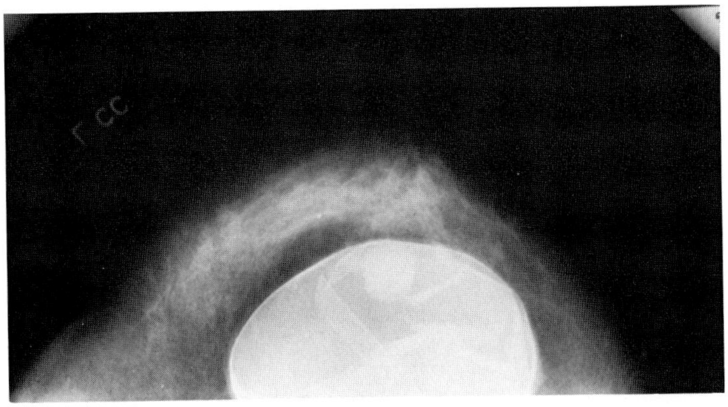

D

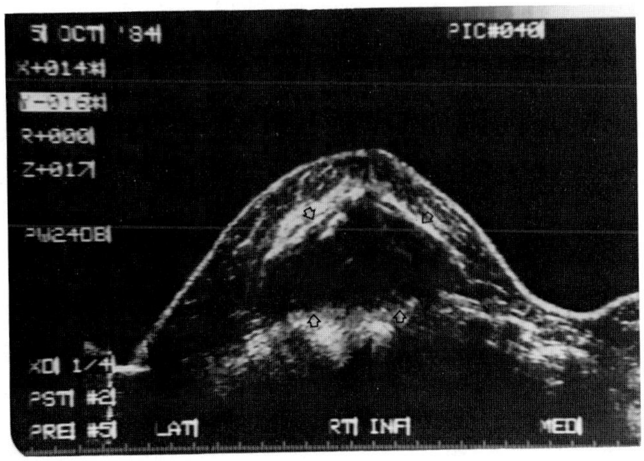

E

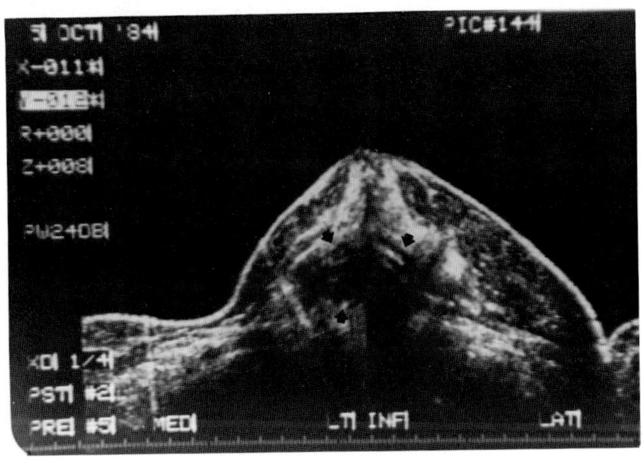

F

Case 8

V.M. is a 30-year-old woman who was referred because of a breast infection. On physical examination there were bilateral implants, lateral in position. Two weeks prior to being seen the patient had had a needle biopsy of the outer right breast, with an infection diagnosed. After a course of antibiotics physical examination showed that there was no residual.

Thermography and diaphanography were essentially normal. Mammography demonstrated bilateral silicone gel implants, with a superior and lateral position bilaterally, especially on the right. There was almost no glandular tissue between the implant on the right and the skin over the lateral aspect of the breast. These findings were also seen on ultrasound (Fig. 18-8).

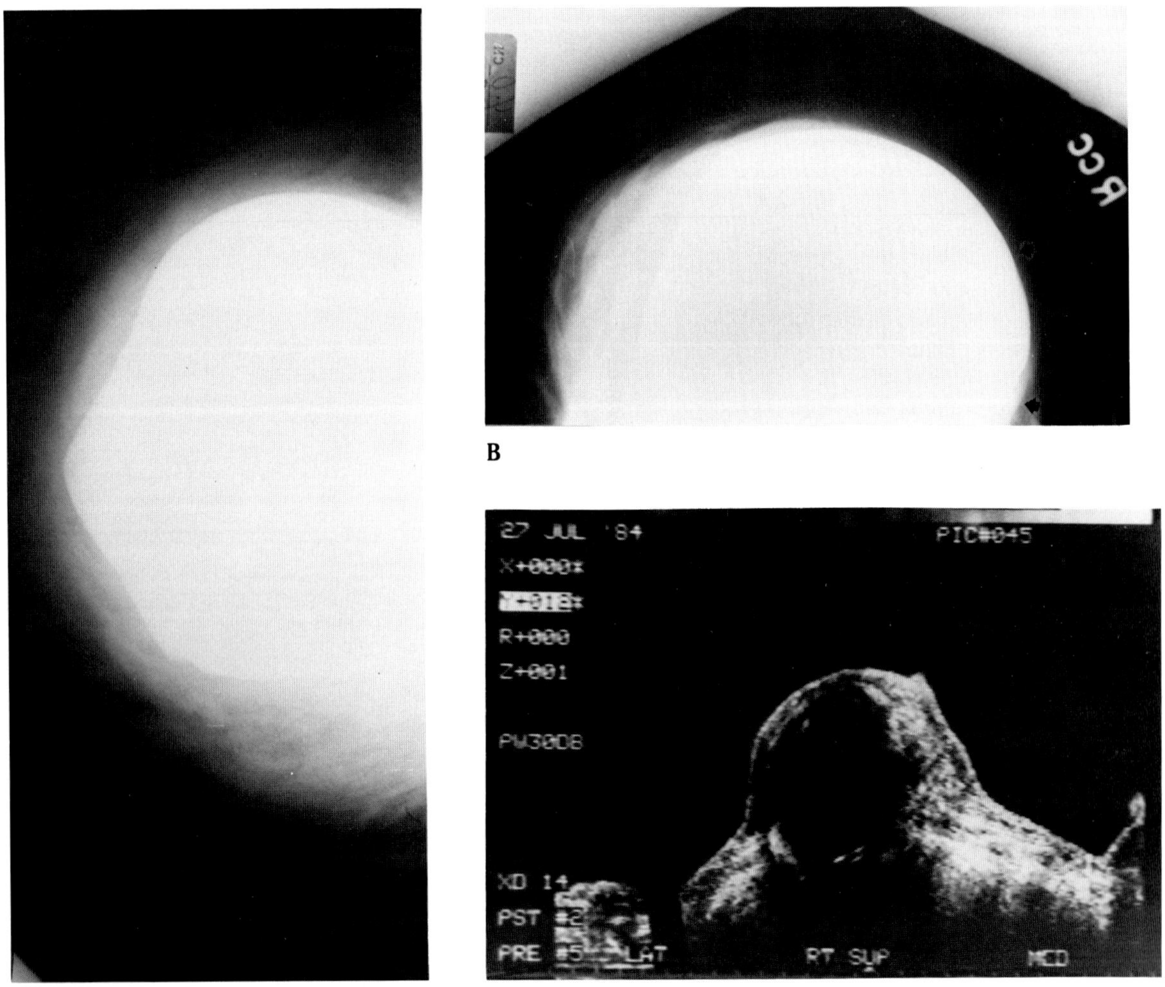

A B C

Fig. 18-8 A: Mammogram, right lateral view. The markedly irregular outline of the silicone gel implant is due to capsular contraction. Compare with the more normal outline seen in Figs. 18-5A and 18-7A, and the minor irregularities in Fig. 18-4. **B:** Mammogram, right CC view, photographed with light contrast to highlight the lack of tissue between the silicone gel implant and the skin laterally (arrows). **C:** Ultrasound. The implant (echo-free area) is eccentrically placed with a relative lack of tissue laterally. Compare with mammogram in **B.**

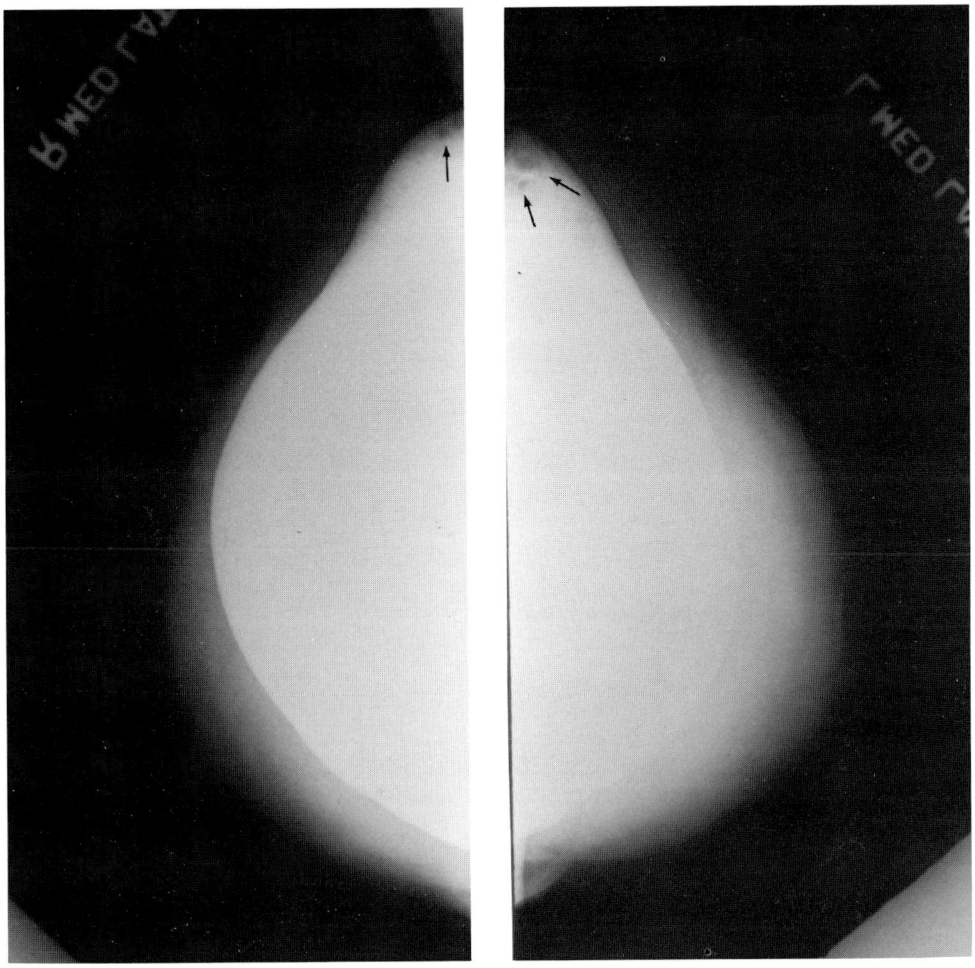

A B

Fig. 18-9 Mammograms, right (**A**) and left (**B**) lateral views. Note the small lucent "bubbles" of unknown etiology in the superior aspect of the implant (thin arrows).

Case 9

A.B. is a 35-year-old woman who was referred for screening. She had had implants inserted many years before. The physical examination was normal.

Thermograms were normal. There was an increase in light transmission through the implants. Mammograms demonstrated bilateral silicone gel implants with small lucencies in the superior portion suggestive of air bubbles (Fig. 18-9). Ultrasound showed the implants but not the air.

Case 10

C.B. is a 41-year-old woman who was referred for evaluation of a breast infection. Three years earlier she had had her initial implants inserted. Two months prior to being seen this time she had had the original implants removed, a breast uplift done, and new implants reinserted. She developed a bilateral infection that was treated with antibiotics for 6 weeks. On physical examination no wound discharge was noted. There was some granulation and crusting in the lower scar on the right.

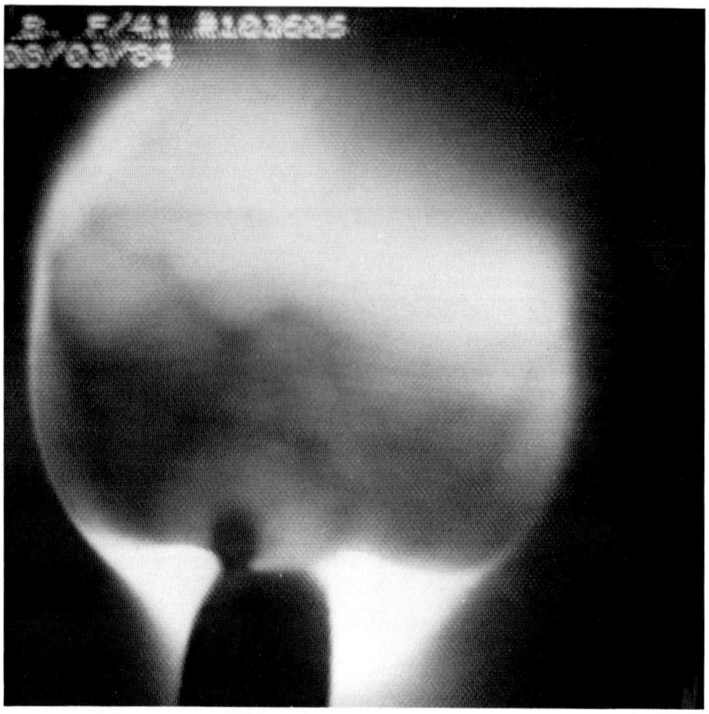

A

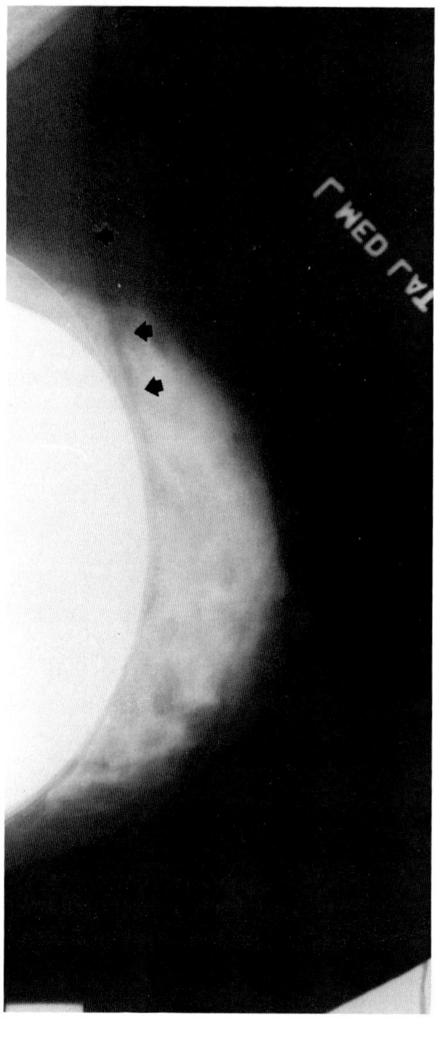

B

Fig. 18-10 **A:** Diaphanography. Note the increased light through the implant with decreased light through glandular tissue anterior and behind the nipple. **B:** Mammogram, left lateral view. Note the double-bag implant behind the pectoralis muscle (arrows).

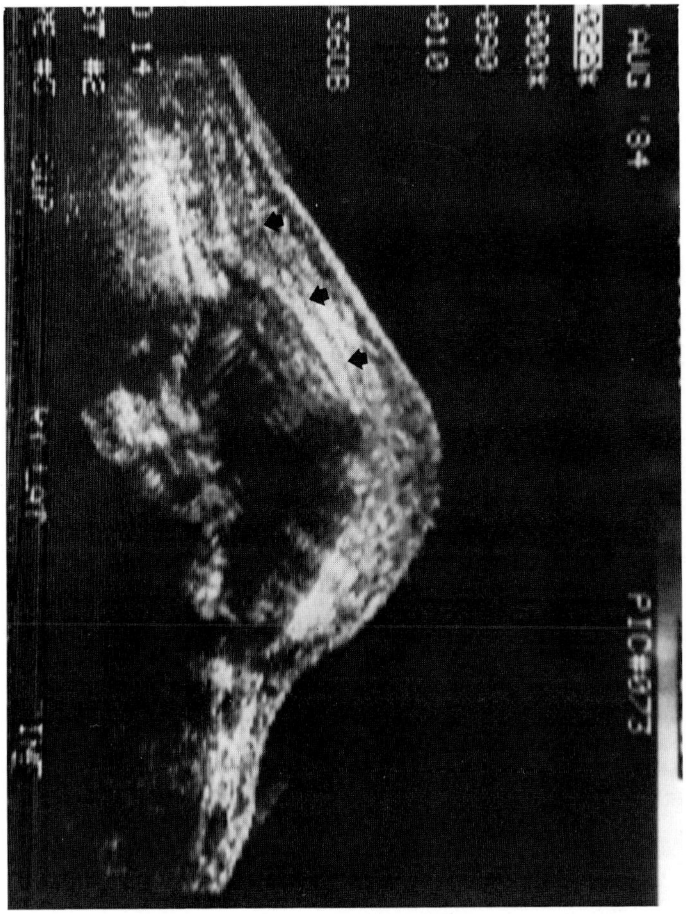

C

Fig. 18-10 **C:** Ultrasound, right longitudinal view. The echoes seen within the implant are a normal finding. Note the pectoralis muscle (arrows) elevated over the implant. The ultrasound has been aligned for viewing so comparison can be made with the mammogram in **B.**

Thermograms were normal. There was decreased light transmission in the anterior inferior portions of both breasts in the area of the scars (Fig. 18-10A). Mammograms demonstrated double-bag implants behind the pectoralis muscle. No masses were seen (Fig. 18-10B). On ultrasound no fluid collections or abscesses could be demonstrated (Fig 18-10C). No site of active infection could be found, especially in view of the negative thermogram. Antibiotic therapy was stopped. The patient has done well since that time, with no recurrence of infection.

Case 11

D.D. is a 58-year-old woman who 20 years earlier had had silicone injections in both breasts for augmentation purposes. On physical examination there were firm silicone masses occupying the upper portions of the breasts and retraction of the lower halves of the breasts.

Thermograms were normal. Diaphanography showed a marked decrease in light transmission in the upper aspects of the breasts, with moderately good light transmission through the lower and medial aspects. On mammography the silicone particles were seen conglomerated in the posterior and superior aspect of the breasts, with silicone scattered in the tissues of the rest of the breast (Figs. 18-11A,B). Ultrasound showed much silicone throughout the breast, primarily posteriorly, and slight duct dilatation anteriorly (Figs. 18-11C,D).

Silicone injections into the breast cause a tissue response with trapping of the silicone particles. Whereas silicone in a gel implant allows increased light transmission, when it is in the tissues there is a marked decrease in light transmission, probably owing to the tissue reaction from the free particles. Mammography cannot penetrate

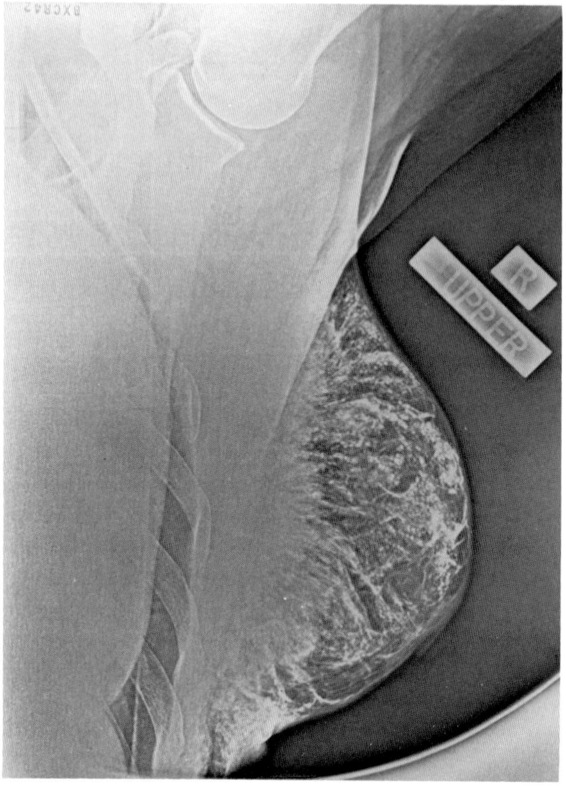

A

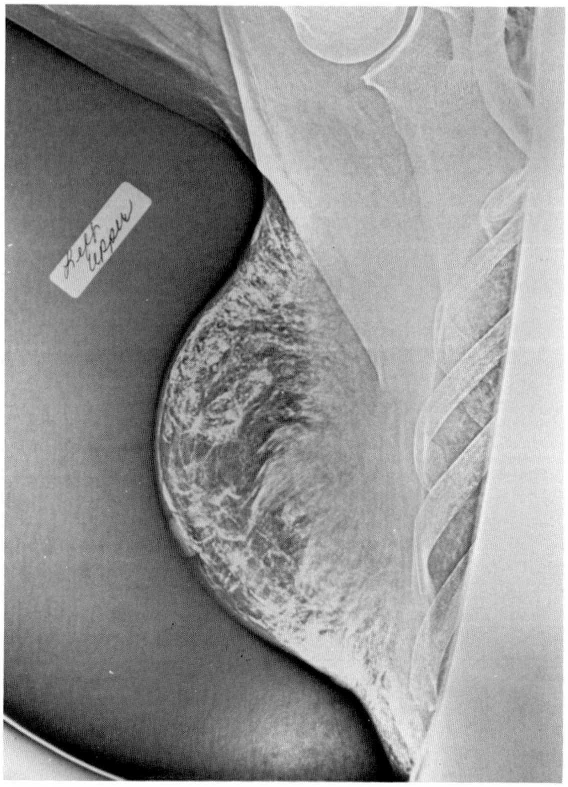

B

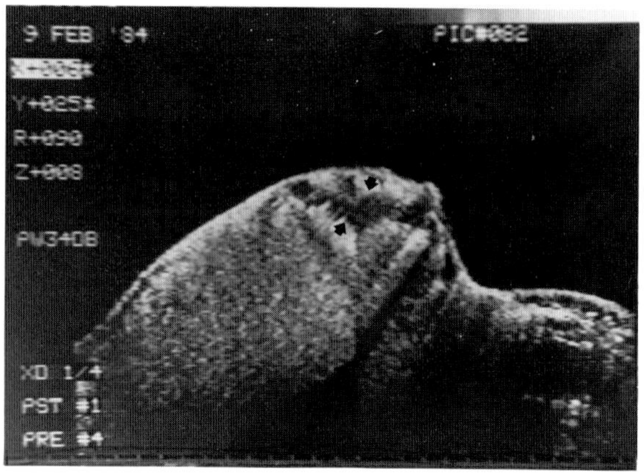

C

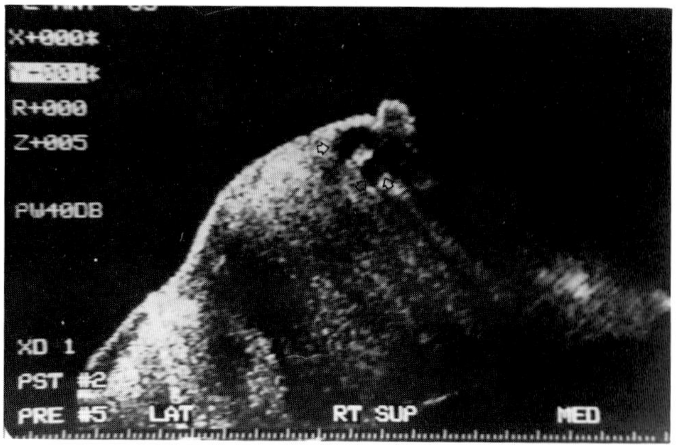

D

Fig. 18-11 Xeromammograms right (**A**) and left (**B**) lateral views. Note the diffuse silicone particles throughout both breasts, most marked posteriorly. **C:** Ultrasound, longitudinal view. The marked echo pattern is consistent with silicone injections. The lucency across the anterior breast (arrows) may represent the separation of the silicone particles into the looser distribution anteriorly and the more compact distribution posteriorly. (This effect has been seen with most ultrasound examinations of silicone-injected breasts.)
D: Ultrasound. Marked duct dilatation is noted in a silicone-injected breast (arrows). Siliconomas can have the same appearance on ultrasound and diaphanography.

the silicone in either form. Ultrasound shows good sound transmission through the silicone gel implants but an inadequacy to penetrate the area when the free particles are encased in the tissue. The retraction in the lower portion of the breast in this case is due in part to a tissue reaction.

Case 12

S.R. is a 35-year-old woman who 17 years earlier had had silicone injected into the breasts for augmentation. The silicone was stable for about 15 years. During the past 2 years there has been an increase in the nodularity extending into the anterior axillary folds and lower axilla. There was nodularity noted in both axillary folds, some of the nodules being more than 1 cm in size.

Thermograms were normal. Diaphanography was unable to penetrate the areas of silicone masses in the breast and was essentially normal in the axillary folds. The large amount silicone present could not be penetrated on mammography. Small silicone particles were noted in both axillary folds (Fig. 18-12).

Migration of the silicone particles is a phenomenon that has been documented over many years in many cases. Silicone particles have been found in the anterior abdominal wall, arms, back, and elsewhere. Why, after 15 years, the migration occurred in this case is not sure. The amount of silicone made it impossible to adequately evaluate the breast with mammography.

Case 13

G.A. is a 38-year-old woman who at age 18 was noted to have a right breast smaller than the left. She had silicone injections into the right breast. About 10 years ago, at age 28, she had a silicone gel implant inserted into the left breast. Over the past few

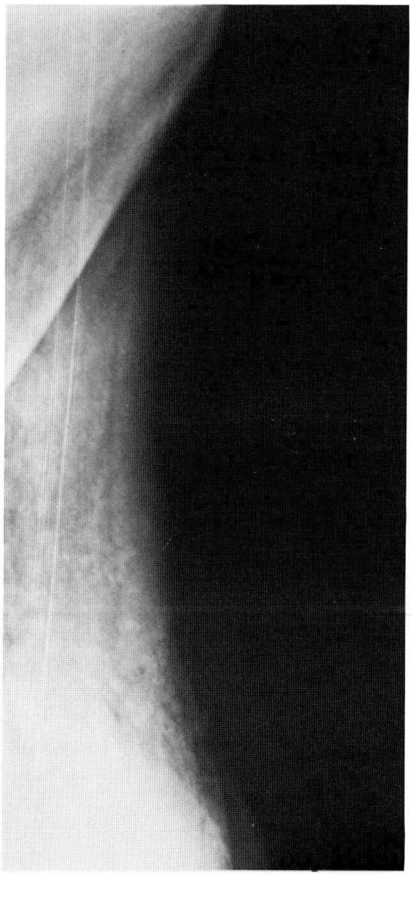

Fig. 18-12 Mammogram, magnified, tail of the breast. Note the whitish silicone particles tracing up along the pectoralis muscle toward the axilla.

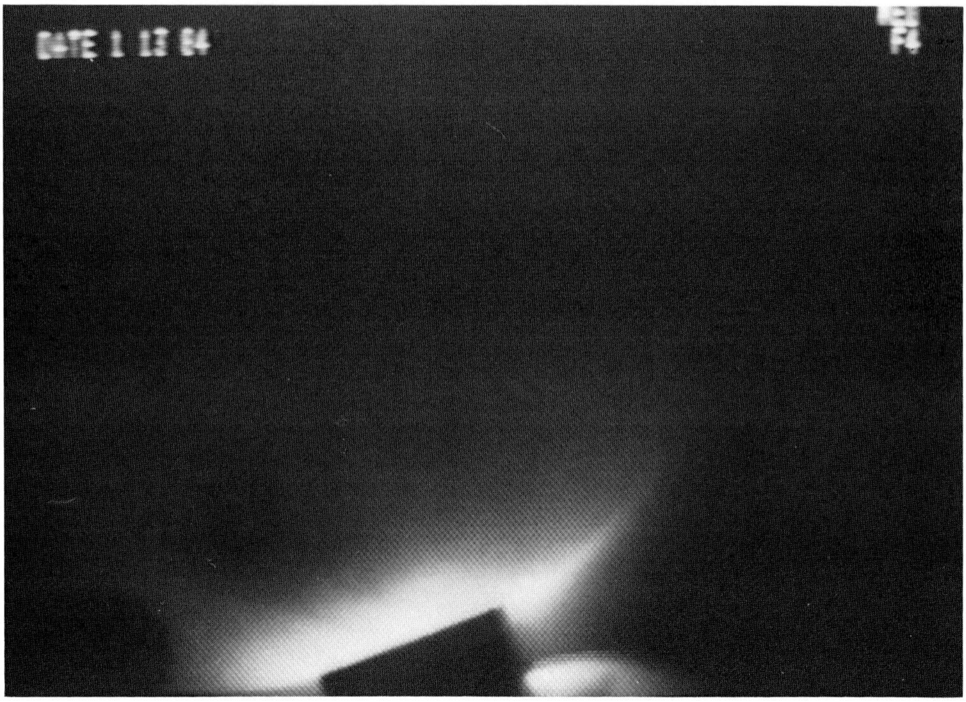

A

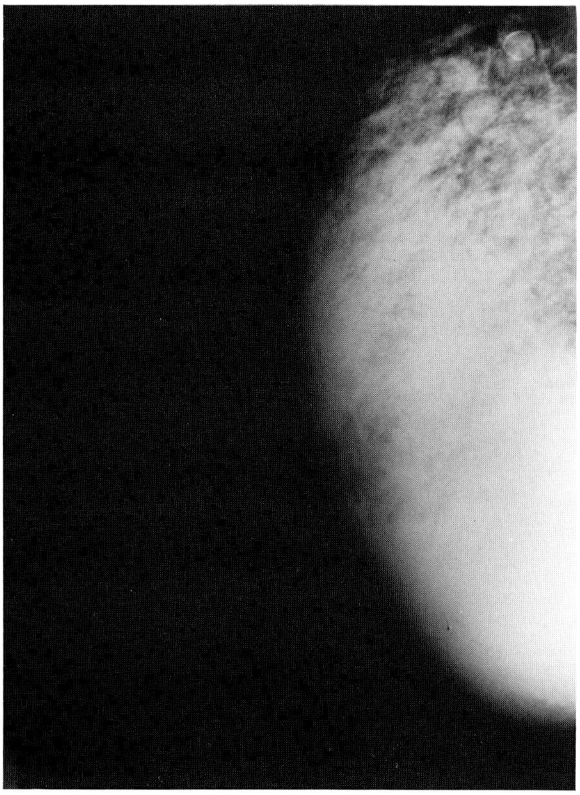

B

Fig. 18-13 A: Diaphanography. Note the inability of light to penetrate the right breast. The light is shining through a small portion of the breast inferiorly, but there is no light through the contracted silicone breast. A skin reaction is present. **B:** Mammogram, right lateral view. There is a marked silicone and tissue reaction, especially in the inferior aspect of the breast.

years the right breast became smaller and firmer, except during a pregnancy when there was apparent recovery of the normal appearance of the breast. On physical examination there was a redness over the mid and lower aspect of the right breast with retraction. The right breast was about one-half the size of the left and was hard and irregular. There was a soft implant on the left.

Thermograms demonstrated increased heat on the left. There was increased light transmission through the left implant, moderate light transmission through the glandular tissue anterior to the implant on the left, and no transmission on the right through the contracted breast (Fig. 18-13A). Mammography showed a silicone gel implant on the left with a thin rim around the implant, questionably representing a fibrous capsule. The implant showed slight flattening anteriorly and inferiorly. On the right there was marked silicone throughout the breast, with skin thickening noted in the inferior aspect (Fig. 18-13B). Ultrasound demonstrated an implant on the left, and marked silicone on the right with a diffuse homogeneous pattern.

This case is an extreme example of a breast undergoing a reaction to the silicone particles with retraction. The redness is caused by the skin reaction to the silicone particles within the skin itself. It is not known why the skin reaction does not cause a positive thermogram. Silicone in the gel implant form can be an insulator that decreases heat transmission from the chest wall and breast, although this author has not noticed this to be true in the free form, as it is with silicone injections.

Case 14

C.B. is a 42-year-old woman who 8 years previously had had silicone injections in the breast. On physical examination there was a 1.5 by 2.5 cm firm nodule in the inner mid-aspect of the right breast. There was diffuse silicone throughout both breasts.

Thermograms were normal. There was surprisingly normal light transmission through the breasts, with diminished transmission through the nodule. Mammography showed many silicone particles but was unable to demonstrate the nodule. The nodule could not be seen distinctly on ultrasound. At biopsy a siliconoma was found with accompanying chronic inflammation and a granulomatous foreign body response.

The formation of nodules of silicone as in this case is not unusual. Such nodules can be found anywhere in the breast, or as in case 12 they may migrate. Diaphanography may demonstrate increased light transmission through these nodules, although not in this case.

Case 15

L.G. is a 60-year-old woman who in 1982 had had a right simple mastectomy for breast cancer. During November 1983 she underwent breast reconstruction, the implant being inserted behind the muscle. One month later 1000 cc of fluid was drained from a seroma. Two days later 70 cc more was aspirated, and 2 days after that another 100 cc was drained. She was referred during August 1984 for right breast swelling.

On physical examination there was a reconstructed breast on the right with the nipple deviated far laterally. There was a very firm implant beneath the skin with a marked fullness in the medial portion of the breast. The left breast was normal.

Thermograms were normal. There was increased light transmission through the implant. Mammograms demonstrated a silicone gel implant behind the pectoralis muscle (Fig. 18-14A). There were many metallic clips in the axilla. Ultrasound showed a fluid collection of about 125 cc behind the implant against the chest wall. The implant was deviated anteriorly (Figs. 18-14B,C).

At surgery a leak in the prosthesis was noted with a globule of free silicone in the tissues. There was a fluid collection behind the implant and marked fibrosis of the tissue surrounding the prosthesis. The prosthesis was removed and a new implant inserted after cleaning out the scar tissue.

A

Fig. 18-14 **A:** Mammogram, right lateral view. Note the silicone gel implant, with slight crumbling, in this reconstructed breast. The implant is behind the pectoralis muscle. **B:** Ultrasound, transverse view. The dense echogenic pectoralis muscle extends over the implant (arrow). Note that there is no glandular tissue in front of the implant (compare with Fig. 18-10C). **C:** Ultrasound. There is a fluid pocket behind the implant (arrows). This finding was also seen on the automated scanner.

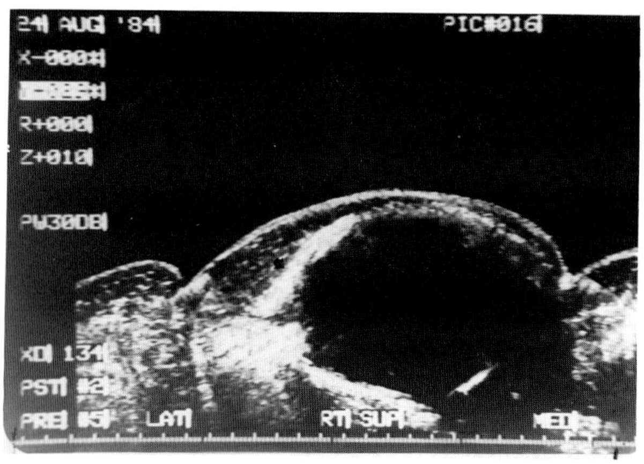

B

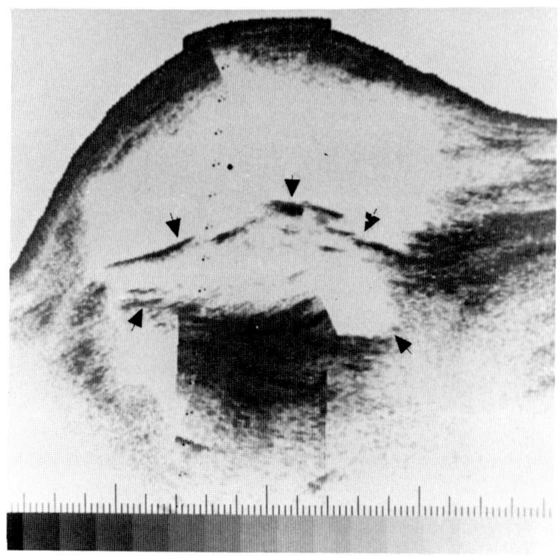

C

Discussion

There are a variety of complications that can occur with implants, primarily related to leakage or a change in contour or position. There can be a partial or complete loss in volume. Infections that occur in the capsule adjacent to the implant may be difficult to treat. If the infection cannot be controlled, removal of the implant may be necessary.

With silicone injections into the breast there is a marked tissue reaction. Unfortunately for the patient, there may be migration of the particles, even extrusion through the skin. Once injected into the breast, there is no good way to rid the breast of the particles and the resultant reaction without surgery. Partial cleanout does not suffice, the best procedure being mastectomy and subsequent reconstruction.

The development of a seroma is unusual but not unknown. The leak of the implant discovered in case 15 was probably due to a knicking of the implant by a needle during drainage of the seroma.

Case Studies: Benign Lesions in Patients with Implants

Case 16

K.J. is a 46-year-old woman who 4 years earlier had had silicone gel implants inserted bilaterally. She then had at least four closed capsulotomies over the next 2 years. On

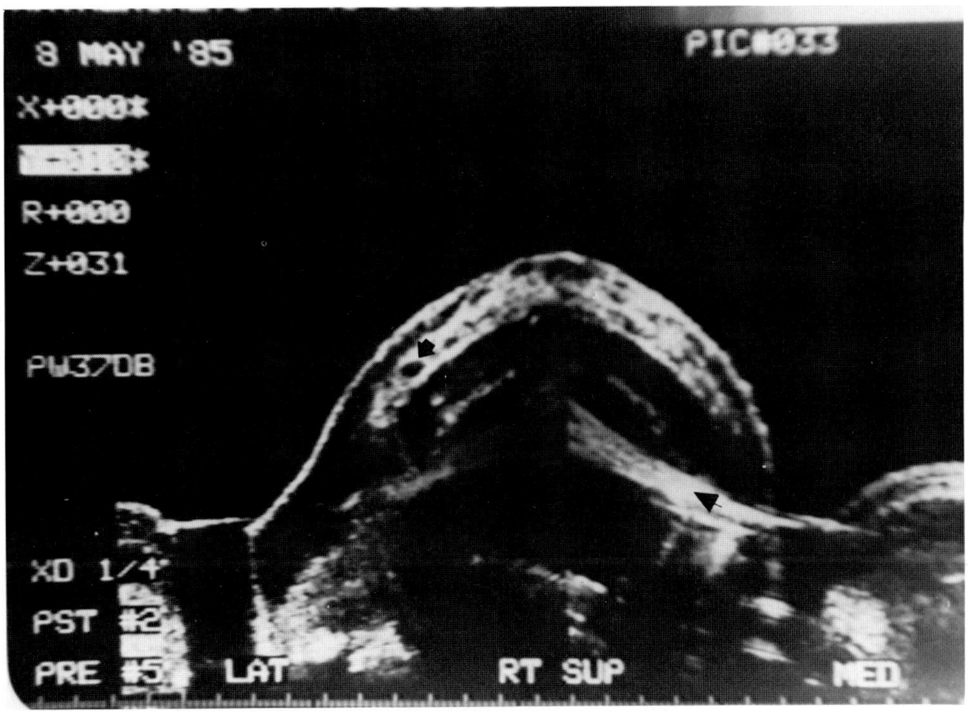

Fig. 18-15 Ultrasound, transverse view. Note the small cystic area (arrow). The dense echogenic areas in the posterior implant are electronically produced rebound artifacts (arrowhead).

physical examination there was moderate firmness to the implants. There was an 8 mm nodule on the lateral aspect of the right breast.

Thermograms, diaphanography, and mammography were essentially normal. On ultrasound there was a 5 mm cyst demonstrated adjacent to the right implant (Fig. 18-15). The nodule was isolated from the implant, and with a 25 gauge needle 0.2 cc of yellow fluid was aspirated, with disappearance of the nodule.

Case 17

B.M. is a 39-year-old woman referred because of breast masses. On physical examination multiple discrete masses were identified throughout both breasts. The masses varied from soft and fluctuant to very firm. There were bilateral implants.

Thermograms were normal. There was an increase in light transmission through the masses bilaterally, as well as through the implants. On mammograms double-bag implants were noted. The masses were not defined because of the marked glandularity of the breasts. On ultrasound there were at least four cysts larger than 1.5 cm on the right and three cysts larger than 2.5 cm on the left as well as many smaller cysts bilaterally (Fig. 18-16A).

Six months later, because of a new mass, a repeat ultrasound examination was done that demonstrated a changed pattern of the cysts. There was now a large multiloculated cyst on the left where separate cysts had been present previously (Fig. 18-16B). The size of many other of the cysts had changed as well, some larger, some smaller. The largest cyst on the left was painful. It was isolated from the implant, and 4 cc of yellow fluid was obtained. No attempt was made to aspirate the other cysts, which were not symptomatic.

One year later, at a follow-up examination, further changes in the cystic pattern were noted, again with some cysts larger, some smaller.

Case 18

D.B. is a 56-year-old woman who has bilateral double-bag implants (silicone implants surrounded by a saline bag). There was a pea-sized (less than 1 cm) nodule at 3 o'clock in the left breast. Thermograms were normal. Diaphanography showed increased light transmission through the implants, the nodule not being evident. Mammograms showed slight crumpling of the upper portion of the left implant. There was somewhat more glandular tissue on the left without a discrete mass. Ultrasound demonstrated implants, but no lesions were seen.

The lesion was thought to be glandular. Seven months later the patient was told by a surgeon that the lesion was definitely suspicious for malignancy, and a biopsy was perfomed. A fibroadenoma and glandular tissue with a foreign body reaction were found.

Discussion

When lesions less than 1 cm in size are discovered, as in case 18, there is difficulty in imaging unless either calcifications or cysts, as in case 17, are present. The fibroadenoma in this case was about 6 mm in size and not evident on diagnostic studies. The foreign body reaction in the adjacent tissue accounted for a portion of the mass. The presence of implants in this case did not play a part in the inability to diagnose the lesion.

Cyst aspiration in patients who have implants can be dangerous unless the cyst can be well isolated from the implant. If this cannot be done, there should be no attempt at aspiration. If the implant is inadvertently punctured, it may cause leakage necessitating removal.

The changing pattern of cysts is demonstrated in case 17. In some patients cysts disappear, whereas in others they continue to grow and enlarge. In this case some of the cysts became conglomerated and merged. Only the symptomatic cyst in this case was aspirated.

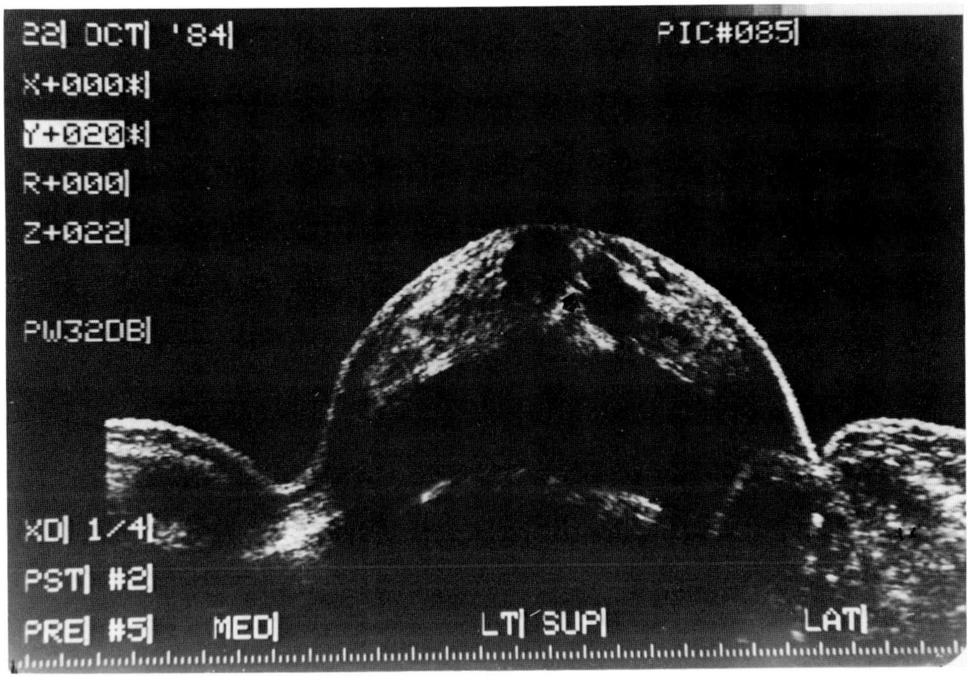

A

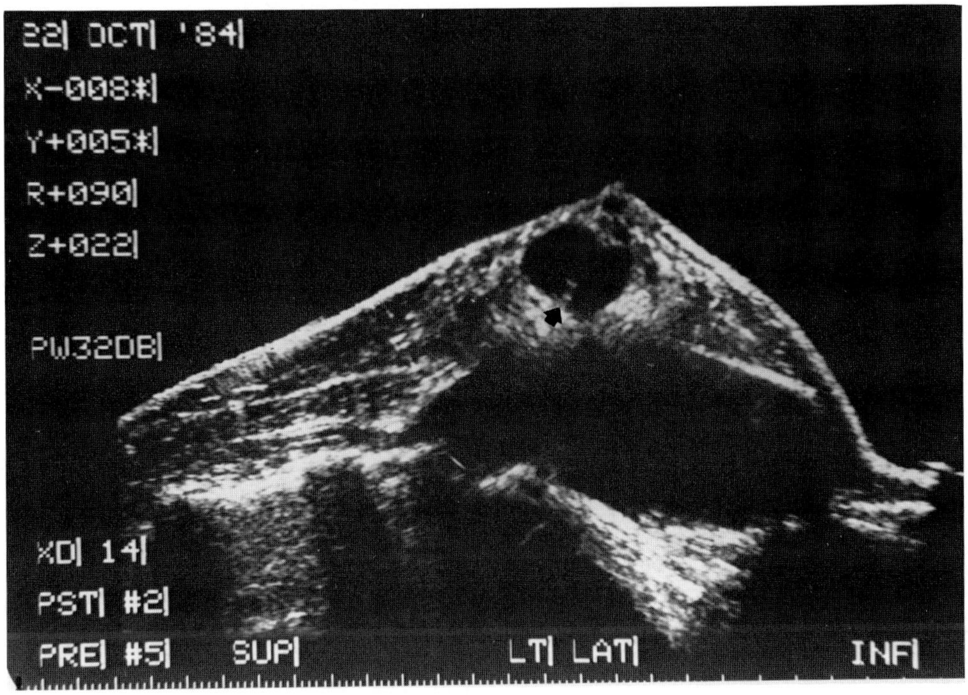

B

Fig. 18-16 **A:** Ultrasound, transverse view. Note the large cysts with ducts (arrows) entering them. Additional dilated ducts are also present. **B:** Ultrasound, longitudinal view. Note the multiloculated cyst with septum (arrow). Dilated ducts are present behind the nipple. Note that the pectoralis muscle ends at the implant (actually dips beneath it) and does not extend over the implant as with a subpectoral implant (Fig. 18-5B).

Bibliography

Augmented Breast

Cole-Beuglet C, Schwartz G, Kurtz AB, et al: Ultrasound mammography for the augmented breast. *Radiology* 1983;146:737–742.

Delage C, Shane JJ, Johnson FB: Mammary silicone granuloma: Migration of silicone fluid to abdominal wall and inguinal region. *Arch Dermatol* 1973;108:105–107.

Kipf EF, Vinnik CA, Bongiovi JJ, et al: Complications of silicone injections. *Rocky Mt Med J* 1976;73:77–80.

Martin, JE: *Atlas of Mammography.* Williams & Wilkins, Baltimore, 1982.

Parsons RW, Thering HR: Management of the silicone-injected breast. *Plast Reconstruct Surg,* 1977;60:534–538.

Picker RH, Jellins J, Kossoff G: The ultrasonic appearances of the breast following surgery and radiotherapy, in Jellins J, Kobayashi T (eds): *Ultrasonic Examination of the Breast.* London, Wiley, 1983, pp 141–147.

Porrath S, Sandhu R, McNeil J: Thermography in the post surgical and post plastic surgery breast. Proceedings American Academy of Thermology, Los Angeles, 1984 (in press).

Benign Lesions in Patients with Implants

Cole-Beuglet C, Schwartz G, Kuirtz AB, et al: Ultrasound mammography for the augmented breast. *Radiology* 1983;146:737–742.

Martin JE: *Atlas of Mammography.* Baltimore, Williams & Wilkins, 1982.

Porrath S, Sandhu R, McNeil J: Thermography in the post surgery and post plastic surgery breast. Proceedings American Academy of Thermology, Los Angeles, 1984 (in press.)

19

Skin and Nipple Lesions

Saar Porrath

It is important to remember that the breast is covered by the same skin as elsewhere on the body and, as such, is predisposed to the same diseases.

Dermatitis involving the breast is common, however. All raw nipples do not represent Paget's disease, although this disease must be ruled out. The nipple and areola may respond with a reaction such as contact dermatitis to a soap or body lotion that for some reason does not affect other skin areas. The offending agent may also come from the pateint's mate, e.g., a particular cologne or mouthwash, the irritation occurring during sexual contact.

There is redness and some swelling of the involved area. Itching and tenderness are usually present, but pain is uncommon. A contact dermatitis responds to stoppage of the offending agent and administration of cortisone creams.

The thermogram often demonstrates increased heat, not as pronounced as with an infection but greater than the normal, uninvolved side. The light scan shows decreased transmission owing to the skin thickening. Mammography and ultrasound are valuable tools for ruling out underlying lesions but are otherwise normal.

Insect bites are localized inflammatory responses and as such appear as infections. The redness and swelling appear suddenly, and there is tenderness and often pain. There may be a small superficial localized mass. The thermogram is very positive, with a marked increase in heat and vascularity. Diaphanography shows a darkened area, often marked in its absorption owing to the increased blood. The mammogram may show slight skin thickening. Attention must be paid to techniques that demonstrate the skin, or this slight skin change will be missed. Ultrasound may show the localized thickening as well.

Melanomas may appear as darkened superficial nevi or raised wartlike lesions. Bleeding or an increase in growth may occur. Although these lesions may be positive on thermography and diaphanography, appear on the mammogram as skin thickening or a distinct skin lesion, and even show skin shadowing on ultrasound, it is usually the dermatologist who makes the diagnosis by biopsy. Our role is to call attention to these lesions and refer them elsewhere.

Metastatic melanoma to the breast is not rare. When a well defined lesion is seen on mammography and ultrasound, this diagnosis is a consideration. In reality, however, it is seldom made unless there is a history of a melanoma having been removed and diagnosed previously.

Skin metastases are not uncommon and can be seen with almost any cancer. They are primarily diagnosed by the physical examination; imaging plays no role except in the unusual case where the primary in the breast may have gone undetected.

Skin cancers, basal cell and squamous, occur and are usually recognized as such on physical examination.

Warts and *sebaceous cysts* are commonly seen. They both present as darkened superficial areas on diaphanography. There may be marked shadowing seen on ultrasound. The thermogram is normal. The mammogram may show a well defined lesion that is seen on tangential views to be superficial. Occasionally talcum powder collects in the folds of the wart and appears on the mammogram as an area of distorted "calcification." The diagnosis is made by observation of the skin lesion.

Lymphedema with skin thickening is seen with a variety of conditions. It may follow radiation therapy or axillary lymph node dissection, or it may be seen post-surgically. It can also occur in congestive heart failure, inflammatory breast cancer, inferior vena caval obstruction, inflammatory conditions of the lymph nodes (e.g., tuberculosis), and other similar conditions. The breast is swollen and may be tender or painful. The skin is thickened, and there may be a peau d'orange effect.

The thermogram is very positive, with diffuse increased global (entire breast) heat and increased vascularity. Diaphanography shows a generalized decrease in light transmission. Both mammography and ultrasound show skin thickening and an increase in the subcutaneous markings reflecting the dilated lymphatics. If there is a deep lesion it may be evident on mammography, ultrasound, or both. The findings may be similar up to a point for any of the causes, although there may be specific changes depending on the diagnosis.

Skin thickening may also be seen in a variety of conditions such as dermatomyositis and scleroderma. Imaging plays no role in the diagnosis, although the skin thickening may be seen on diaphanography, mammography, and ultrasound.

Rashes are common and can be extensive. Their observation is basically clinical, and although imaging plays no role in the diagnosis the thermogram and diaphanography may be positive because of them.

Paget's disease is a clinical presentation of a ductal carcinoma. A portion of or the entire nipple may be raw and irritated. The initial presenting complaint may be blood on the brassiere. There is seldom a palpable mass, and pain is unusual.

The thermogram is variable, the involved nipple often demonstrating increased heat. Light scanning may be normal. Mammography may demonstrate a mass or malignant calcification deeper in the breast. Ultrasound may demonstrate a tumor. These tests may be normal and no tumor demonstrable. A smear from the nipple occasionally shows malignant cells. If hydrocortisone cream is used, the nipple may temporarily clear, but the redness and raw area usually recur. Any raw area of the nipple must be considered Paget's disease until proved otherwise.

Keratosis of the nipple is common, especially in women over age 40. It presents as a darkened firm deposit usually in the slight concavity of the center of the nipple. It can be removed with a little pressure, and a slightly raw area of the nipple is seen below it. It is not pathologic and should be recognized as such.

Most *biopsy scars* are now placed in the periareolar area for cosmetic purposes. These scars occasionally present a slight problem on ultrasound and mammography. The site of the superficial scar may not correspond on the site of the deeper scar. There may be shadowing on ultrasound and spiculization on mammography in the upper outer quadrant, although the evident scar on the breast is periareolar. This picture represents a superficial entry near the nipple, dissection under the skin to the site of the lesion, and the actual biopsy far removed from the skin incision. When there is a question, the patient should be asked the location of the original lesion.

Keloids not uncommonly form in scars, especially in Black women. They vary greatly in size and extent. Clinical findings are usually sufficient to establish the diagnosis. The thermogram is normal. The light scan may show either increased or decreased light transmission, and there may be marked shadowing on ultrasound. The mammogram shows increased skin thickness, some spiculization, and rarely calcification.

Benign skin calcifications are not uncommon. They may be apparent only on one view of a mammogram unless special attention is paid to skin detail. Care must be taken so that these calcifications are not sent to biopsy.

Redness and irritation of the skin secondary to the superficial location of *free silicone particles* may be seen in patients who underwent silicone injection into the breast as a form of augmentation. The silicone particles tend to migrate and can cause skin breakdown and occasionally even extrusion of the free silicone. More commonly there may be discrete silicone nodules formed in the skin.

Suture granulomas are a reaction to the foreign body, the suture, and may form a small, firm, superficial nodule in the area of a scar. Imaging again plays no role, the diagnosis established by excision.

Nipple papillomas are solitary papillomas that may present as a small mass extruding from the nipple. They are discussed in Chapter 17.

Accessory nipples are common, the nipples forming along the milk line, which extends from the axilla to the mid-inguinal canal. The usual presentation is a small brownish nodule of 3 to 4 mm located in the six o'clock position between the nipple and the inframammary fold. It is important to be aware of the normality of this formation.

The presentation of *accessory glandular tissue in the axilla* with a nipple and ducts is not unusual. It is thought that this area may be at higher risk for the development of breast cancer. In the lactating patient it may cause a cosmetic problem with constant leakage of milk. It usually subsides after lactation ceases. The area shows up on diagnostic tests as a dense glandular area filled with milk and hence is very dark on diaphanography. The mammogram shows glandular tissue. The thermogram may be positive. Ultrasound also shows glandular tissue and may demonstrate the dilated ducts seen with lactation. On very rare occasions there may be an accessory duct with an orifice in the areola or, more rarely, in the accessory nipple, which presents with discharge or milk on lactation. (The reader is referred to the section on axillary breasts, Chapter 20.)

Small *skin tags* extending from the nipple are not uncommon and are not pathologic, although some patients complain of the cosmetic appearance.

Bifid nipples are common, the appearance being a cleft through the center of the nipple. They may cause a problem during lactation because of the constant moisture that accumulates in the cleft that results in irritation, sometimes forcing the patient to stop nursing from that breast. Bifid nipples can be unilateral or bilateral.

Nipple inversion is a finding that must be investigated to rule out the possibility of an underlying cancer. Some patients have unilateral or bilateral inversion that has been present for years or since puberty. Occasionally inversion occurs and persists after a duct infection or nursing. Inversions of long standing are usually of no significance.

The nipple and areolar area in patients who have undergone plastic surgery may show slight distortion. *Nipple reconstruction* done in patients who have had previous mastectomy appears different on the imaging procedures. This subject is discussed further in Chapter 18.

Montgomery's glands are found surrounding the nipple throughout the areola. They vary in number, distribution, and size, and are often the site of infections (see Chapter 15).

Skin retraction carries the ominous possibility of an underlying carcinoma. Most skin retractions are not cancer-related, however. The commonest benign cause is previous surgery, with the retraction seen adjacent to a superficial scar. It occurs most frequently in the inferior periareolar area but can be seen anywhere. There may also be retraction at the site of the actual biopsy, even though the superficial scar may be periareolar in location. It is caused by the undermining of the tissues as the surgeon tunnels under the skin to reach the area distant from the periareolar entry site. Retraction can also be seen in Mondor's disease, thrombophlebitis of the vein (see Chapter 16). If fat necrosis is superficial, this entity can also create dimpling not dissimilar to that seen with carcinoma. Occasionally in obese patients who have lost a great deal of weight there are small areas, especially in the upper outer aspect of the breast, that show slight skin irregularity, not quite dimpling. This change results from the attachment of Cooper's ligaments with the loss of tissue between them.

Case Studies

Case 1

D.B. is a 23-year-old woman who was referred because of a brownish discharge from the nipple of the right breast. On physical examination there was scaling and crusting of both nipples, most marked on the right. There was oozing from the right nipple area with no real discharge. The oozing is what the patient thought was a discharge.

Liquid crystal thermograms demonstrated increased nipple heat and vascularity on the right (Th III thermogram). Diaphanography and ultrasound were normal. Mammography was not done.

The patient was treated with hydrocortisone cream, with complete resolution of the findings. There has been one recurrence that also resolved with treatment. The oozing was thought to represent a contact dermatitis, although in this case the causative agent was not identified.

Case 2

L.G. is a 46-year-old woman who was referred because of the discovery of a light brownish discharge found on her brassiere. On physical examination the right nipple was swollen with some scaling and a raw oozing inferior border at the base of the nipple. It was from this area that the brownish fluid was obtained. There was no true nipple discharge. There were extensive eczematous changes over the inner aspect of the elbows, shoulders, and other parts of the body.

Thermograms were normal. Diaphanography showed decreased light transmission over the right nipple itself but was otherwise normal. Mammograms and ultrasound were noncontributory.

The patient complained of itching of the right nipple similar to that of the eczematous areas. A smear of the fluid was normal. It was thought the patient had an eczema of the right nipple and was prescribed cortisone creams, with resolution of the dermatitis.

Case 3

C.R. is a 24-year-old woman who had had chronic boils in both axillary areas for many years, more marked on the right. There were many scars in both axillae from previously lanced boils. She had had a similar condition in both groin areas as well, now under control. No tests were done. She was referred to a dermatologist as a case of chronic hidradenitis suppurativa.

Case 4

T.D. is a 44-year-old woman who was referred because of a reddened area on the left breast, seen on physical examination, about 2 cm from the edge of the areola. There was some firmness in the mid-portion of the area, the total area measuring 3 cm. It had been present for 4 days.

Thermograms were markedly positive on the left with increased heat and vascularity. The area was also very evident on diaphanography, with marked light absorption. The other tests were essentially normal. The reddened area was thought to represent an insect bite. It cleared with warm packs within 4 days.

Case 5

B.H. is a 64-year-old woman who was seen at a local HMO because of a lump in the inner lower aspect of the right breast. Mammograms had demonstrated a poorly defined density of uncertain origin. She has a sister who had breast cancer, and despite the fact that she was assured that this was a benign lesion she presented with fear. On physical examination she had a 1 cm sebaceous cyst in the area in question.

Thermograms were normal. There was a marked decrease in light transmission. A 19 gauge needle was inserted into the mass and with manual pressure grumous whitish material was expressed consistent with a sebaceous cyst. The area drained for 10 days and then cleared. This patient needed reassurance greater than to be told the lesion was nothing to worry about.

Case 6

N.T. is a 22-year-old woman who was referred because of a reddened area in the under aspect of the right breast adjacent to the scars from a prior breast reduction. Liquid crystal thermograms demonstrated increased nipple heat and vascularity on the right. (Color Fig. 7). Diaphanography showed decreased light transmission from the scar areas and the reddened area. Whole breast ultrasound demonstrated the scars and glandular tissue.

Interestingly, the warm water in the automated water-path ultrasound brought the reddened area to more prominence. It turned out to be a "pimple," which was subsequently squeezed. The area cleared.

Discussion

The physical examination and history are the most important parts of the evaluation of dermatologic conditions. Thermography plays a role in the determination of infectious or inflammatory conditions. Most dermatologic findings with skin thickening are positive on diaphanography. Mammography and ultrasound play a minor or no role in the diagnosis.

There is often a nipple discharge reported by the patient, which, as in cases 1 and 2, is really a dermatologic problem with involvement of the nipple and oozing, rather than a real discharge. The imager can aid in establishing the correct diagnosis and obtaining proper therapy.

Bibliography

Barth V: *Atlas of Diseases of the Breast.* Stuttgart, Georg Thieme-Stratton, 1979.

Egan RL, McSweeney MB: Breast sonography—interpretative criteria, in Jellins J, Kobayashi T (eds): *Ultrasonic Examination of the Breast.* London, Wiley, 1983, pp 307–318.

Haagensen CD, Bodian C, Haagensen DE: *Breast Carcinoma; Risk and Detection.* Philadelphia, Saunders, 1981.

Kopans DB, Meyer JE, Proppe KH: The double line of skin thickening on sonograms of the breast. *Radiology* 1981; 141:485–587.

Martin JE: *Atlas of Mammography.* Baltimore, Williams & Wilkins, 1982.

Paulus DP: Benign diseases of the breast. *Radiol Clin North Am* 1983;21(1):27–50.

Porrath S, Sandhu R, McNeil J: Thermography in the post surgery and post plastic surgery breast. Proceedings American Academy of Thermology, Los Angeles, 1984 (in press).

Tabár L, Dean PB: *Teaching Atlas of Mammography.* New York, Thieme-Stratton, 1983.

20

Other Entities

Saar Porrath

Case Studies: Postoperative Changes

Case 1

T.W. is a 43-year-old woman who had had breast reduction surgery 3 years prior to being seen this time. On mammography there was a mild glandular pattern (Wolfe P1). Behind and medial to the right nipple was a small area of tissue with two rounded calcifications and some irregular calcifications thought to be benign. Anterior to this was a 1 cm thin-walled, rounded calcification (Fig. 20-1). None of these calcifications was present on mammograms done prior to the reduction surgery. They are thought to represent postoperative calcifications, possibly in areas of postoperative fat necrosis, although this is unproved.

Case 2

D.P. is a 75-year-old woman who was referred because of right-sided breast pain. She had had three previous biopsies in the right breast, one below the nipple area and two above it. There was moderate retraction associated with the scars above the nipple, with the retraction extending between the scars and being adjacent to the lower scar. No nodules were felt. The left breast was approximately twice the size of the right, the decrease in size thought to be due to the multiple biopsies. There was some tenderness associated with the scar in the lower right breast.

Liquid crystal thermograms showed a marked increase in the heat over the right breast and an edge sign, thought to be due to the surgical deformity (Color Fig. 8). Diaphanography demonstrated normal light transmisssion. On mammograms there was atrophy of the glandular tissue (N1 pattern), a spiculated area above the nipple on the right, and the two areas of retraction (Fig. 20-2). The retractions, spiculated area, and the slight tenderness were all thought to be due to postoperative changes, as was the thermographic picture.

Case 3

M.S. is a 43-year-old woman who 10 days before had undergone an aspiration attempt of a nodular area in the inner aspect of the left breast, with no fluid obtained. Now, on physical examination there was an ecchymotic area overlying an ill-defined glandular-feeling density in the upper inner aspect of the left breast.

Thermograms were normal. Diaphanography showed decreased light transmission through the bruised area but was otherwise normal. On mammography there was moderate glandularity present (P2 pattern); no discrete nodule was seen. Ultrasound demonstrated glandular tissue and a small amount of fluid in the tissues probably secondary to a small bleed from the recent aspiration (Fig. 20-3). The glandular area gradually regressed.

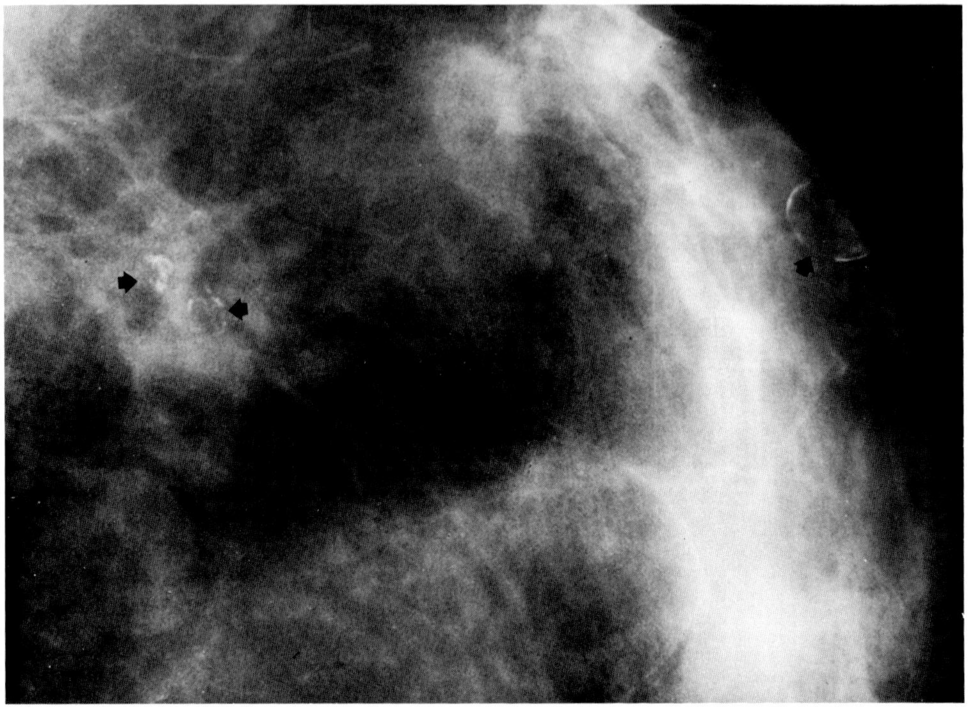

Fig. 20-1 Mammogram. The large rounded calcification at the outer edge of the breast and benign rounded calcifications (arrows) are consistent with postoperative changes.

Case 4

M.R. is a 26-year-old woman who was referred because of a breast nodule. Three months previously she had had a biopsy of the outer aspect of the right breast with a diagnosis of collagenization of mammary gland tissue. This was her second biopsy in the same area. On physical examination there was a hard, movable, slightly irregular nodular density encompassing the area of the two adjacent scars.

Liquid crystal thermograms showed markedly increased heat over the periareolar and outer area of the right breast (Th IV thermogram) (Color Fig. 9). There was decreased light transmission through this area. A single-view mammogram demonstrated marked glandularity, without a mass. On ultrasound there was shadowing from the area of the scar and nodule, without a discrete mass (Fig. 20-4).

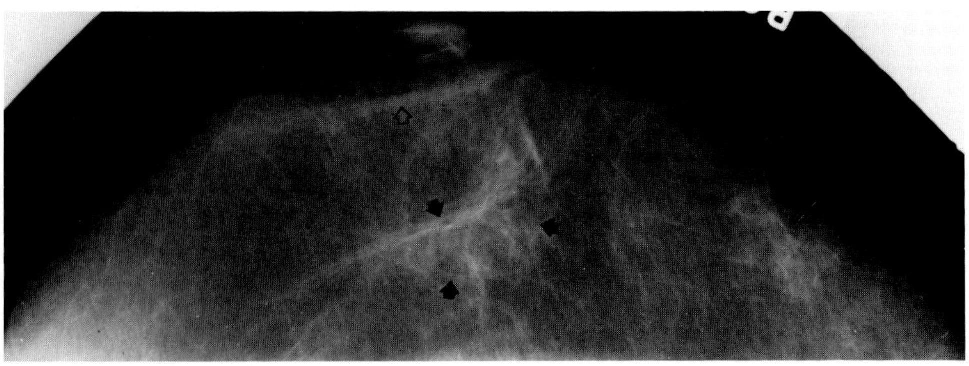

Fig. 20-2 Mammogram, CC view. The irregular density at mid-breast is a scar (arrow). There is an area of retraction (open arrow) behind the nipple.

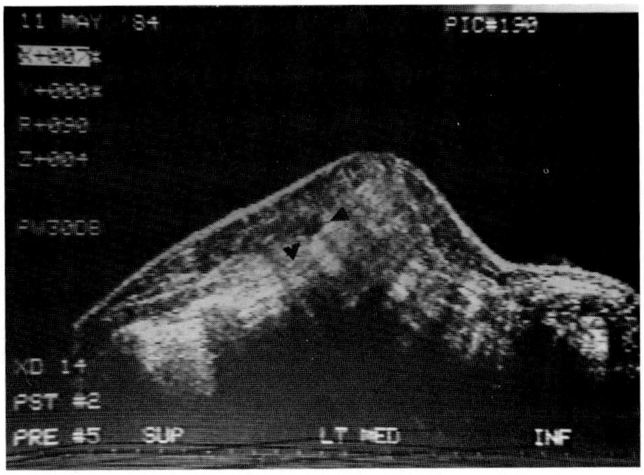

Fig. 20-3 Ultrasound. Note the low-level echo area with slightly increased through transmission (arrows).

When seen 4 months later there was a freely movable 1 cm nodule at the medial end of the scar and a decrease in the thickening previously noted. Thermograms were still positive, but there was a decrease in the heat and vascularity (Th III thermogram). One year later there was no change in the 1 cm nodule, thought to possibly represent a suture granuloma. The thickening otherwise had resolved. The thermogram was normal.

Discussion

A variety of postoperative changes have been presented. Case 1 demonstrates mammographic changes of fat necrosis, with thin-walled areas of calcification. In case 2 there is retraction and spiculization from previous biopsies. In case 3 there were acute changes of a recent aspiration, shown most vividly on diaphanography, with a small hemorrhagic fluid collection seen on ultrasound. Case 4 demonstrates the length of time a thermogram may remain positive because of resolving postoperative changes. The reader is referred to the case studies on fat necrosis (Chapter 11) and postoperative hemorrhage (Chapter 14) for other examples of postoperative changes that may occur.

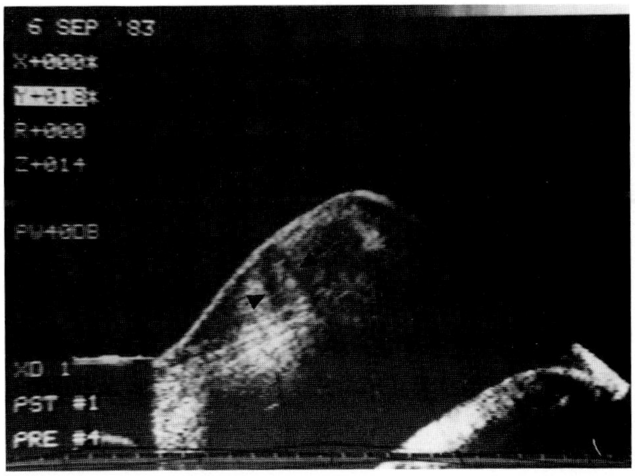

Fig. 20-4 Ultrasound. Note the shadowing from the scar (arrowheads).

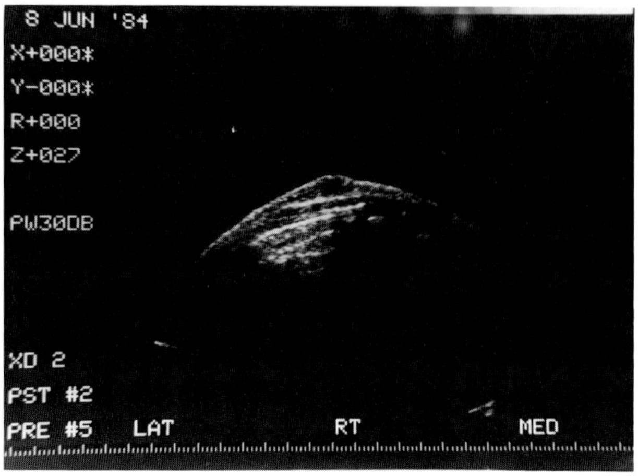

Fig. 20-5 Ultrasound. Note the shadowing behind the nipple and glandular tissue present on either side of the nipple shadow. There is a prominent pectoralis muscle.

Case Study: Prepubescent Breast

Case 5

A.M. is an 8.5-year-old girl who presented with slight inversion of the right nipple and a tender, firm mass beneath the nipple. On physical examination there was minimal inversion of the mid-portion of the nipple but not the areola. There was a 3 cm nubbin of tissue, circular in appearance, behind the nipple that was somewhat tender. The thermogram showed increased heat in the area of the right nipple compared to the left (Color Fig. 10). Automated ultrasound showed a small amount of glandular tissue and slight shadowing behind the nipple (Fig. 20-5).

This case represents early development of one breast. The tenderness is from the developing glandular tissue. It is not known why there was slight inversion of the nipple. On close inspection there was very early pubic hair present. Six months later there was equal development of both breasts, and the tenderness disappeared.

Discussion

Unequal early development of one breast is not uncommon, although this patient was younger than usual. Assurance should be given to the patient and her parents that this situation is not abnormal and that development of the other breast usually soon follows. On occasion, one breast becomes much larger than the other, necessitating plastic surgery. Mammography in this age group is unjustified unless there is a very strong suspicion of a tumor, an unlikely occurrence. Ultrasound usually shows the small nubbin of glandular tissue. Diaphanography can be difficult because of the small breast size. Thermography showed the increased heat generated by the active glandular tissue.

Case Studies: Axillary Breasts

Case 6

T.C. is a 27-year-old woman who 1 week prior to being seen lost a 5-month pregnancy. This was her third pregnancy, all ending in abortions. The first was lost during the first month 3 years ago. The second pregnancy was aborted at 7 months approximately 2 years ago. She had a dilatation and curettage (D&C) following the third abortion, the abortions occurring for unknown causes. The axillary areas were swollen and tender during this latest pregnancy but became acutely enlarged after D&C. There was minimal swelling with the 7-month pregnancy and none with the first. She normally felt some tenderness, without a mass, premenstrually in the axillary areas.

On physical examination there were moderate-sized breasts with a milky discharge elicited from multiple ducts bilaterally. Moderate glandularity was present with slight tenderness. In the right axilla there was a 3 cm glandular-feeling mass with a very small nipple; no milk was elicited. On the left there was a 2.5 cm glandular-feeling mass also with a very small nipple and no milk.

Thermography demonstrated a vascular pattern bilaterally consistent with the recent pregnancy. There was increased heat in the axillary areas. Diaphanography showed a diffuse decrease in light transmission throughout both breasts consistent with pregnancy or lactation. There was a decrease in the axillary areas corresponding to the masses felt clinically, the light transmission being about equal to the denser areas of the breasts (Fig. 20-6A).

A single-view oblique mammogram of each breast showed marked glandularity consistent with a Wolfe DY pattern. There was a dense glandular area noted in each axilla (Fig. 20-6B). Ultrasound showed glandular tissue extending into the axilla with very small ducts identified in the area, not extending to the small nipples that were present (Fig. 20-6C). The patient was reassured that this was breast tissue in the axilla, and it resolved within 2 weeks.

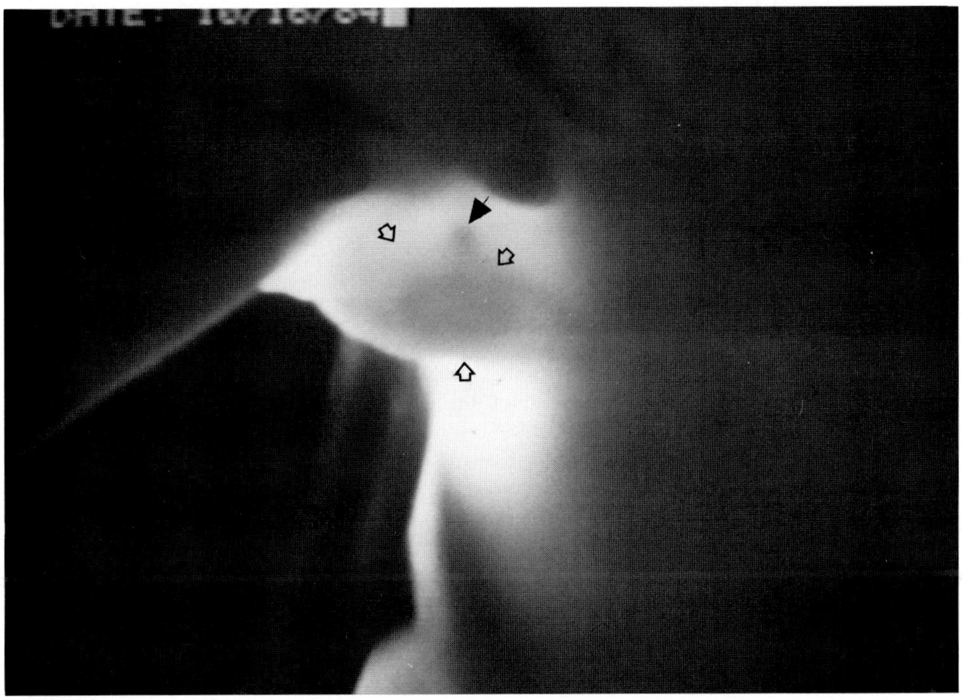

A

Fig. 20-6 A: Diaphanography. Note the decreased light transmission over the glandular area in the axilla (open arrows). The dark area above represents the ectopic nipple (arrow).

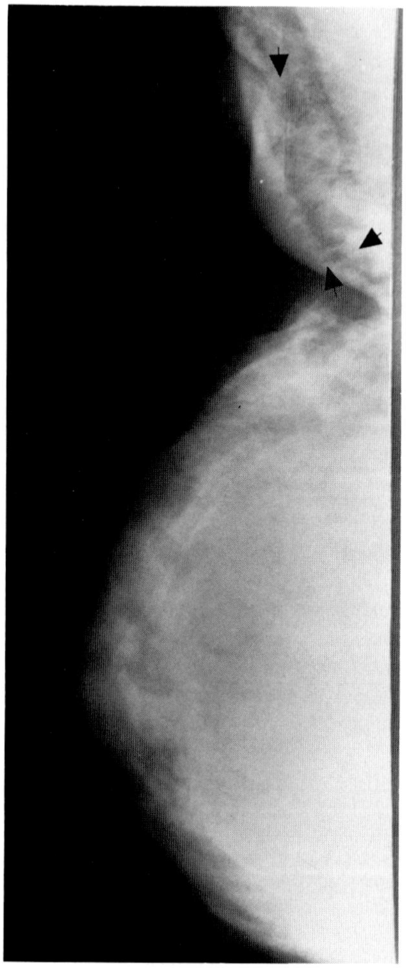

B

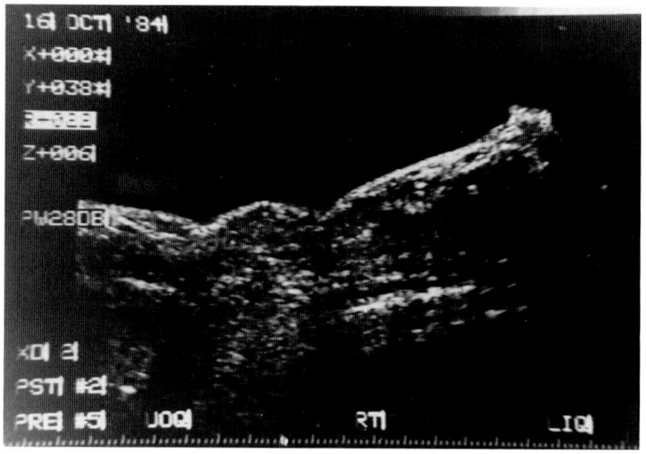

C

Fig. 20-6 **B:** Mammogram. Note the dense glandular tissue in the axilla (arrows). **C:** Ultrasound. The hump in the contour represents the axillary breast. Fine glandularity is noted. A duct is seen extending into the axillary breast (arrows).

Case 7

G.K. is a 41-year-old white woman who was referred for routine screening. On physical examination she had marked glandularity to the breasts with some fullness in the axillary areas associated with moderate tenderness. She was premenstrual and related having pain in the axilla, especially the left, prior to her menstrual periods.

Thermograms, ultrasound, and diaphanography were essentially normal. On mammography there was a small collection of glandular tissue seen in each axilla (Fig. 20-7). The pain and tenderness in the axilla was secondary to the hormonal stimulation of the glandular tissue in the axilla.

Case 8

M.L. is a 34-year-old woman who was referred for screening because of a positive family history of breast cancer. On physical examination there was prominent tissue in the upper axilla extending into the upper arm, more marked on the right. The patient claimed that these areas became very sore with her cycles and a previous pregnancy. On mammography, with views taken to encompass the area of the upper arm, a small amount of glandular tissue was noted to extend from the upper axilla to the upper arm and was more marked on the right (Fig. 20-8).

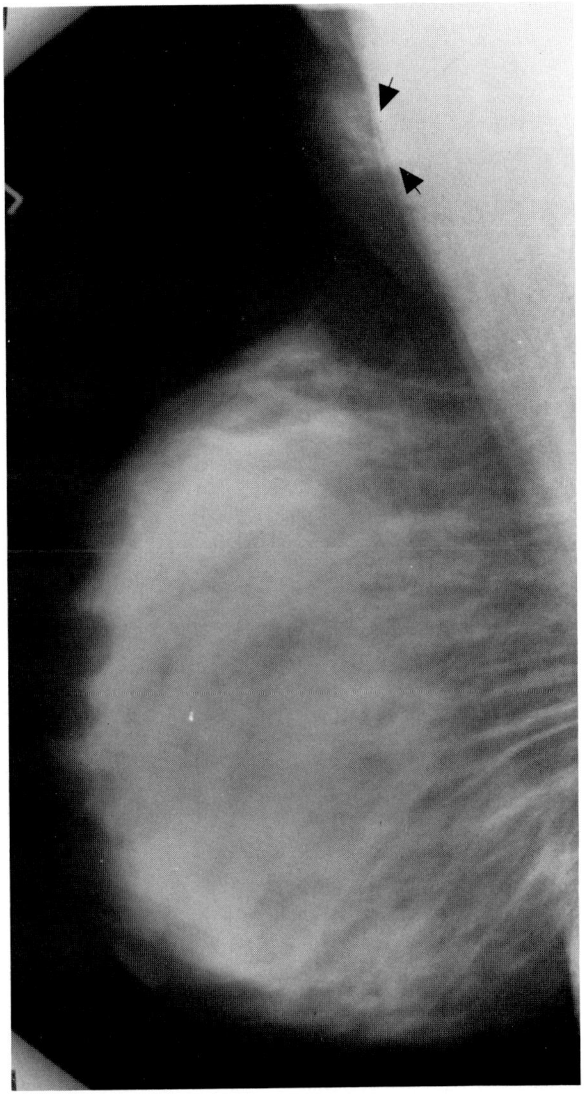

Fig. 20-7 Mammogram. The nubbin of glandular tissue in the axilla (arrows) is consistent with an axillary breast.

Case 9

D.K. is a 57-year-old woman who was seen in consultation. She had had a mass in the axillary area which over the period of a year had grown from 1 cm to 4 cm. The breast examination and mammograms were negative preoperatively other than the mass. At surgery the mass was fluid-filled and ruptured as it was being resected. The slides prepared were reported as adenoid cystic carcinoma involving a lymph node, with necrosis.

The question that arose was what further surgery was indicated. It was decided to have the patient undergo an axillary node dissection and blind biopsy of the tail of the breast. A focus of intraductal carcinoma was found in an additional lymph node; the tail of the breast was negative. She has had no additional treatment.

Case 10

N.N. is a 48-year-old woman seen in consultation. She had a 1 cm nodule resected from the left upper arm that revealed a differentiated adenocarcinoma. She subsequently underwent left axillary node dissection and blind biopsy of the tail of the left breast. The remaining nodes were negative, although a microscopic focus of lobular carcinoma in situ (lobular neoplasia) was found in the tail of the breast.

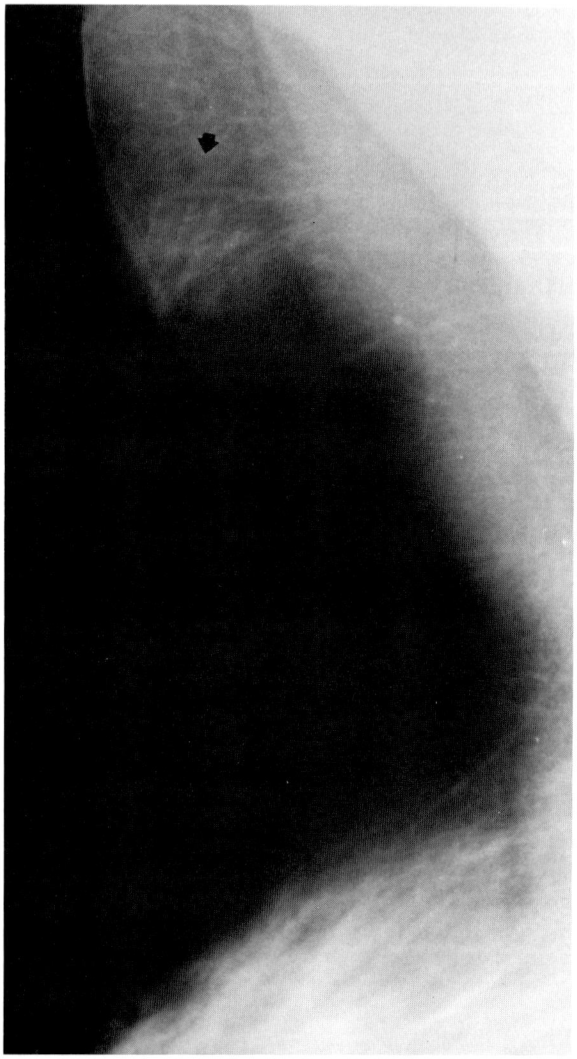

Fig. 20-8 Mammogram, magnified: axilla. Note the small amount of glandular tissue in the upper arm (arrow).

The adenocarcinoma in the nodule appears to be an isolated carcinoma arising in an ectopic breast. No further therapy would be indicated if it were not for the finding of the lobular neoplasia in the tail of the breast. The patient had been advised to obtain a blind biopsy of the opposite breast and, if negative, close follow-up on a regular basis. One surgeon advised bilateral mastectomy, and another recommended bilateral subcutaneous mastectomy.

The patient has been advised by an eastern cancer center to do nothing further except obtain frequent checkups. The patient has decided on this course.

Discussion

Accessory nipples are not uncommon, and accessory breast tissue can be seen, much less commonly, anywhere along the milk line extending from the axilla to the groin. Martin reported a case of carcinoma occurring in ectopic breast tissue of the vulva. Breast tissue not infrequently extends into the lower axilla. There have been cases of lactating breast tissue complete with nipples from which milk could be expressed, creating a problem for the patient because of the size of the axillary breasts and the constant milk flow. In these patients the flow ceased with the cessation of nursing.

The presence of glandular tissue in the upper axilla extending into the upper arm as in case 8 is unusual. This situation also occurred in case 10, where a cancer developed in the ectopic tissue.

Barth mentioned that there is believed to be an increased tendency to tumor formation in the accessory breast tissue and related that consideration should be given to prophylactic removal because of this fact. It is difficult to imagine a large enough series to validate this recommendation. The two cases of cancer in axillary breasts that this author has seen in consultation (cases 9 and 10) are unusual in presentation and complexity.

Case Studies: Breast During Pregnancy and Lactation

Case 11

S.J. is a 29-year-old woman who was 4 weeks' pregnant. On physical examination there was a tender ridge in the outer aspect of the right breast. Liquid crystal thermograms showed a very prominent vascular pattern bilaterally. There was a slight decrease in light transmission through the entire breast, greater in the periareolar areas. Mammography was not done. On ultrasound there was marked glandularity bilaterally with slight duct dilatation. The ridge was thought to represent glandular tissue, it blended into the breast as the pregnancy progressed and was absent postpartum.

Case 12

D.C. is a 31-year-old woman who was 3 months' pregnant. On physical examination there was fullness to both breasts with 1.5 cm nodules present bilaterally in the upper breasts. The patient related that the mass on the right presented when she went off birth control pills just prior to her becoming pregnant.

Thermograms showed a marked vascular pattern consistent with pregnancy. There was a moderate decrease in light transmission through the breast. Mammography was not done. On ultrasound there was marked glandularity. There were 1 cm cysts in the location of the masses bilaterally, as well as other smaller cysts and dilated ducts bilaterally (Fig. 20-9). The cysts were aspirated, with disappearance of the masses following the aspiration.

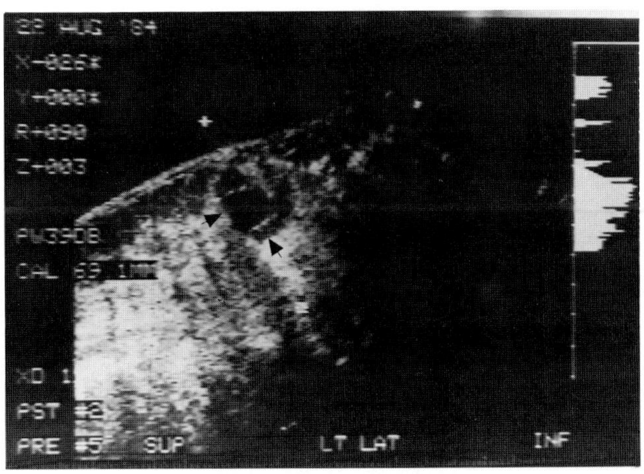

Fig. 20-9 Ultrasound. Cysts are present with increased through transmission (arrows). Note the echo-free areas on this A-mode picture.

Case 13

M.D. is a 32-year-old woman who was referred for screening because of a positive family history. The patient was lactating. Thermograms showed marked vascularity consistent with lactation (Color Fig. 11). It was impossible to penetrate the breast with diaphanography. On ultrasound there was marked glandularity and duct dilatation bilaterally. The patient was advised to return for evaluation to include mammography 2 months after cessation of nursing. At that time all studies were normal.

Case 14

H.W. is a 33-year-old woman who on physical examination was found to have an 8 mm nodule in the right breast. She has a positive family history of breast cancer and when seen was lactating. She has bilateral implants. Thermograms were very vascular, consistent with lactation. There was a marked decrease in light transmission through the breasts. Mammograms demonstrated bilateral silicone gel implants and marked glandularity (DY pattern); the nodule not seen. On ultrasound there was a 5 mm fluid area consistent with a cyst or dilated duct. There was marked glandularity and duct dilatation seen bilaterally as well as the implants (Fig. 20-10). The nodule subsequently regressed.

Case 15

N.P. is a 30-year-old woman who, during the fifth month of pregnancy, had a bloody discharge from a single duct on the right. A month later she also began to have a bloody discharge from a single duct on the left as well. Smears were negative for malignancy. There was a family history of a mother who had breast cancer at age 52. On physical examination there was a nipple discharge from many ducts bilaterally that was clear to milky, and a reddish discharge from a single duct from each nipple.

Liquid crystal thermograms demonstrated a vascular pattern bilaterally, consistent with pregnancy (Color Fig. 12). Diaphanography showed marked diminution of light transmission. A single-view mammogram, with the abdomen shielded, showed marked glandularity and duct dilatation, with no mass or calcification noted (Fig. 20-11). On ultrasound there was marked glandularity and slight duct dilatation.

This case is thought to represent "physiologic" bleeding seen with pregnancy. The fact that there is bilateral bloody discharge makes it very unlikely that there is a malignancy. Occult blood was found in a significant percentage of pregnant women studied by Kline and Lash. Haagensen et al. reported on a series of 14 patients with similar bleeding during pregnancy. The author has consulted on two additional cases of bleeding during pregnancy, with no lesion found.

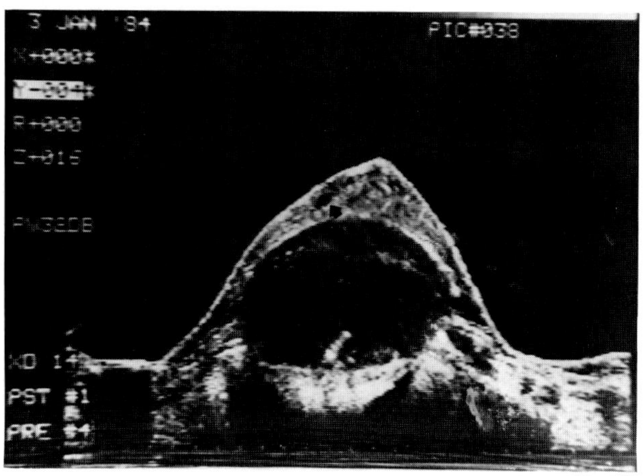

Fig. 20-10 Ultrasound. Note the dilated duct or cystic area (arrows), as well as other dilated ducts behind the nipple.

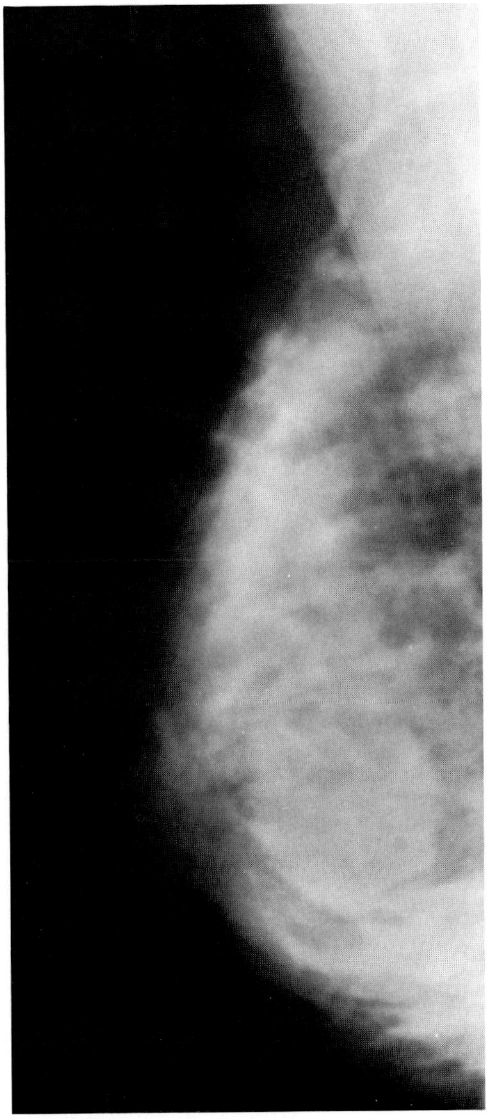

Fig. 20-11 Mammogram, lateral view. Note the marked glandularity and ductal prominence.

Discussion

During pregnancy and lactation there is a marked increase in the density of the breast. The thermographic pattern is markedly vascular. On diaphanography there is an increasing density to the breast as the pregnancy progresses. On mammography this density diminishes the accuracy of the examination, unless calcifications are present. Ultrasound demonstrates a marked increase in glandular tissue and duct dilatation. The cases above were chosen to demonstrate the "normal" appearance of the breast on these examinations.

Any suspicious lesion must be investigated. Even though pregnancy and lactation increase the difficulty of imaging masses, it is possible to diagnose cancer in these patients.

Case Study: Chronic Ductal Disease

Case 16

J.C. is a 60-year-old woman who was referred because of a brownish discharge from her left breast. By history she had had many episodes of inflammation while nursing her children 40 years earlier. On physical examination no discharge was noted.

Thermograms were normal. On diaphanography there was a diffuse decrease in light transmission above the nipples bilaterally (Fig. 20-12A). Mammograms demonstrated marked ovoid ductal calcifications throughout both breasts (Fig. 20-12B,C).

The benign-appearing ductal calcifications probably occurred in the areas of inflammation. The material in the duct dried and eventually calcified, the calcifications occurring in the duct itself, not in the duct wall.

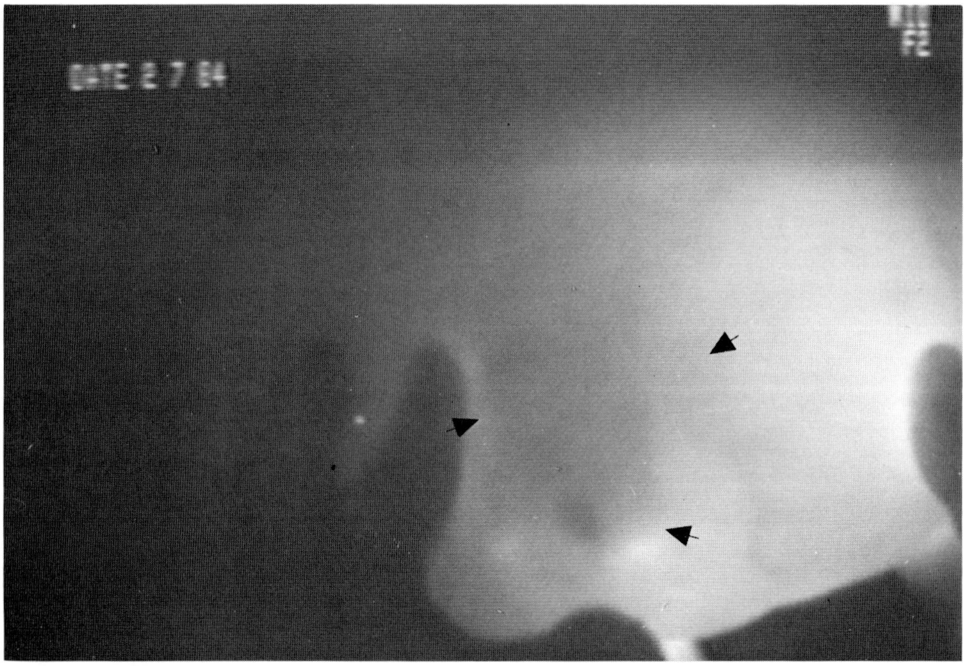

A

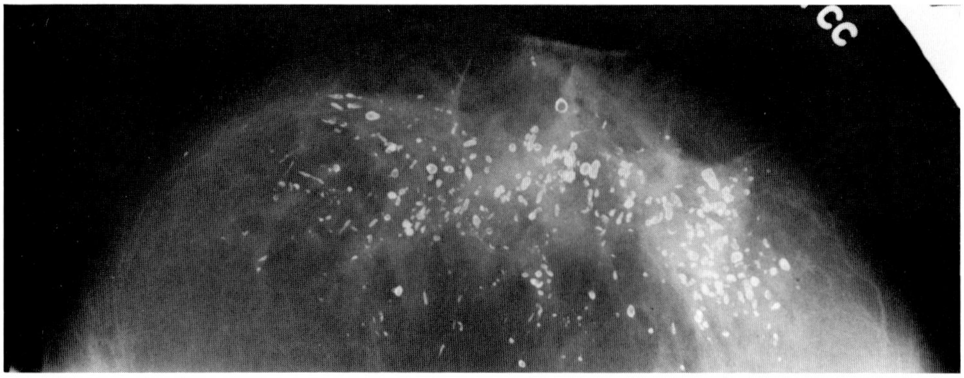

B

Fig. 20-12 A: Diaphanography. Note the poorly defined, slightly decreased light transmission above the nipple area (arrows). **B:** Mammogram, right CC view.

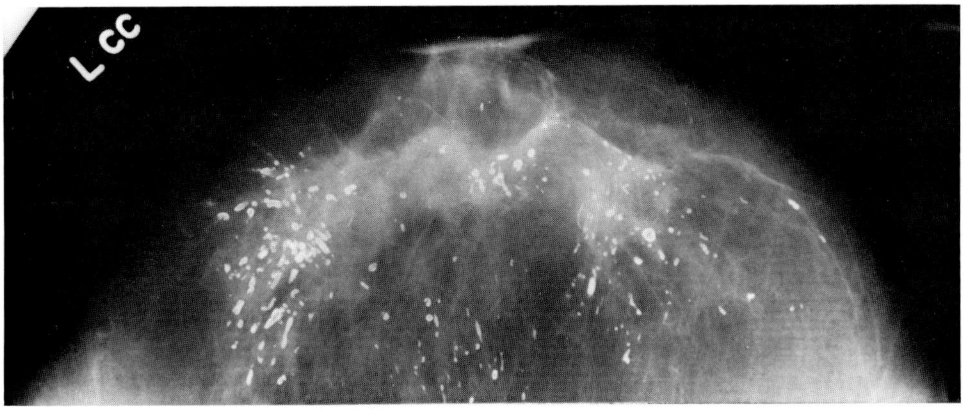

C

Fig. 20-12 **C:** Mammogram, left CC view. Note the diffuse calcifications (rounded, oblong, and linear, representing duct material that has saponified and calcified).

Case Studies: Intramammary Lymph Nodes

Case 17

J.D. is a 50-year-old woman originally referred for screening. Physical examination was normal. Thermograms and diaphanography were normal. There was atrophy of the glandular tissue (N1 pattern) on mammography, with a 5 mm well defined nodule present in the outer aspect of the right breast. Repeat mammograms 16 months later demonstrated that the nodule was 8 mm in size. Review of a mammogram done 6 years earlier showed the nodule to be about 4 mm.

It was thought that the nodule represented a benign lesion, but because of the growth in its size biopsy was recommended. Preoperative localization was done. At surgery an intramammary lymph node was found.

Case 18

J.B. is a 36-year-old woman who was referred because of a left breast mass that had been present for 15 months. The nodule appeared while the patient was nursing and had a right breast infection. Four months after she stopped nursing the nodule decreased to about one-half its former size, and it has been unchanged since. On physical examination there was a round, firm, 1 cm nodule in the outer left breast.

Thermograms and diaphanography were normal. On mammography there was a well defined 1 cm nodule without calcification (Fig. 20-13). On ultrasound the nodule was not distinguishable from the underlying tissue.

A needle biopsy revealed inflammatory cells and keratinized material. The nodule was unchanged 9 months later. Because of the patient's concern a biopsy was done, and an intramammary lymph node with reactive hyperplasia was found.

Discussion

Intramammary lymph nodes are usually incidental findings seen on mammography. They are often well defined, most often kidney-bean-shaped with a fatty hilum. If the lesion grows, as in case 17, biopsy is mandatory to rule out a slow-growing malignancy. In case 18 the breast infection probably caused the lymph node to grow reactively, shrinking when lactation was over. Even though there was a normal needle biopsy and no growth over a 13-month period, the patient's concern justified biopsy.

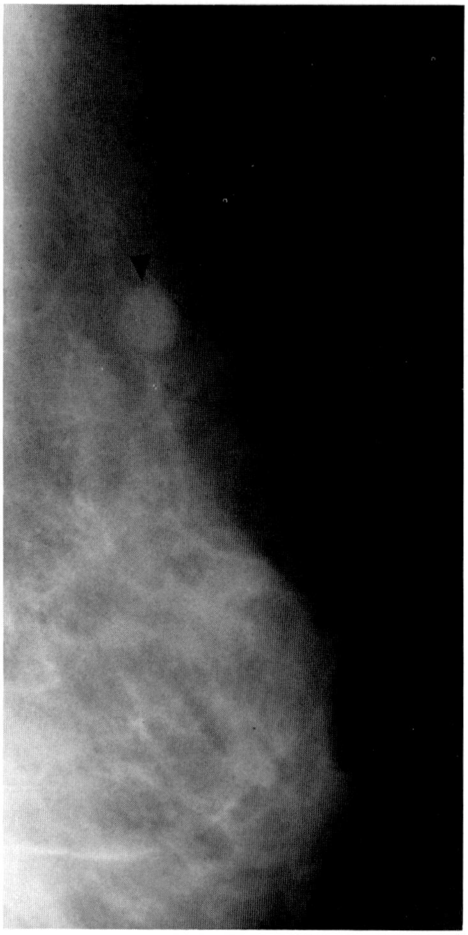

Fig. 20-13 Mammogram, lateral view. Note the well defined nodule in the tail of the left breast (arrow).

Bibliography

Postoperative Changes

Barth V: *Atlas of Diseases of the Breast.* Stuttgart, Georg Thieme, 1979.

Bassett LW, Gold RH, Mirra JM: Nonneoplastic breast calcifications in lipid cysts: Development after excision and primary irradiation. *AJR* 1982;138:335–338.

Egan RL, McSweeney MB: Breast sonography—interpretative criteria, in Jellins J, Kobayashi T (eds): *Ultrasonic Examination of the Breast.* London, Wiley, 1983, pp 307–318.

Grant EG, Richardson JD, Cigtay OS, et al: Sonography of the breast: Findings following conservative surgery and irradiation for early carcinoma. *Radiology* 1983;147:535–539.

Homer JJ: Cardiopulmonary pathology masquerading as primary breast disease. *Breast* 1984;10(2):6–9.

Klein DL, Sickles EA: Effects of needle aspiration on the mammographic appearance of the breast: A guide to the proper timing of the mammography examination. *Radiology* 1982;145:44.

Kopans DB, Meyer J, Proppe KH: The double line of skin thickening on sonograms of the breast. *Radiology* 1981;141:485–487.

Martin JE: *Atlas of Mammography.* Baltimore, Williams & Wilkins, 1982.

Paulus DP: Benign diseases of the breast. *Radiol Clin North Am* 1983;21(1):27–50.

Picker RH, Jellins J, Kossoff G: The ultrasonic appearances of the breast following surgery and radiotherapy, in Jellins J, Kobayashi T (eds): *Ultrasonic Examination of the Breast.* London, Wiley, 1983, pp 141–147.
Porrath S, Sandhu R, McNeil J: Thermography in the post surgery and post plastic surgery breast. Proceedings American Academy of Thermology, Los Angeles, 1984 (in press).
Tabár L, Dean PB: *Teaching Atlas of Mammography.* New York, Thieme-Stratton, 1983.

Prepubescent Breast

Barth V: *Atlas of Diseases of the Breast.* Stuttgart, Georg Thieme, 1979.
Martin JE: *Atlas of Mammography.* Baltimore, Williams & Wilkins, 1982.
Reeve TS, Jellins J, Kossoff G, et al: Classification of the sonographic appearance of the normal breast, in Jellins J, Kobayashi T (eds): *Ultrasonic Examination of the Breast.* London, Wiley, 1983, pp 149–156.
Sandison AT, Walker JC: Diseases of the adolescent female breast. *Br J Surg* 1968;55(6):443–448.

Axillary Breasts

Barth V: *Atlas of Diseases of the Breast.* Stuttgart, Georg Thieme, 1979.
Haagensen CD, Bodian C, Haagensen DE: *Breast Carcinoma; Risk and Detection.* Philadelphia, Saunders, 1981.
Klose H, Sebening W: Die Chirurgie der Brustdruse, in Kirchner M, Nordmann O (eds): *Chirurgie*, ed 1. Berlin, Urban & Schwarzenberg, 1941, vol 5.
Martin JE: *Atlas of Mammography.* Baltimore, Williams & Wilkins, 1982.
Schwargen M, Herfarth Ch: Erkrankungen der Brustdruse, in Schwalm H, Doderlein G (eds): *Klinik der Frauenheilkunde und Geburtshilfe.* Munich, Urban & Schwarzenberg, 1967, vol 7.

Breast During Pregnancy and Lactation

Barth V: *Atlas of Diseases of the Breast.* Stuttgart, Georg Thieme, 1979.
Haagensen CD, Bodian C, Haagensen DE: *Breast Carcinoma: Risk and Detection.* Philadelphia, Saunders, 1981, p 152.
Jellins J, Kossoff G, Reeve TS: Detection and classification of liquid-filled masses in the breast by Gray scale echography. *Radiology* 1977;125:205–212.
Leis HP, Cammarata A, La Raja RD: Nipple discharge: Significance and treatment. *Breast* 1985;11(2):6–12.
Martin JE: *The Breast in Pregnancy. Atlas of Mammography.* Baltimore, Williams & Wilkins, 1982, pp 288–294.
Rifkin MD, Pasto ME: Normal breast parenchymal patterns identified by ultrasound mammography, in Leopold GR (ed): *Ultrasound in Breast and Endocrine Disease*, New York, Churchill Livingstone, 1984, pp 1–24.
Schwartz GF: Benign neoplasms and "inflammations" of the breast. *Clin Obstet Gynecol* 1982;25(2):373–385.

Chronic Ductal Disease

Barth V: *Atlas of Diseases of the Breast.* Chicago, Year Book, 1979.
Leis HP, Cammarata A, La Raja RD: Nipple discharge: Significance and treatment. *Breast* 1985;11(2):6–12.
Matallana R, Orenberg C: Ultrasound diagnosis of mammary duct ectasia, in Jellins J, Kobayashi T (eds): *Ultrasonic Examination of the Breast.* London, Wiley, 1983, pp 319–324.

Tabár L, Dean PB: *Teaching Atlas of Mammography*. New York, Thieme-Stratton, 1983.
Tabár L, Dean PB, Pentek Z: Galactography: The diagnostic procedure of choice for nipple discharge. *Radiology* 1983;149:31–38.

Intramammary Lymph Nodes

Egan RL, McSweeney MB: Intramammary lymph nodes. *Cancer* 1983;51:1838–1842.
Meyer JE, Kopans DB: Stability of a mammographic mass: A false sense of security. *AJR* 1981;137:595–598.
Tabár L, Dean PB: *Teaching Atlas of Mammography*. New York, Thieme-Stratton, 1983.

Section III

Malignant Disease

21

Cancer

Saar Porrath

Because of the myriad of presentations it is very difficult to present a succinct description of carcinoma of the breast. So much depends on the size, location, and type of cancer.

To define a cancer as nonpalpable is deceptive. The tumor could be millimeters or centimeters in size and still be unpalpable. In a patient with very large glandular breasts it is possible for a lesion, benign or malignant, of many centimeters in diameter, deep within the breast to go undetected on physical examination, whereas that same lesion in a fatty, atrophic breast or a small breast would cause a large bulge. Similarly, if a lesion is only a few millimeters in size and very superficial it may be palpable, whereas that same lesion, if deep, may go undetected by any test until it is larger.

The cancer, if palpable, may be hard and well defined or soft and poorly defined. In general, colloid and medullary cancers are softer and less defined than intraductal carcinomas. If there is an increased amount of fibrous tissue reaction, as with the "scirrhous" variety of ductal carcinoma, the tumor may feel very hard when palpated. Most cancers feel larger, as much as twice their actual size, because of the surrounding tissue reaction.

If the tumor is superficial and affects Cooper's ligaments, there may be retraction of the skin even with small lesions, whereas if deep and large there may be no retraction. The same is true of nipple retraction. If the adjacent ducts and ligaments are affected early the nipple may be deformed, whereas if deep and large without a "pull" on the ducts there may be no change.

Nipple discharges are variable. Most of the discharges noted are not bloody but serous or watery. On rare occasions there is a whitish, almost cheesy discharge noted in comedocarcinoma. Pain and tenderness, although not always present, are common enough that the old admonition, "If it hurts, it isn't cancer" is not true and should not be relied on.

Skin changes such as redness or peau d'orange (orange peel) appearance are usually late evidence of inflammatory carcinoma. These changes do not indicate a true infection but result from plugging of the lymphatics by tumor cells, and in essence represent lymphedema of the adjacent skin. There is increased heat, skin thickening, and an overall firmness to the skin that can be localized or involve almost the entire breast. The changes noted are not specific to inflammatory carcinoma and can be seen with any lesion or disease that decreases lymphatic drainage of the breast, e.g., marked congestive heart failure, obstruction of the vena cava, after lymph node dissection of the axilla (unusual), postradiation therapy in the early stages of recovery, and tuberculosis and other inflammatory diseases of the axillary nodes.

Thermography is variable. In lesions less than 1 cm in size there may be increased heat or vascularity in more than 50 percent of cases. As the size of the lesion increases, so does the incidence of positive thermograms, approaching 80 percent. The thermogram is nonspecific in that it does not demonstrate the location of the cancer but reflects the metabolic activity of the tumor. A deep-seated tumor may show an increase in nipple heat because of the conduction of this heat through the ductal system, the tumor being far removed from the area of the increased superficial heat.

Isard, Amalric and Gautherie have shown that in cancers with a marked thermographic response the survival rates are decreased. The experience of some thermographers is that a positive thermogram may precede detection of the cancer by many years (see Chapter 5).

Diaphanography is more specific for locating cancers than thermography. The tumor may appear as an area of diminished light transmission. In some cases there is increased vascularity. The closer the tumor is to the surface of the breast, the more the size on diaphanography approximates the actual tumor size. The larger the tumor, the easier it is to see on the light scan; however, there are reports of nonpalpable tumors being found on diaphanography and not on other imaging studies. The greater the vascularity of the tumor and the greater the amount of dense fibrotic material, the more positive is the diaphanography.

Ultrasound of the breast has proved to be a valuable adjunct in the detection of breast cancer. Originally promoted as a screening device, it has now been shown to be inconsistent in the detection of cancers less than 1 cm in size; however, it can find cancers undetected by mammography in a significant percentage of cases. McSweeney and Egan reported that 7 percent of their cancers were found by ultrasound only. Montalava reported that the addition of ultrasound to mammography increased accuracy to 98 percent.

The lesion is usually an area of low-level echoes. The borders, although well defined in some cancers such as a medullary cancer, are usually irregular. There may be minimal or marked shadowing seen behind the tumor or just from the edges of the lesion. Whole breast ultrasound with the breast hanging free within the waterbath is very sensitive for showing minimal skin dimpling or retraction. Cooper's ligaments, when involved, may appear as thickened echoes on the scan. There may be increased echoes seen in the subcutaneous tissues and occasionally skin thickening.

Mammography is still the best test for demonstrating the presence of cancers. Whereas most mammographers report an accuracy between 80 and 85 percent, others have shown an ability to detect almost 95 percent of the cancers. In addition, mammography has been shown to be the only examination that can detect minimal breast cancer with any degree of consistency. In the Breast Cancer Detection Demonstration Project (BCDDP) approximately 45 percent of the cancers were found by mammography alone, with a negative physical examination. The development of grids and magnification has increased the ability to find cancers earlier.

Approximately 40 percent of cancers have malignant calcifications, which have been described as small (punctate) and irregular, with a variation in size. They may also be rodlike or branching. The number of calcifications may vary greatly from three to innumerable. As the number increases, so does the likelihood of malignancy. Calcifications are more common in colloid, intraductal, and ductal carcinomas, although they may appear with any malignancy.

If evident on mammography, the mass may be well defined, as with medullary carcinoma, or irregular and poorly defined with indescript borders. The density of the lesion is usually increased with respect to the surrounding tissue. Many tumors show tenacles of tumor extending into the surrounding tissue, described as spiculization. If involved, Cooper's ligaments may be thickened and straightened, and skin retraction and thickening may be evident.

The signs on mammography may be very subtle. An area of asymmetry may signal an early cancer. Comparison with previous mammograms, when possible, may be very helpful. With the better and more advanced mammography and magnification views now available, it is possible to see some areas with better definition. Care should be taken when calling an abnormality a new finding; however, if we are to err, it should be on the side of aggressiveness and biopsy, as the consequences of a missed cancer are greater than those of a benign biopsy. Another subtle sign may be dilatation of a single or a small group of ducts. Although important at any age, it is more important in the older patient. Most often at surgery there are dilated but empty ducts, probably secondary to a sloughed area of papilloma; however, an intraductal or ductal carcinoma is found often enough to warrant investigation.

Lymph nodes are frequently seen on the mammogram. Usually they are small and shotty, and represent old inflammatory nodes. When a large node is seen, the possibility of lymphoma or active infection is considered. Occasionally malignant calcifications are seen in a node. On rare occasions lymph node masses become necrotic, and on ultrasound may appear cystic.

Ideally, the cancer is found before it is palpable and before there are lymph node metastases. In order for this to happen on a greater scale than is now prevalent, screening asymptomatic patients is necessary. Although thermography or diaphanography may prove in the future to be helpful, mammography currently offers the best means of this early detection. Every effort should be made to obtain the best possible films, with good detail and compression.

Case Studies: Infiltrating Ductal Carcinoma

Case 1

L.M. is a 37-year-old woman who presented with a 6 mm nodule in the right breast of 3 weeks' duration. Prior to the current presentation a surgeon had attempted aspiration of the nodule, with no fluid obtained.

On physical examination the nodule was firm and movable. Thermograms, diaphanography, mammography, and ultrasound were all normal.

It was thought that this might be a glandular nodule. The patient returned 1 month later, and the nodule was slightly larger. A biopsy revealed infiltrating ductal carcinoma. She underwent lumpectomy, axillary node dissection (with all nodes negative), and a course of radiation therapy. At 36 months there has been no evidence of recurrence.

Case 2

M.L. is a 53-year-old woman who was seen 6 months earlier at a university breast clinic with a left breast mass. Mammograms done at that time were reported as showing marked glandularity without a discernible mass. No further studies or biopsy were performed.

On physical examination there was a 1.5 cm hard, firm mass in the upper outer left breast. Liquid crystal thermograms demonstrated increased vascularity on the left (Th III thermogram) (Color Fig. 13). Diaphanography showed a marked decrease in light transmission through the mass (Fig. 21-1A). Mammograms showed an asymmetry with an increase in glandular tissue in the upper outer left breast without a discrete mass or calcifications (Fig. 21-1B,C). There was no change from the mammograms done 6 months earlier. Ultrasound showed shadowing in this area without a discrete mass (Fig. 21-1D).

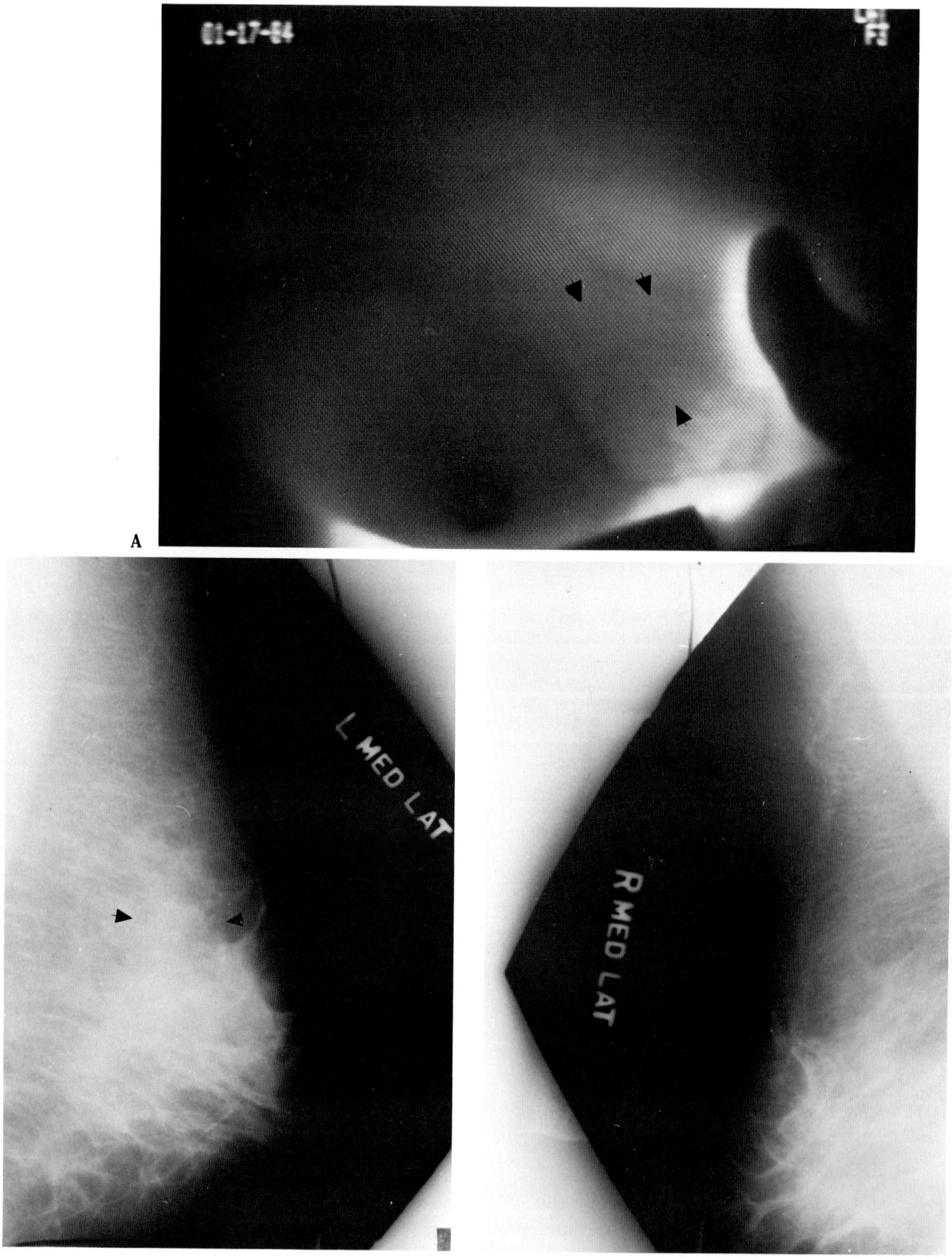

Fig. 21-1 A: Diaphanography. Note the decreased light transmission over the lateral left breast (arrows). **B:** Mammogram, left lateral view. There is increased tissue density in the upper outer left breast (arrow). Compare with **C**. **C:** Mammograph, right lateral view. Normal glandularity. *(Figure continues.)*

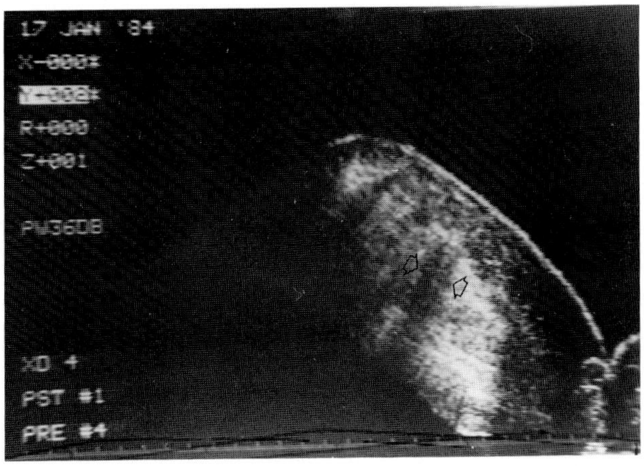

D

Fig. 21-1 D: Ultrasound. Note the area of shadowing (open arrow); there is no mass.

A needle biopsy demonstrated cells suspicious for malignancy. A formal biopsy demonstrated an infiltrating ductal carcinoma. Subsequently the patient underwent a modified radical mastectomy, and all nodes were negative.

Case 3

S.C. is a 47-year-old woman who was self-referred for a screening breast examination because of her family history: Her mother had had breast cancer at age 51. On physical examination no abnormality was detected. Liquid crystal thermograms demonstrated increased nipple heat and vascularity on the right (Th III thermogram) (Color Fig. 14). Diaphanography was normal. Mammograms showed benign calcifications on the lower right and a group of rodlike calcifications at 12 o'clock on the right without a mass (Fig. 21-2). Ultrasound was normal.

Following preoperative mammographic localization a biopsy was performed, and a 5 mm area of intraductal carcinoma was found. On reexamination of the slides a

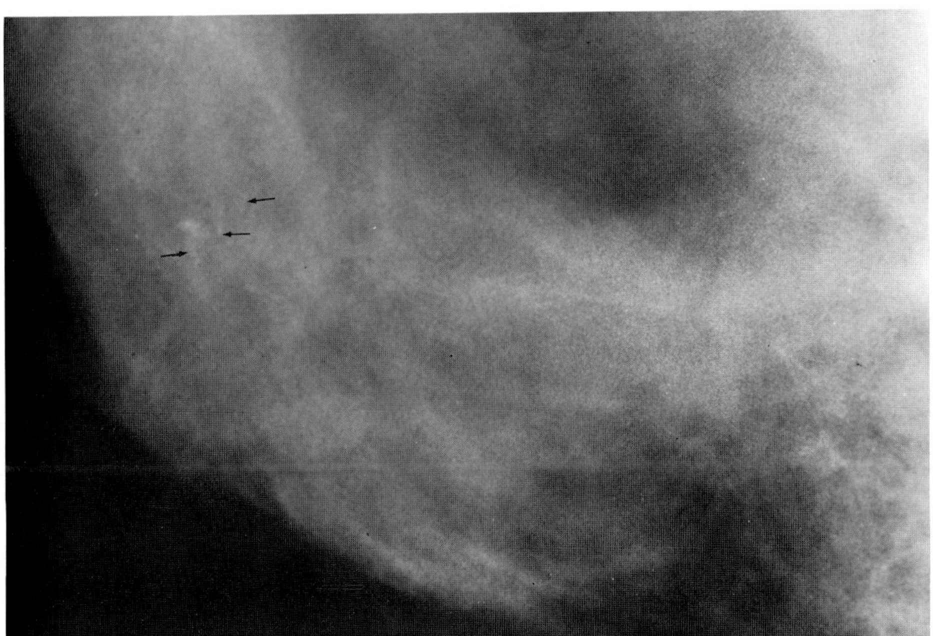

Fig. 21-2 Mammogram, magnified. Rodlike calcifications (arrows) are present without a mass.

single area of microinvasion was seen. Because of the very minimal invasion it was elected not to do an axillary dissection. The patient was treated with lumpectomy and irradiation. There has been no recurrence at 24 months.

Case 4

R.W. is a 41-year-old woman who was referred because of a ropey area in the upper outer right breast, thought to be glandular tissue by the primary physician.

On our physical examination there was an irregular area which felt somewhat ropey in nature. There was very slight retraction over the area when the patient's arms were extended forward. Liquid crystal thermograms were very positive on the right (Th IV pattern), with a diffuse increase in heat (Color Fig. 15). Diaphanography demonstrated a slight decrease in light transmission over the area. Mammograms showed a dense glandular breast (P2 pattern), with multiple microcalcifications in the tail of the right breast (Fig. 21-3A). Ultrasound showed skin thickening, retraction, and an increase in the echo pattern in the subcutaneous tissues. No discrete mass was seen (Fig. 12-3B).

A biopsy revealed extensive intraductal carcinoma and an infiltrating ductal carcinoma, primarily comedo type. The patient underwent a lumpectomy, axillary node dissection (all nodes negative), and radiation therapy. There has been a recurrence at 24 months.

Case 5

L.L. is a 56-year-old woman who was referred because of a left breast lump. On physical examination there was a 1 by 2 cm somewhat ovoid density in the inner aspect of the left breast which felt like a ridge when the patient was erect and like a mass when she was supine.

Thermograms demonstrated a slight asymmetry with some increased heat on the left, but within normal limits. Diaphanography was normal. On mammography there was moderate glandularity (P2 pattern), with malignant-type calcifications within a poorly defined mass in the inner aspect of the left breast (Fig. 21-4A). Ultrasound showed an area of decreased echoes with shadowing (Fig. 21-4B).

Biopsy revealed infiltrating ductal carcinoma arising in a comedocarcinoma. On axillary node dissection 1 of 28 nodes was positive. The patient has refused further therapy. There has been no recurrence at 2 years.

Case 6

K.C. is a 48-year-old woman who hit her breast against the side of a dresser. The breast subsequently became inflamed and swollen. She presented, self-referred, a month later. On physical examination there was a hard, firm 2 by 4 cm mass in the lower outer aspect of the left breast. In addition, there was a 3 cm firm, rounded mass in the lower axilla.

Liquid crystal thermograms showed the presence of an abnormal draining vein in the inferior portion of the left breast, making this a positive Th III thermogram (Color Fig. 16). On diaphanography there was a very slight decrease in light transmission (Fig. 21-5A). Mammography showed a 1 by 2 cm somewhat poorly defined mass, with the posterior borders not seen owing to overlying glandular tissue. There was a well defined 3 cm mass in the left axilla thought to represent a lymph node (Fig. 21-5B). Ultrasound demonstrated a poorly defined mass with low-level echoes (Figs. 21-5C, D).

Because of the traumatic incident the possibility that this lesion represented an area of fat necrosis with a reactive node in the axilla was raised, although the possibility of cancer was considered. A biopsy revealed a 1.5 cm infiltrating ductal carcinoma. The node was involved with tumor. One additional node of 18 was positive. The patient underwent lumpectomy, node dissection, and radiation therapy. There has been no recurrence at 24 months (Color Fig. 17; Fig. 21-5E).

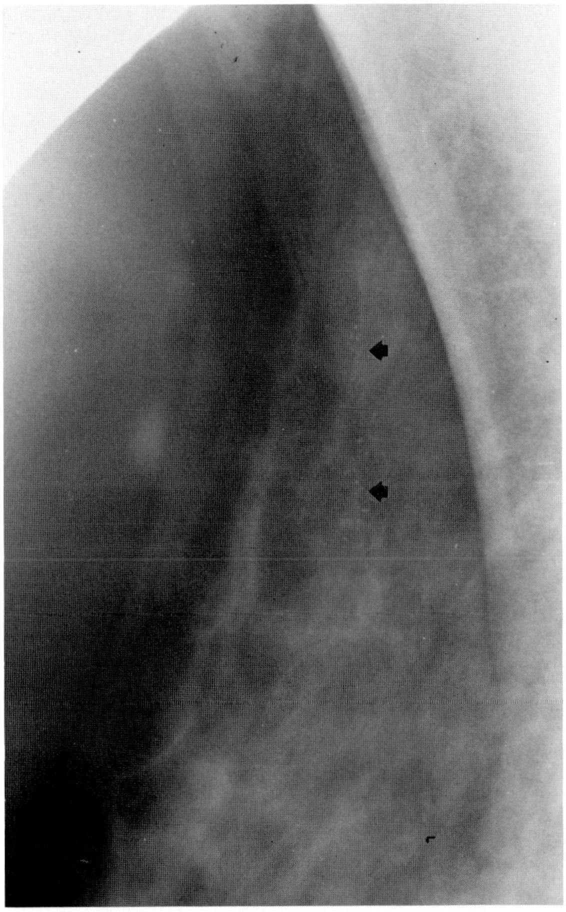

A

Fig. 21-3 **A:** Mammogram, magnified. Note the diffuse punctate calcifications in the tail of the right breast (arrows). **B:** Ultrasound. Note the skin thickening and slight skin retraction (arrows). Skin thickening shows as a double line.

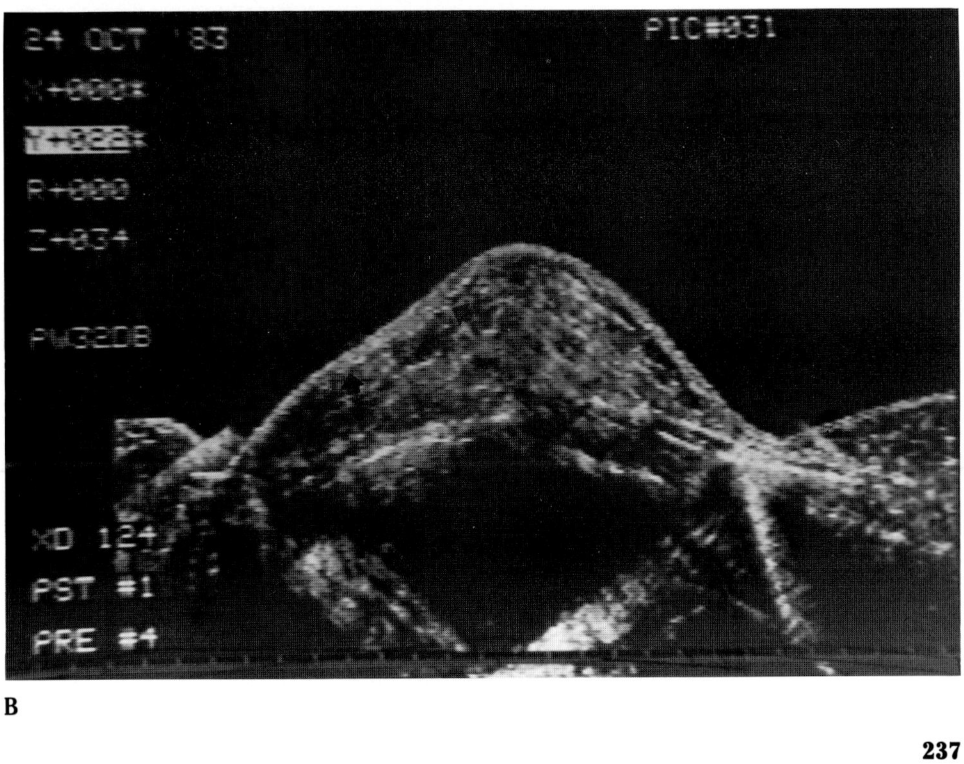

B

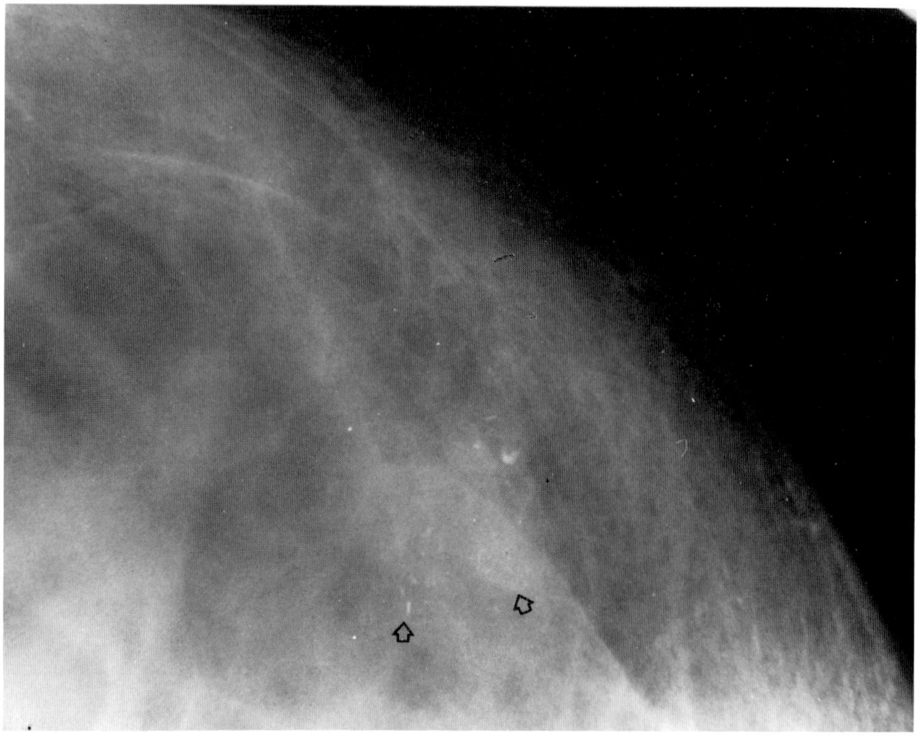

A

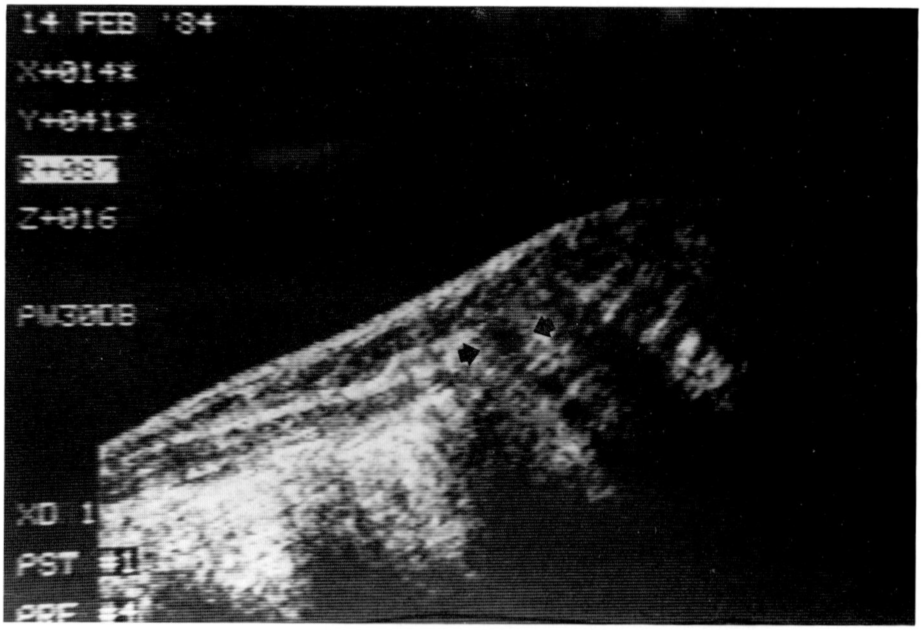

B

Fig. 21-4 **A:** Mammogram, magnified. Malignant calcifications (arrows) are seen. **B:** Ultrasound. Note the low-level echo area (open arrows) with shadowing.

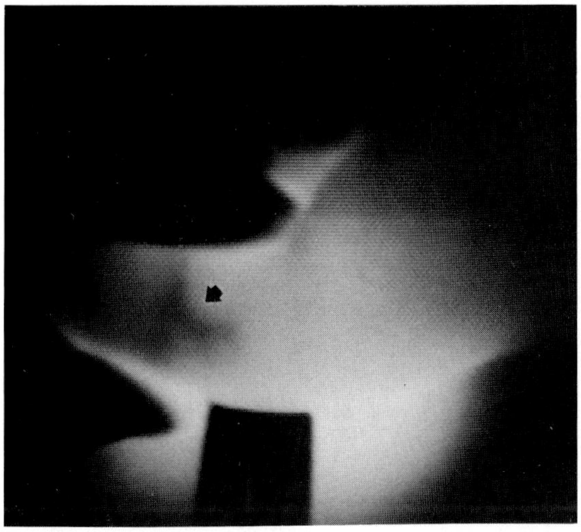

A

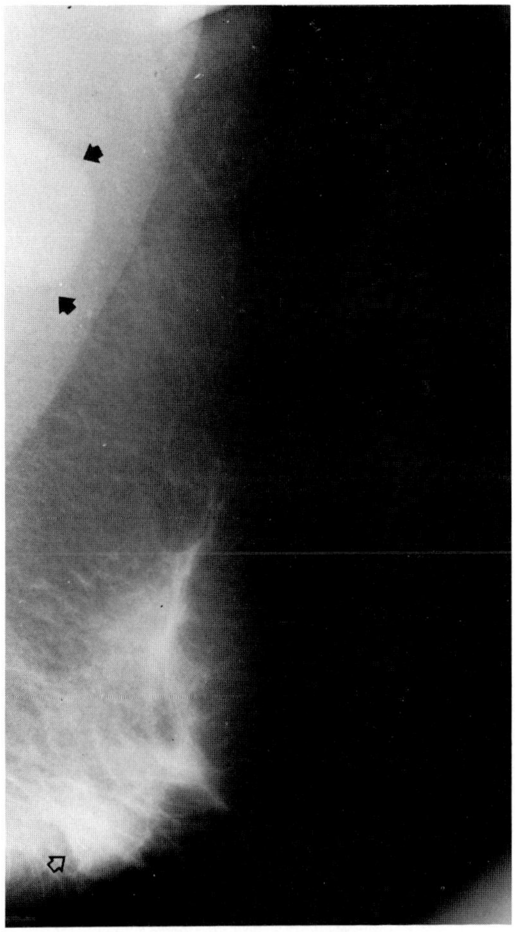

B

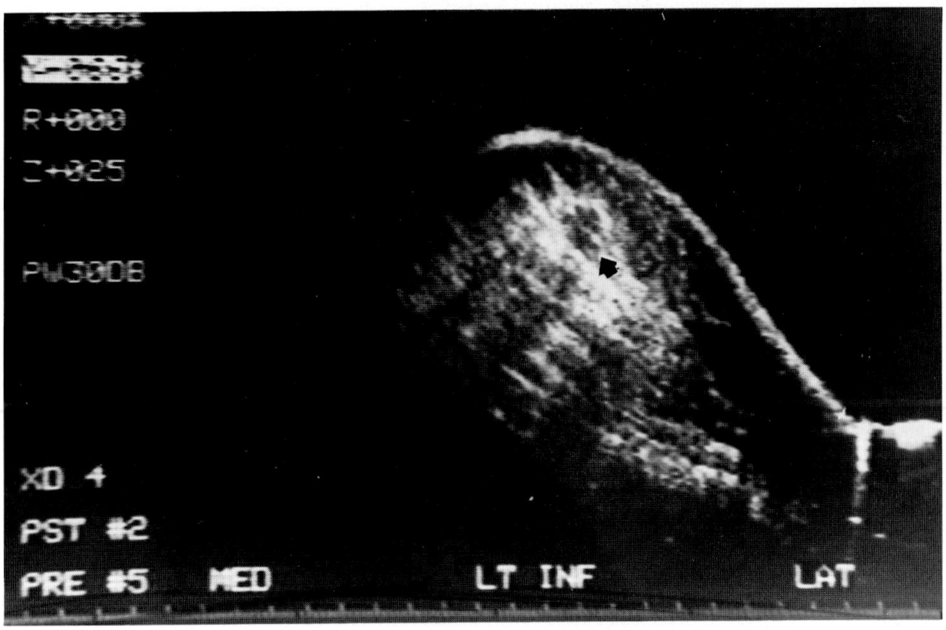

C

Fig. 21-5 **A:** Diaphanography. Note the area of decreased light transmission and the prominent superficial vein (arrow). **B:** Mammogram. Note the large lymph node in the axilla (arrows). There is a well defined mass inferior to the nipple (open arrow). **C:** Ultrasound. There is an irregular low-level mass (arrow) with some edge shadowing. *(Figure continues.)*

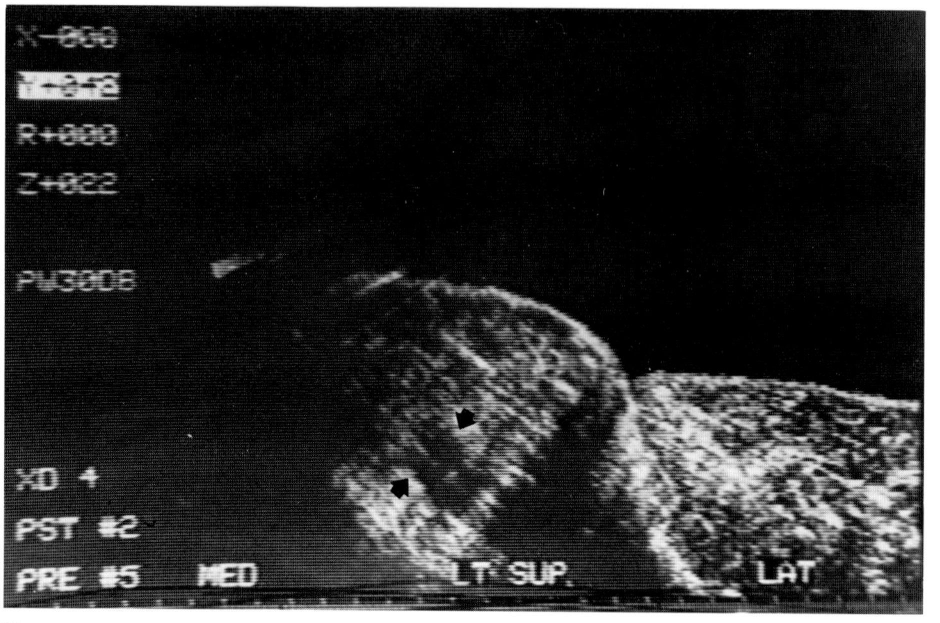

D

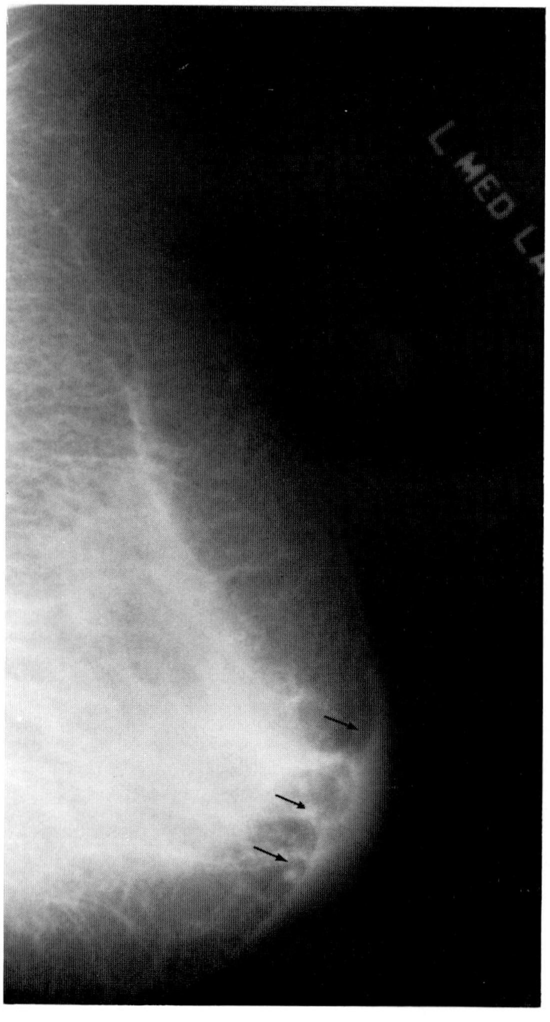

E

Fig. 21-5 D: Ultrasound, axillary lymph node. Note the low-level echo mass (arrows) with slightly increased through transmission. The marked shadowing is due to an axillary skinfold.
E: Postirradiation mammogram. Note the skin thickening near the nipple (arrows). Masses are absent.

Case 7

V.D. is a 57-year-old woman who was referred because of a left breast mass of 9 months' duration. On physical examination there was an ill-defined, approximately 3 cm mass in the lower outer aspect of the left breast. There was retraction over the mass, with deviation of the nipple laterally.

Liquid crystal thermograms demonstrated an abnormal vascular pattern (Th IV thermogram). On diaphanography there was marked light absorption in the area of the mass (Fig. 21-6A). Mammograms showed an irregular 2 by 3 cm mass with spiculization and stringing extending toward the deformed nipple (Fig. 21-6B).

Biopsy revealed a 2.4 cm infiltrating, focally necrotic, ductal carcinoma. At mastectomy there was a separate focus of infiltrating ductal carcinoma. Two of 15 nodes were positive.

Case 8

S.S is a 76-year-old woman who 7 years earlier had had a carcinoma of the right breast treated with a modified radical mastectomy. She was referred because of a questionable left breast mass. On physical examination there was a diffuse hardness in the upper portion of the left breast extending to behind the nipple; no discrete mass was identified. There was a slight retraction just below the nipple when the patient had her hands on her hips and used pectoralis pressure. In addition, there was a profuse serous discharge from the mid-nipple.

Liquid crystal thermograms demonstrated an abnormal vascular pattern. On diaphanography there was a diffuse decrease in light transmission throughout the mid-portion of the breast (Fig. 21-7A). Mammograms demonstrated punctate calcifications posteriorly and in the mid-portion of the breast (Fig. 21-7B). Ultrasound showed the presence of a poorly defined 1 cm mass against the chest wall where the calcifications were seen. In addition, there was slight flattening just behind the nipple, with a suggestion of an additional mass (Fig. 21-7C,D).

At biopsy and subsequent mastectomy there were multiple foci of intraductal carcinoma and an infiltrating ductal carcinoma against the chest wall. In addition, there were florid fibrocystic changes, and beneath the nipple area was a large intraductal papilloma. The patient underwent a modified radical mastectomy.

Case 9

B.M. is a 66-year-old woman referred for screening. On physical examination there were large breasts without a mass. Liquid crystal thermograms demonstrated increased nipple heat and vascularity on the left (Th III thermogram). Diaphanography was normal. On mammography there was atrophy of the glandular tissue (N1 pattern). There was a 1 cm spiculated lesion with questionable small calcifications in the upper portion of the left breast. On review of outside mammograms obtained 8 years earlier, the lesion was present and 5 mm in size (Fig. 21-8A,B).

At surgery a 1 cm infiltrating ductal carcinoma was found. The patient underwent lumpectomy and radiation therapy. (Interestingly, she has been angry that a cancer was found and has refused to return for checkups.)

Discussion

The cases presented have been chosen to demonstrate the wide clinical range of infiltrating ductal carcinoma, as well as the variety of presentations seen on the various imaging procedures.

In case 1 there was a small palpable nodule with all imaging procedures normal. This picture is similar to the presentation of the lobular carcinoma in case 31. With nodules that small it may not be possible to visualize these nodules with presently available imaging procedures. That is why the physical examination plays an essential part in the discovery of cancer and must not be ignored. This is further

A

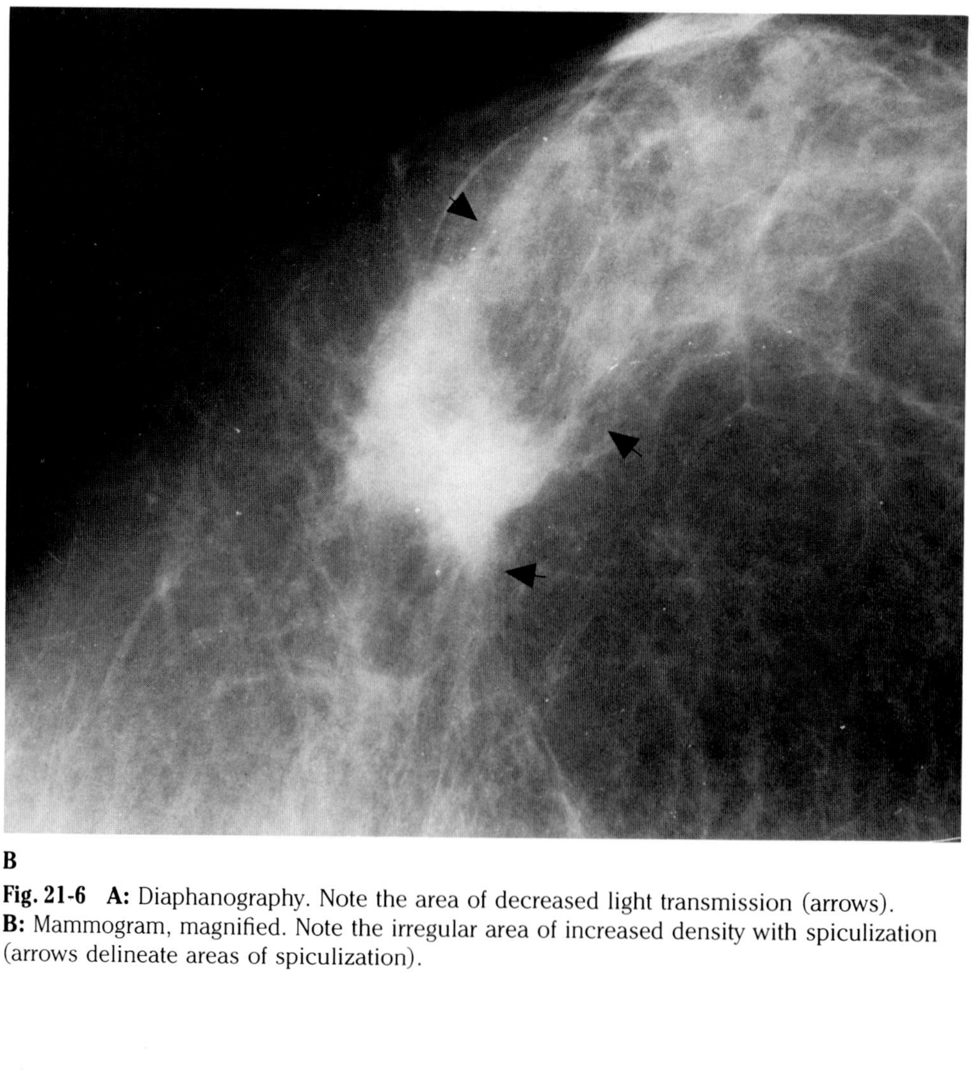

B

Fig. 21-6 **A:** Diaphanography. Note the area of decreased light transmission (arrows). **B:** Mammogram, magnified. Note the irregular area of increased density with spiculization (arrows delineate areas of spiculization).

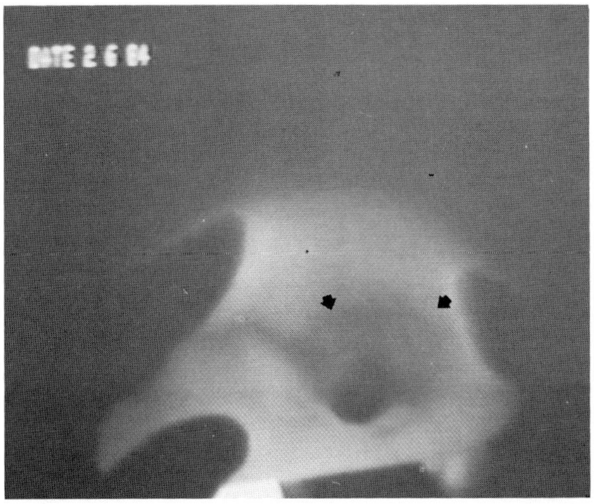

A

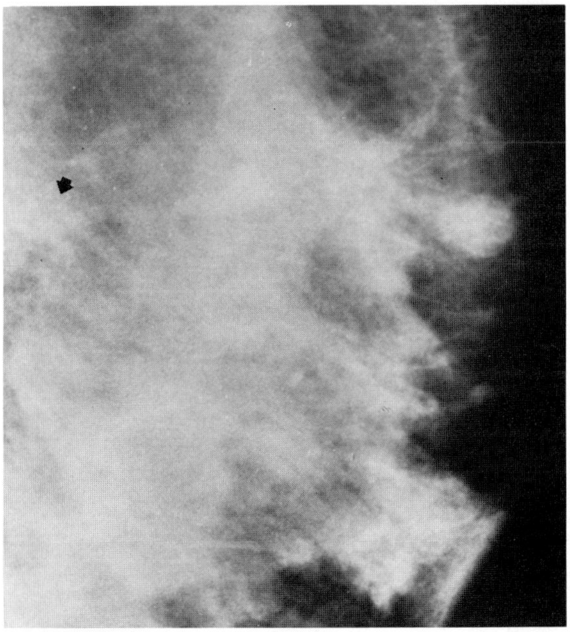

B

Fig. 21-7 **A:** Diaphanography. Note the area of decreased light transmission above and behind the nipple (arrows). **B:** Mammogram, magnified. Punctate calcifications (because of the photographic process they appear amorphous) (arrow) are present. There are scattered groups of calcification between the posterior calcification and the nipple. **C:** Ultrasound. There is marked nipple shadowing. The area of widening of nipple shadows (arrow) represents carcinoma. **D:** Ultrasound, slightly more lateral view. The irregular echo-free area represents another portion of the carcinoma seen in **B.**

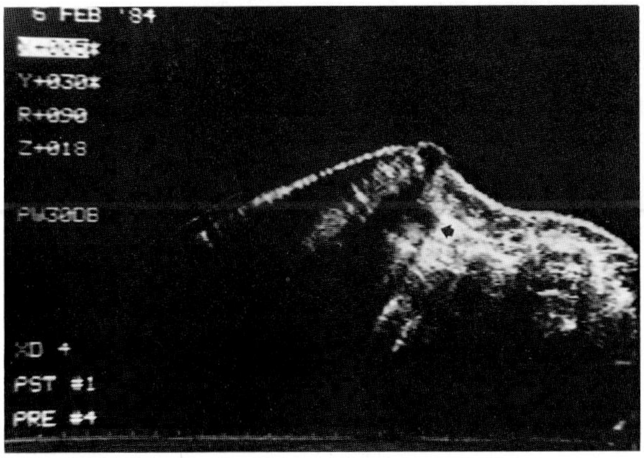

C

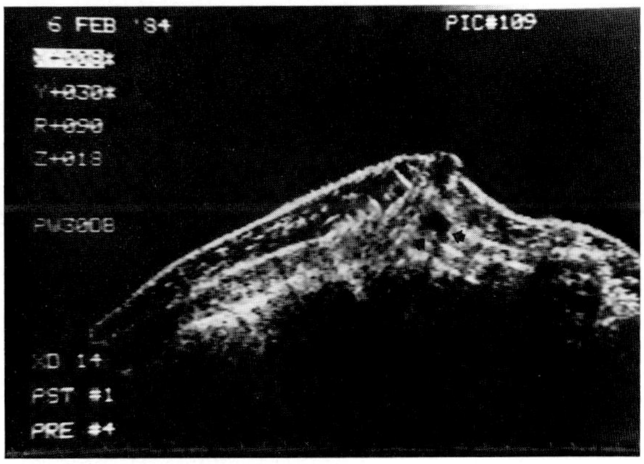

D

A

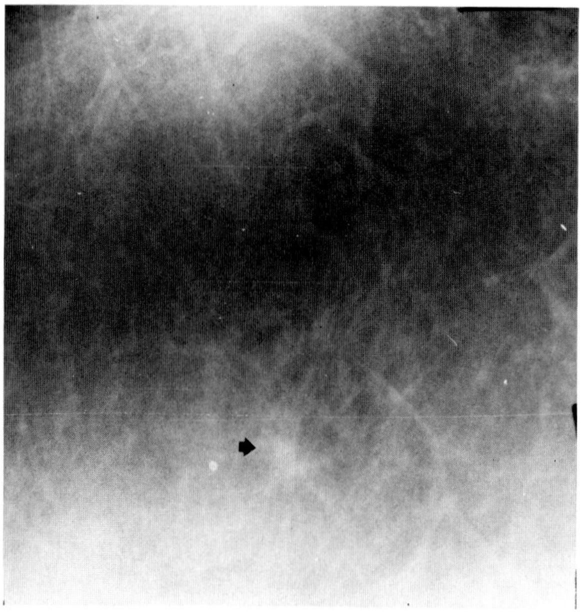

B

Fig. 21-8 **A:** Mammogram, magnified, 1976. Note the 5 mm poorly defined slightly spiculated area (arrow). Detail has been lost in trying to show the area because of the relative lack of contrast in this old film. **B:** Mammogram, magnified, 1984. Note the spiculated 8 mm lesion (arrow).

demonstrated in case 2 where there was a mass present. The minimal asymmetry on the mammogram was not appreciated. In cases where a mass is present, even if the studies are normal, biopsy is essential. (See case 33 in the section of medullary carcinoma.

Case 3 showed a positive thermogram and mammogram whereas other studies were normal, and in case 2 the thermogram and diaphanography were positive and the mammogram and ultrasound were only slightly suggestive. The physical examination was positive in most of the cases, although it was negative in case 3 and only minimally suggestive in case 4.

Case 8 demonstrated the presence of two abnormal areas on mammography and ultrasound. The more posterior of these two was a carcinoma, whereas the anterior mass was a large papilloma. The profuse nipple discharge was probably due to the papilloma, although it could have been caused by either lesion, or both.

Case 9 is unusual in that the carcinoma was seen in retrospect on mammograms 8 years earlier. This growth rate is extremely slow.

Case Studies: Multicentric Carcinoma In The Same Breast

Case 10

K.P. is a 45-year-old woman who was referred because of a 1 cm movable density at 12 o'clock in the right breast. On physical examination a very slight skin retraction was also noted inferomedially on the right with some thickening.

Liquid crystal thermograms demonstrated increased nipple heat on the right (Th III thermogram). Diaphanography showed a slight decrease in light transmission over the right nodule. No change could be seen in the area of retraction. Mammograms showed a moderately glandular breast (P2 pattern). There was a spiculated lesion with calcifications in the upper right, multiple areas of clumped calcifications on the right, and an asymmetrical area of glandularity in the inferior right breast with some thickening of Cooper's ligaments (Fig. 21-9A). On ultrasound there was shadowing from the density superiorly and a poorly defined area inferiorly (Fig. 21-9B).

The patient subsequently underwent a modified radical mastectomy. A multifocal carcinoma with infiltrating ductal carcinoma was found superiorly, and infiltrating lobular carcinoma was found inferiorly. At 11 months an 8 mm skin nodule appeared on the chest wall that was found to be recurrent ductal carcinoma.

Case 11

H.M. is a 72-year-old woman who presented with a 5 cm mass of 2 months' duration in the outer inferior portion of the right breast. In addition, there was a 2 cm poorly defined mass in the upper inner right breast. The breasts were somewhat "pancake" in configuration.

On thermography there was increased vascularity inferiorly and an edge sign on the right (Th IV thermogram) (Color Fig. 18). On diaphanography there was diminished light transmission in the upper right area and a dark rim and dark center with a relative increased light area otherwise within the large right mass (Figs. 21-10A,B). Mammograms demonstrated a spiculated irregular mass with calcifications in the inner upper right breast, and a 7.5 cm mass with a slightly irregular border in the outer lower portion of the right breast (Fig. 21-10C). Ultrasound over the upper mass demonstrated a low-level mass with posterior shadowing (Fig. 21-10D). The larger mass was primarily fluid with a solid portion posteriorly, with poor through transmission (Fig. 21-10E).

The larger mass was aspirated, and brownish fluid was removed. A pneumocystogram was performed. Not all the fluid has been removed, so the air formed bubbles within the mass. The air was noted not to fill the posterior area of the mass, and on the magnification views for the pneumocystogram spiculization was noted posteriorly (Fig. 21-10F).

The patient subsequently underwent biopsy and mastectomy. The upper lesion was an infiltrating ductal carcinoma. The larger mass was a hemorrhagic cyst, the posterior margin of which contained a second primary of infiltrating ductal carcinoma arising within an area of intraductal carcinoma. All nodes were negative.

Case 12

C.C. is a 42-year-old woman who presented with a 1.5 cm hard nodule in the inner aspect of the right breast almost adjacent to the skinfold. Thermograms were slightly positive on the right. There was a marked decrease in light transmission over the nodule (Fig. 21-11A). Mammograms demonstrated a P2 pattern. There was an irregular mass with calcifications medially. In addition, there was a group of microcalcifications oriented along a duct in the mid-portion of the breast (Figs. 21-11B,C). Ultrasound showed marked shadowing behind the medial density; the area of calcifications was not identified (Fig. 21-11D).

At biopsy the nodule was found to be in situ (intraductal) and infiltrating ductal carcinoma. After mammographic localization the calcifications were within multiple foci of well differentiated ductal carcinoma. The patient underwent a modified radical mastectomy, and all nodes were negative. There has been no recurrence at 2 years.

Case 13

N.F. is a 46-year-old woman who presented with a hard nodule, just under 1 cm in size, at 12 o'clock on the right. On the left, high on the chest wall at 12 o'clock there was a tender 1.5 cm nodule and just below this area a larger density somewhat discrete from the glandularity of the breast. The thermograms and diaphanography were within normal limits. Mammograms demonstrated marked glandularity (P2 pattern), an irregular density in the upper left breast with spiculated borders, and a separate additional mass also with irregular borders just above this against the chest wall (Fig. 21-12A). The lesion on the right was not seen mammographically. On ultrasound there was a

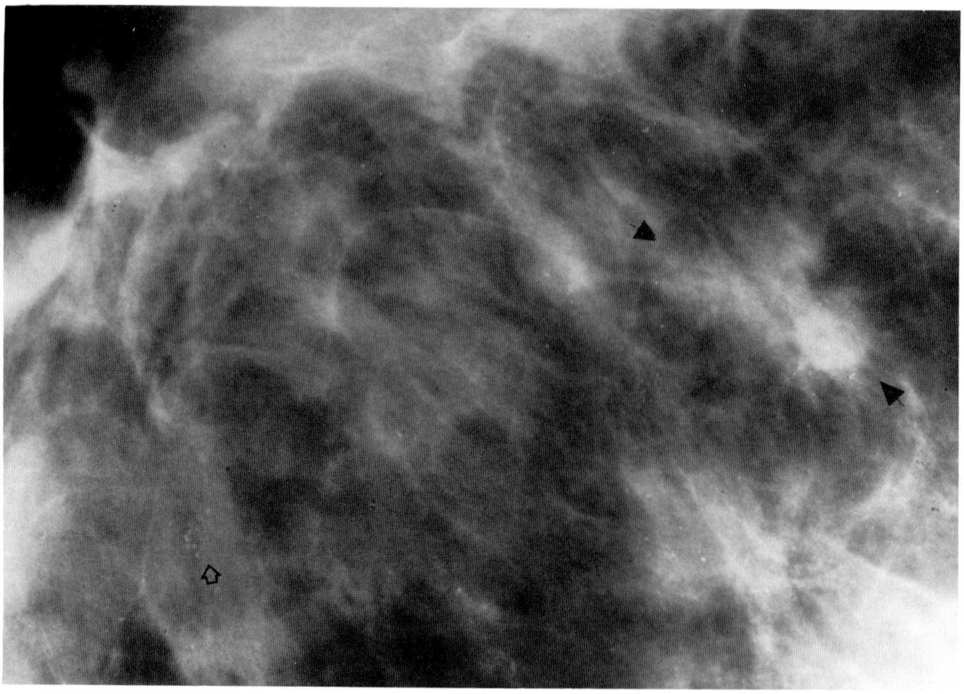

A

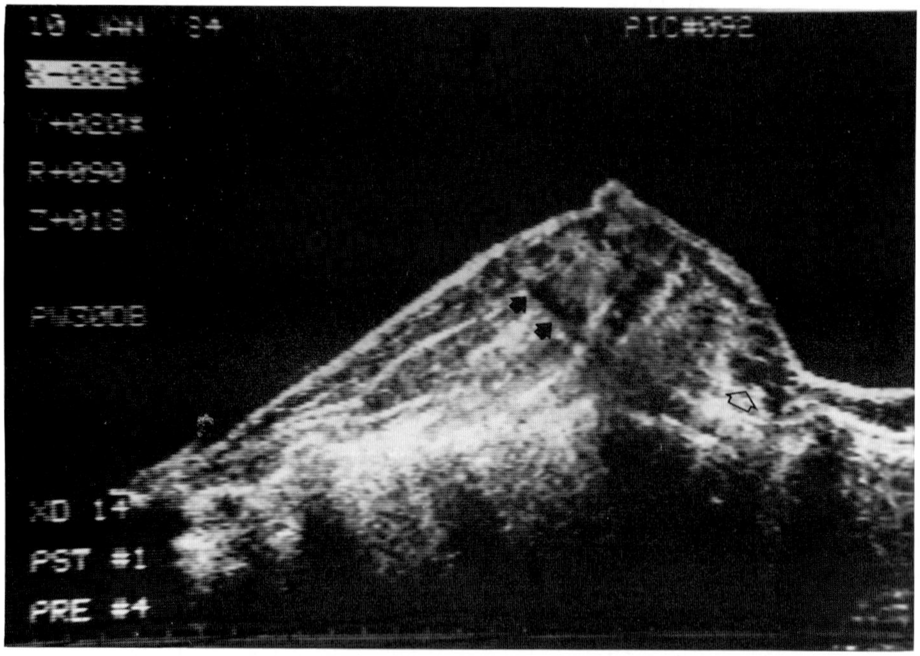

B

Fig. 21-9 A: Mammogram, magnified. Note the dense spiculated lesion with small calcifications (arrows); clumped calcifications are probably within a lobule (open arrow). **B:** Ultrasound. Note the shadowing from a spiculated lesion (arrows) superiorly and the low-level echo area inferiorly (open arrow). Both areas were cancers.

A
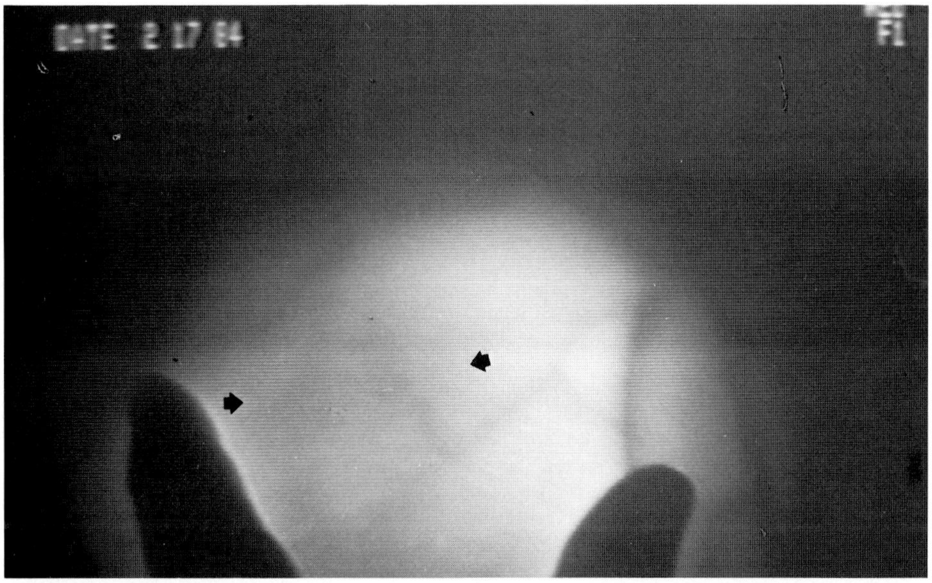

B
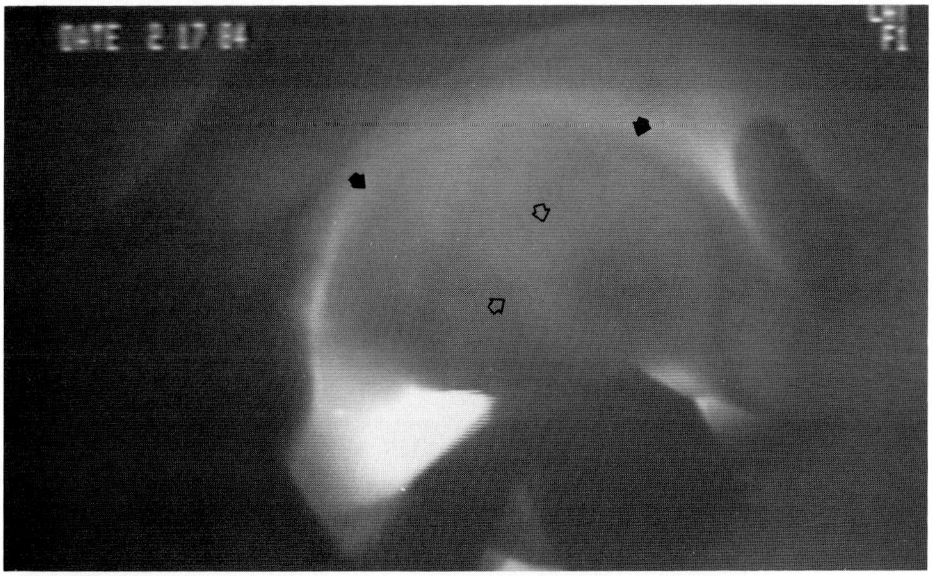

C
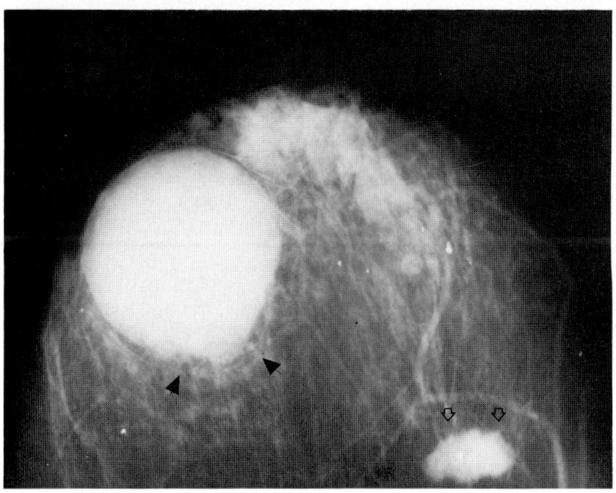

Fig. 21-10 A: Diaphanography. There is a slight decrease in light transmission over the upper lesion (arrows).
B: Diaphanography. There is a marked decrease in light transmission over the large mass (arrows) with slightly increased light transmission in the center of the mass (open arrow).
C: Mammogram, CC view. Note the smaller lesion (open arrows) with spiculization and the larger mass with a slightly irregular posterior border (arrows). *(Figure continues.)*

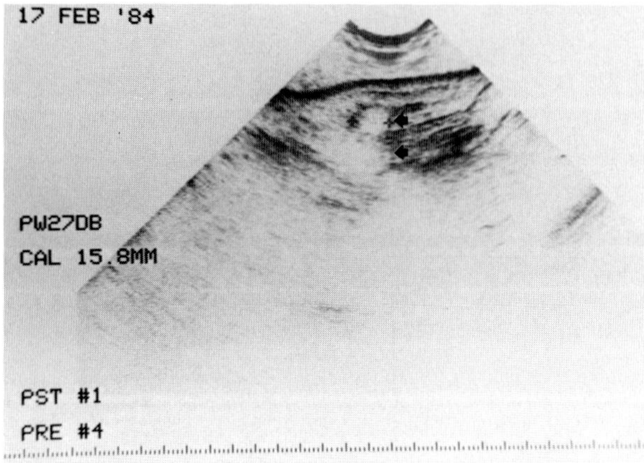

D

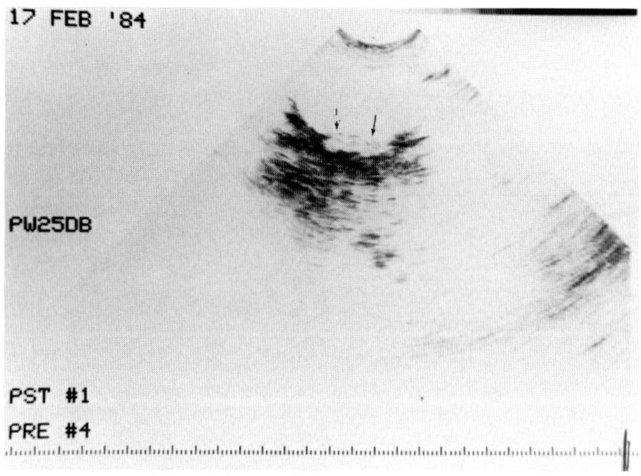

E

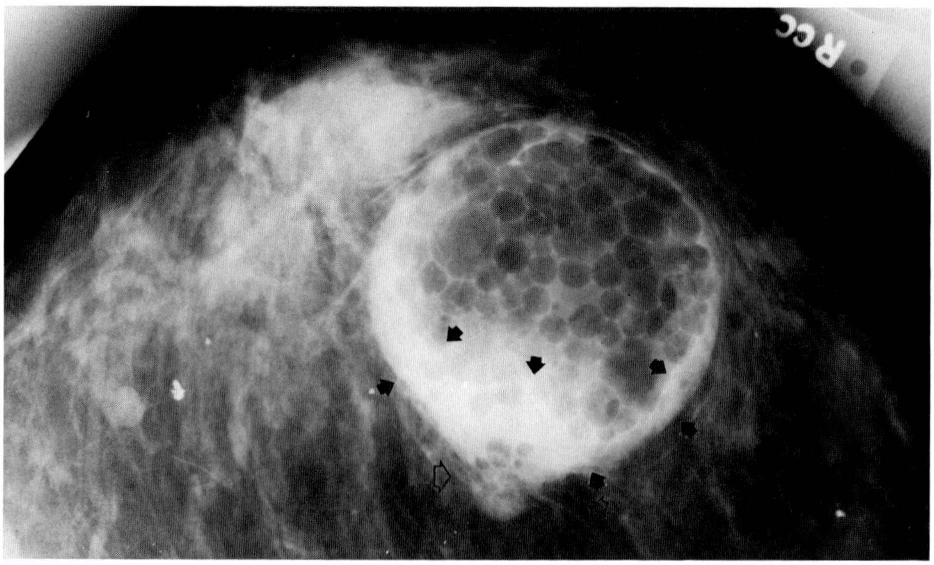

F

Fig. 21-10 D: Ultrasound: upper mass. Note the low-level echo mass with posterior shadowing (arrows).
E: Ultrasound. The fluid portion of the mass is echo-free, superiorly. Note also the solid posterior portion of the mass (arrows).
F: Pneumocystogram, magnified. Diffuse air bubbles occupy most of the mass. The air bubbles are due to incomplete emptying of the fluid and a mixture of the air and fluid. Note the thick wall of the mass posteriorly (arrows) and the spiculated lesion extending off the posterior aspect of the mass (open arrows). This could not be appreciated in **C.**

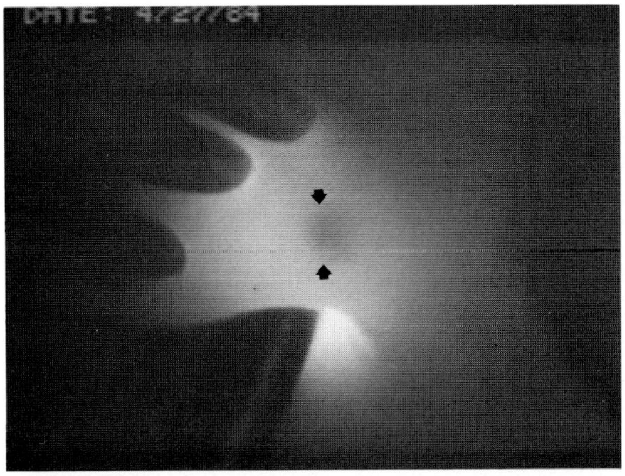

A

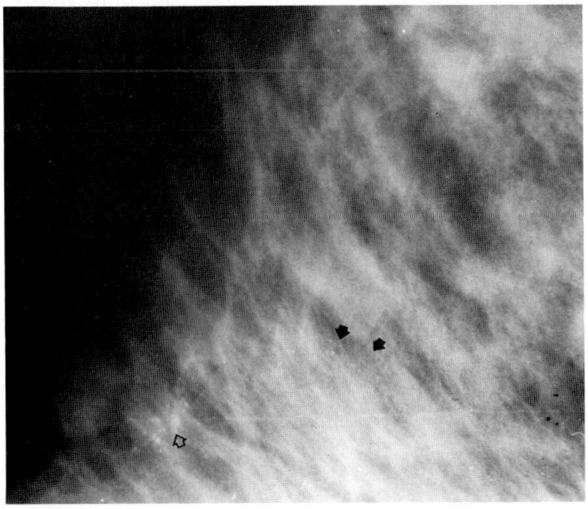

B

Fig. 21-11 A: Diaphanography. Note the small area of decreased light transmission (arrows) in the medial aspect of the right breast. **B:** Mammogram, magnified, inferior aspect, lateral view. Microcalcifications are noted along the duct (arrows), as is an irregular mass with calcifications (open arrow). **C:** Mammogram, CC view, inner aspect of the right breast, magnified. There is an irregular lesion with microcalcifications (arrows). **D:** Ultrasound, medial aspect of the right breast. Note the irregular density with shadowing (arrows).

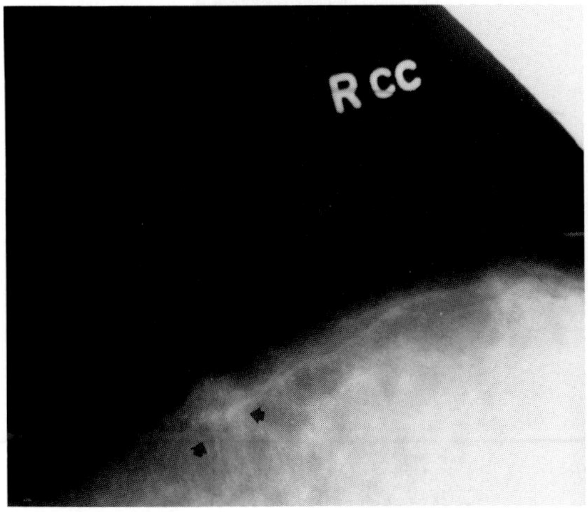

C

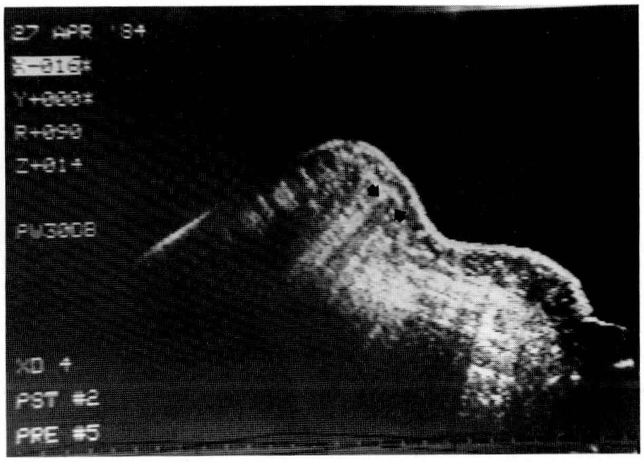

D

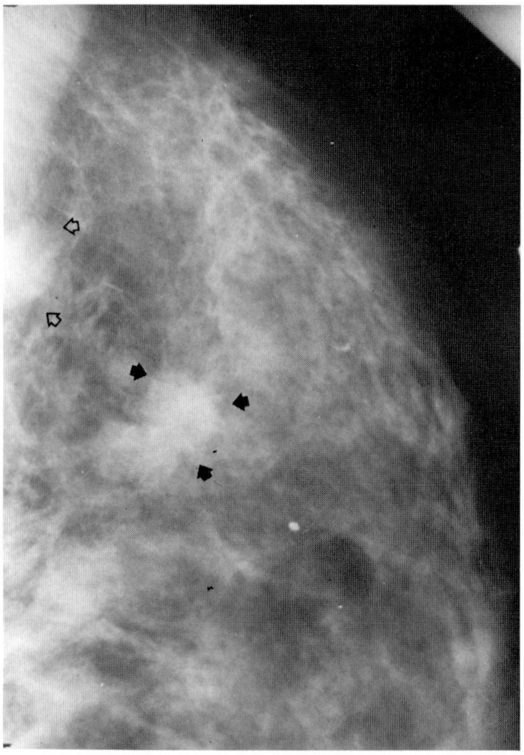

A

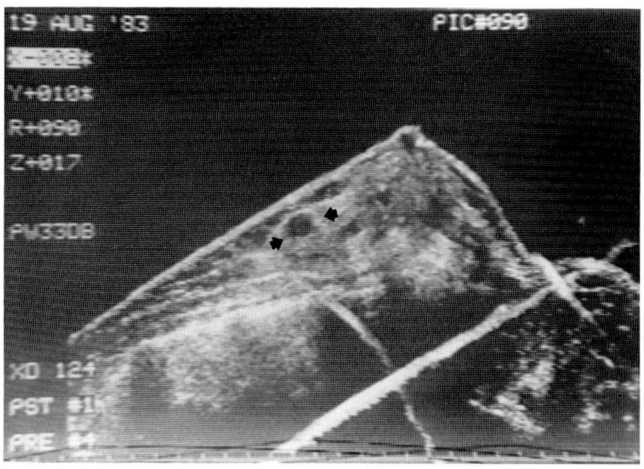

B

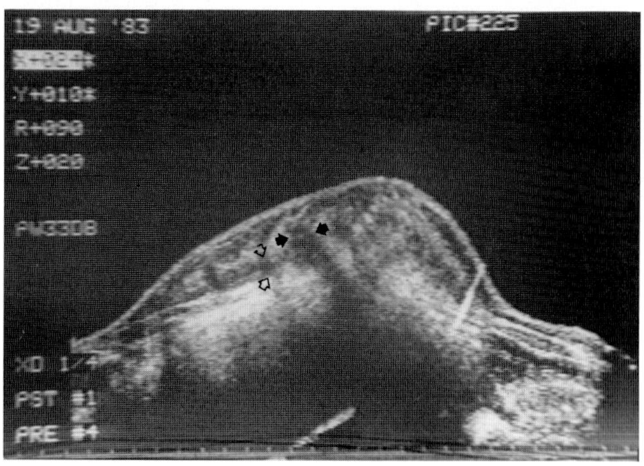

C

Fig. 21-12 **A:** Mammogram, magnified, upper left breast, lateral view. Bilobed mass with spiculization (arrows). There is an irregular dense mass (open arrows) against the pectoralis muscle. **B:** Ultrasound, longitudinal view, right breast. There is a well defined low-level echo mass (arrows) with no increased through transmission. It is a fibroadenoma. **C:** Ultrasound, longitudinal view, left breast. There is a mass with shadowing (arrows) and a second mass, appearing as a low-level echo area against the pectoralis muscle (open arrow).

smooth, well defined, low-level density on the right with some shadowing (Fig. 2A-12B). On the left there were two poorly defined densities with shadowing (Fig. 21-12C). It was thought that the patient has two carcinomas on the left and a fibroadenoma on the right.

At biopsy there were two distinct areas of infiltrating ductal carcinoma on the left. The patient refused mastectomy despite the multicentricity and underwent a course of radiation therapy. All nodes were negative. A later biopsy on the right demonstrated a fibroadenoma.

Follow-up a year later demonstrated radiation changes to the left breast but no evidence of recurrent tumor. At 18 months there has been almost complete resolution of the radiation changes.

Discussion

The development of multicentric carcinomas within the same breast is not unusual or unexpected when it is realized that the factors responsible for the development of breast cancer act on all of the breast tissue, not just one area. These factors are also responsible for the bilaterality. Multicentricity is considered a contraindication to lumpectomy and radiation therapy, and an indication for mastectomy, although the patient in case 13 has done well with this therapy. With the current push toward breast-saving procedures when possible, it is important for the imager to detect any questionable areas.

The multiple foci of cancer are not always the same cell type, as can be seen in case 10.

Case Studies: Bilateral Breast Cancer

Case 14

B.T. is a 61-year-old woman who presented with a 3 cm mass adjacent to the left nipple and slight flattening of the overlying skin. There was an additional 1 cm tender nodule in the upper outer right breast.

Thermograms were positive on the left with increased vascularity. Diaphanography demonstrated diminished light transmission over the left mass (Fig. 21-13A). Mammograms showed the presence of a spiculated lesion on the left with rodlike calcifications (Fig. 21-13B). On the right, in the tail of the breast, was an irregular lesion with spiculization (Fig. 21-13C).

The patient underwent bilateral mastectomy. Infiltrating lobular carcinoma with two foci was found on the left; all of eight nodes were negative. Infiltrating scirrhous carcinoma with focal tubular differentiation (one of eight nodes positive) was found on the right.

Case 15

H.H. is a 60-year-old woman who presented with a hard, somewhat fixed, 2.5 cm mass at 3 o'clock in the left breast. There was skin retraction below the mass.

Thermograms showed increased vascularity and nipple heat on the left. Diaphanography was normal. Mammograms demonstrated marked glandularity (P2 pattern). On the left there was a poorly defined mass deep in the breast (Fig. 21-14A), with marked thickening of the ductal structures and suspensory structures extending toward the skin with retraction of the skin in this area. On the right there was a group of small calcifications without a mass (Fig. 21-14B). No calcifications were seen on the left. Ultrasound on the left showed a mass of diminished echogenicity and slight shadowing on the right without a mass. Bilateral biopsy was advised. A bilateral ductal carcinoma was found. All nodes were negative following a bilateral mastectomy.

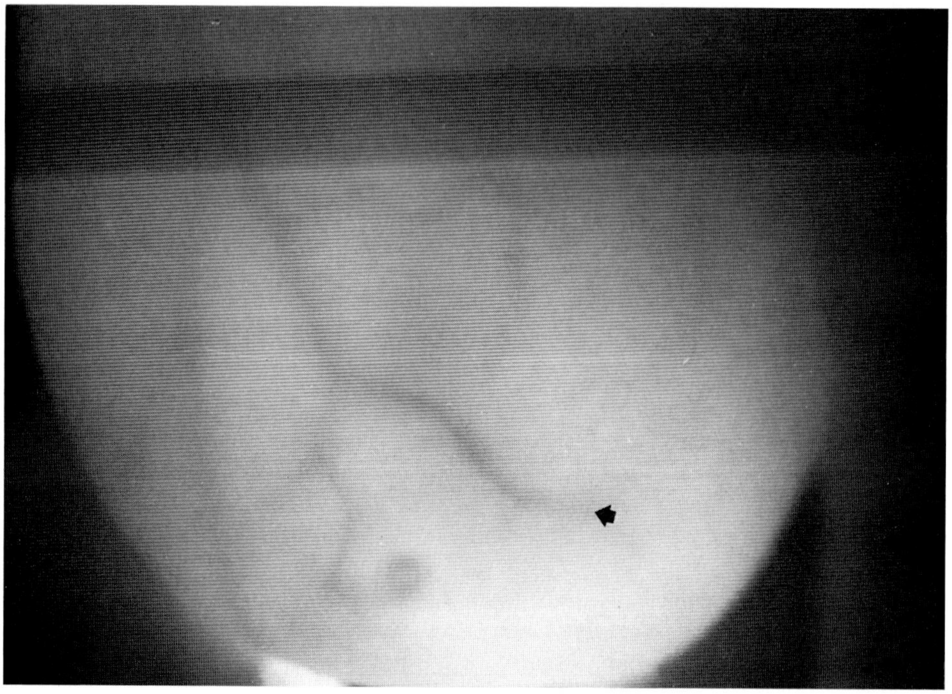

A

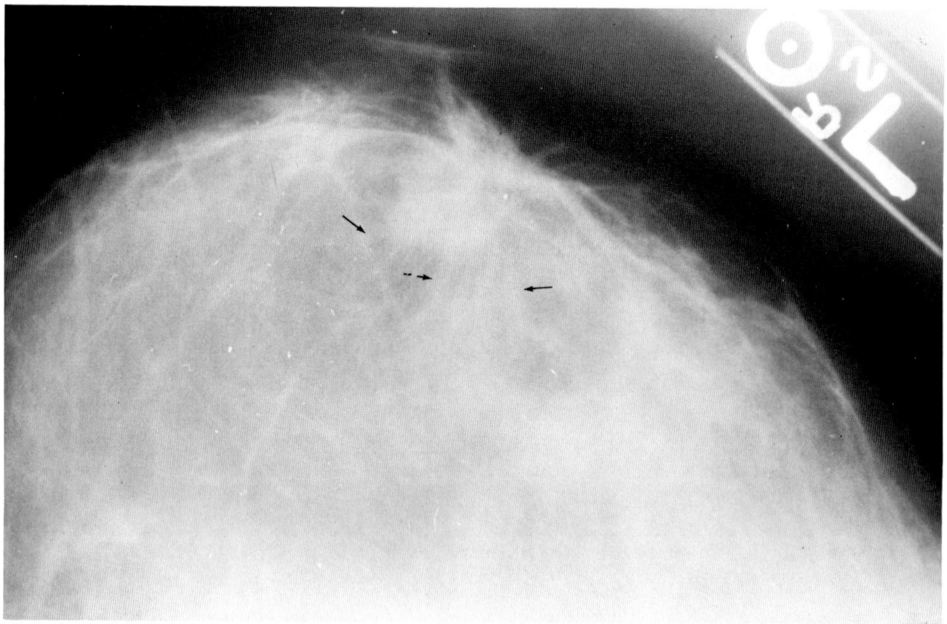

B

Fig. 21-13 A: Diaphanography. Note the abruptly ending vein (arrow) with a very small area of decreased light transmission. **B:** Mammogram, left CC view. Large spiculated (arrows) lesion. Calcifications are not apparent here. *(Figure continues.)*

C

Fig. 21-13 C: Mammogram, magnified, right axillary tail. This is an irregular lesion (arrows).

Case 16

D.H. is a 52-year-old woman who presented with a 2 cm, freely movable nodule at 12 o'clock in the left breast. In addition, there was a tender ridge noted at 9 o'clock on the right.

Thermograms and diaphanography were both normal. Mammograms showed an irregular density with three small calcifications in the area of the mass on the left and diffuse punctate calcifications in the outer portion of the right breast (Fig. 21-15A). Ultrasound demonstrated shadowing in both areas and a poorly defined mass on the left (Figs. 21-15 B,C).

The patient had biopsies and a subsequent bilateral modified radical mastectomy. There was an infiltrating ductal carcinoma found on the left and a predominantly intraductal comedo carcinoma with rare microfoci of infiltration on the right. All nodes were negative.

Discussion

All three of the patients discussed were referred because the primary care physician had found a unilateral mass. In none of the cases was the cancer in the opposite breast appreciated prior to our examination. This does not mean to imply that the masses would not have been delineated by the surgeon prior to surgery. These cases demonstrate the necessity for mammographic examination, at the least, prior to biopsy of a dominant mass in patients over age 30 (see case 30, below).

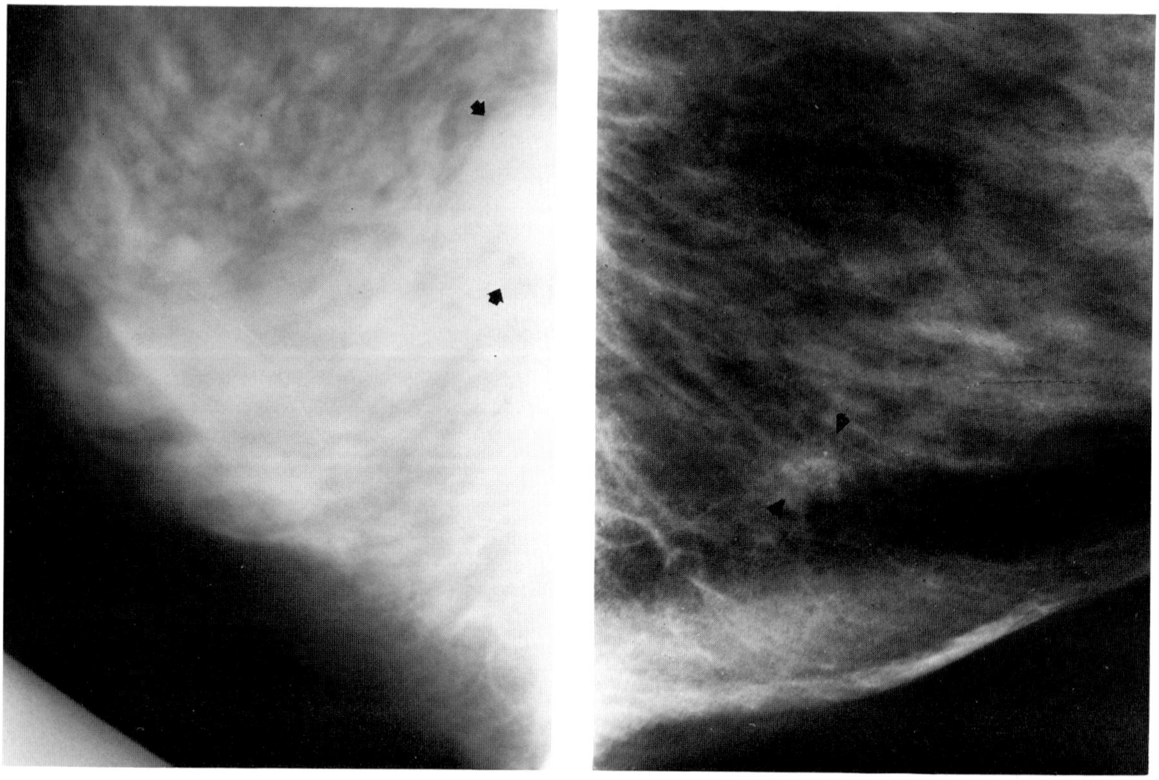

A B

Fig. 21-14 **A:** Mammogram, left lateral view. Note the poorly defined mass in the posterior aspect of the breast (arrows). **B:** Mammogram, magnified, right breast. There is a group of small calcifications with a slight suggestion of a mass (arrowheads).

The bilaterality of breast cancers has been reported to be between 15 and 20 percent during the lifetime of the patient, with about 5 percent of the patients presenting with synchronous cancers. These statistics point out the need for careful initial examinations as well as follow-up in breast cancer patients. It is probable that as we find earlier carcinomas the number of synchronous cancers may decrease.

Case 14 demonstrates that bilateral cancers may be of different cell types. The larger lobular carcinoma was node-negative, whereas the smaller tubular cancer (an early form of infiltrating ductal carcinoma) was node-positive. The size of the tumor does not always reveal the nodal status. (See also case 10, above.)

Case Studies: Paget's Disease of the Breast

Case 17

D.H. is a 53-year-old woman referred because of bilateral breast pain and nipple discharge. She had a slightly elevated prolactin level. When seen, no nipple discharge could be elicited. She was large-breasted. There was no discrete mass, but there was a slightly raw area in the center of the left nipple.

Liquid crystal thermograms demonstrated increased nipple heat and increased vascularity on the left (Th IV thermogram) (Color Fig. 19). Light scanning was normal. Mammograms demonstrated a fatty breast without a lesion. A nipple biopsy was advised. Because the prolactin level was borderline abnormal, it was decided to repeat this test at a later time, and if it was still elevated a microadenoma would be sought.

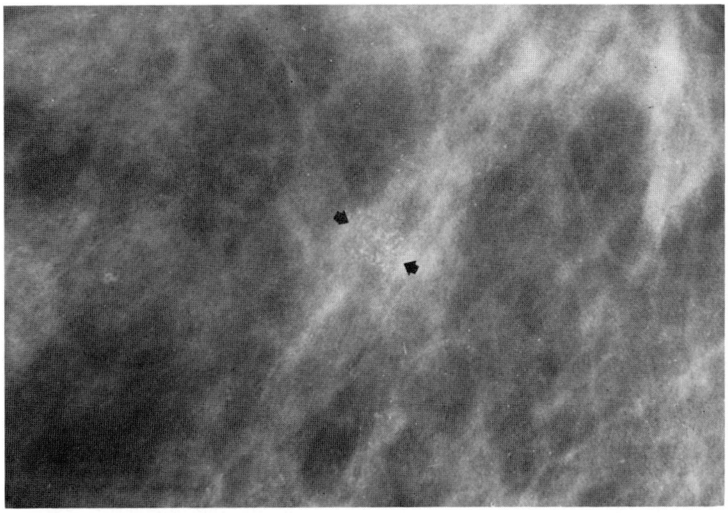

A

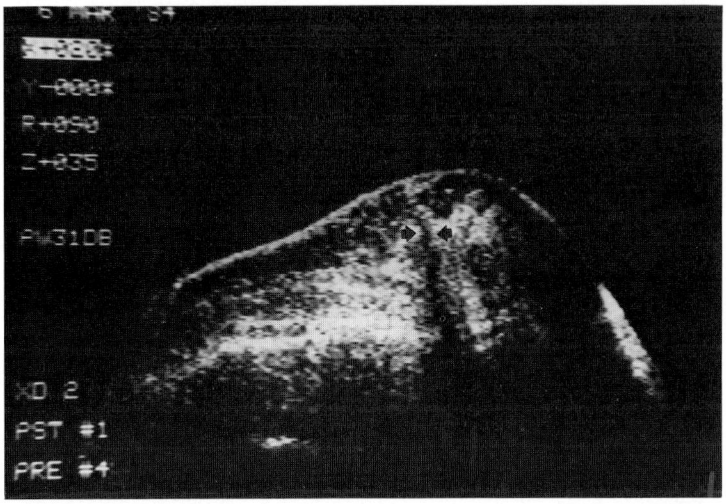

B

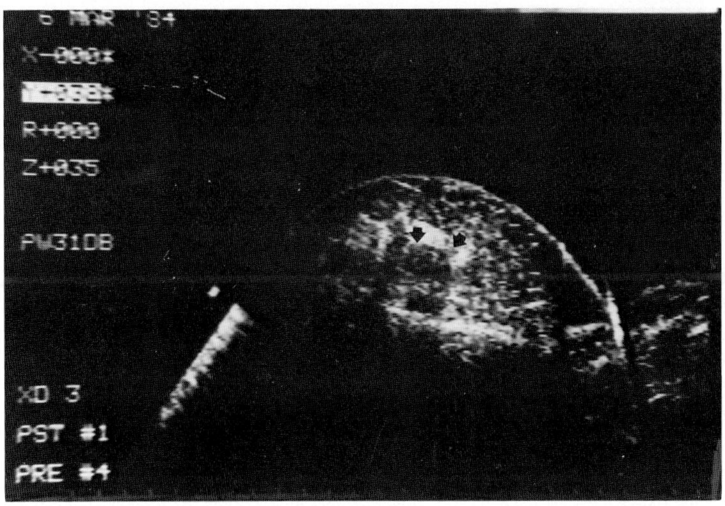

C

Fig. 21-15 **A:** Mammogram, magnified, right breast. Note the diffuse punctate and irregular calcifications (arrows). **B:** Ultrasound. There is shadowing in the area of the calcifications (arrows). **C:** Ultrasound. There is a low-level echo mass (arrows) with posterior shadowing.

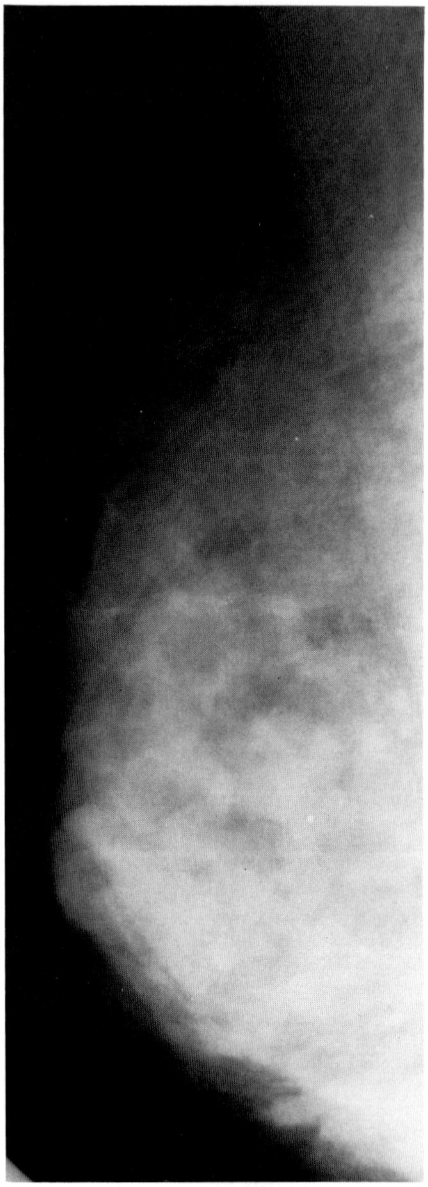

Fig. 21-16 Mammogram, right lateral view. There is marked glandularity but no mass.

At biopsy a carcinoma involving the ducts immediately behind the left nipple was found. The patient had a resection of the anterior left breast and a course of radiation therapy. There has been no recurrence at 18 months. The nipple discharge has again occurred on the right and is being followed by her primary physician.

Case 18

P.B. is a 47-year-old woman who presented with a raw bleeding area occupying 60 percent of the right nipple. She denied trauma or irritation to the nipple. Glandularity was felt in the breasts without a mass.

Thermograms and diaphanography were normal. Mammography demonstrated marked glandularity in the breasts (DY pattern), without a mass (Fig. 21-16). There was a group of somewhat benign-appearing calcifications beneath and behind the right nipple.

A smear of the nipple demonstrated cancer cells, and an infiltrating ductal carcinoma was found behind the right nipple. The patient underwent a modified radical mastectomy.

Case 19

M.B. is an 85-year-old woman who was referred because of a bleeding right nipple. Three months earlier a biopsy of that nipple had shown Paget's disease with an infiltrating ductal carcinoma. She had refused mastectomy and was started on a course of radiation therapy; she had received about 2000 rads to the breast when she stopped radiation therapy about 6 weeks prior to our seeing her.

On physical examination the right nipple and periareolar area were hard and indurated. Multiple bruised and raw areas were noted on the right breast from abrasions. There was a hard, firm area in the axilla thought to be due to radiation changes. The left breast was normal.

Thermograms showed a marked increase in heat and vascularity on the right (Th V thermogram). Mammograms demonstrated benign calcifications within fat on the left. On the right there was marked thickening of the periareolar area with spiculization extending from this area (Figs. 21-17A, B). No mass was seen otherwise.

The patient was advised to undergo mastectomy. She has refused any further therapy. She related by phone 6 months later that the bleeding had stopped and the raw areas on the breast had cleared.

Case 20

L.R. is a 60-year-old woman who 3 years earlier had undergone a wide excision biopsy for an infiltrating ductal carcinoma of the right breast. She refused any further therapy and went on a regimen of Chinese herbs.

On physical examination the right breast was about twice the size of the left breast, and the right nipple was raw and reddened and three times the size of the left nipple. There were ill-defined masses above and below the right nipple.

There was a marked increase in the heat of the entire right breast (Th IV thermogram) and a slight decrease in light transmission. On mammography there were diffuse malignant calcifications throughout the entire right breast, extending into the nipple (Fig. 21-18). Ultrasound demonstrated disruption of the normal glandularity, with multiple areas of shadowing. The patient was advised to undergo mastectomy. Diffuse ductal carcinoma was found.

Discussion

As demonstrated in cases 17 and 18, any raw area on the nipple must be considered Paget's disease until proved otherwise. It is unusual (as in case 18) to obtain cancer cells on a nipple smear.

In case 19 the findings are the result of the cancer and the partial course of radiation therapy. The radiation was responsible for the raw areas on the skin, and both the cancer and the radiation account for the marked spiculization behind the nipple.

Case 20 is an unusual presentation of Paget's disease. There was a known ductal carcinoma that had been resected but had recurred. The growth of the tumor into the nipple area accounted for the raw and reddened nipple as well as the increased nipple size.

Case Studies: Ulcerating and Necrotic Carcinomas

Case 21

A.J. is a 68-year-old woman who presented with an autoamputation of the anterior third of the right breast. The nipple area and anterior breast were absent (Color Fig. 20). There were rolled edges and a mass extending toward the axilla. Retraction was present just below the axilla, and lymph nodes were felt in the axilla.

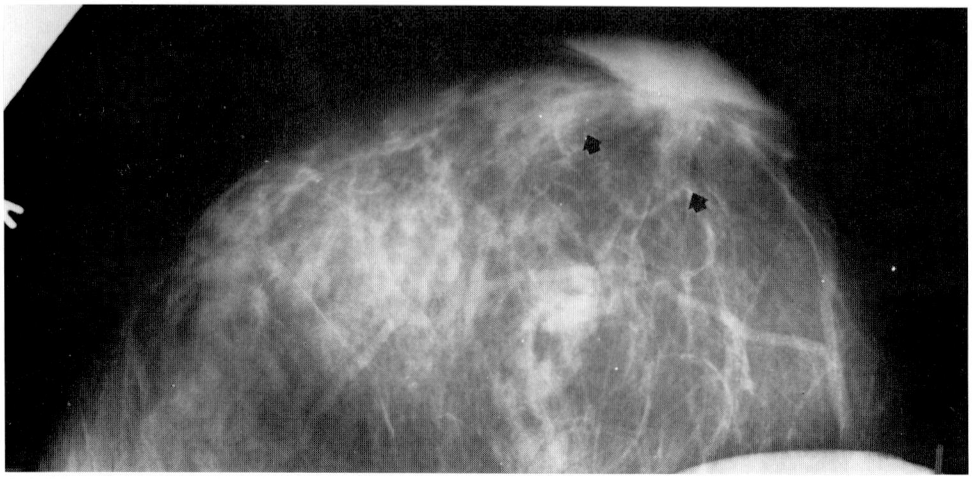

A

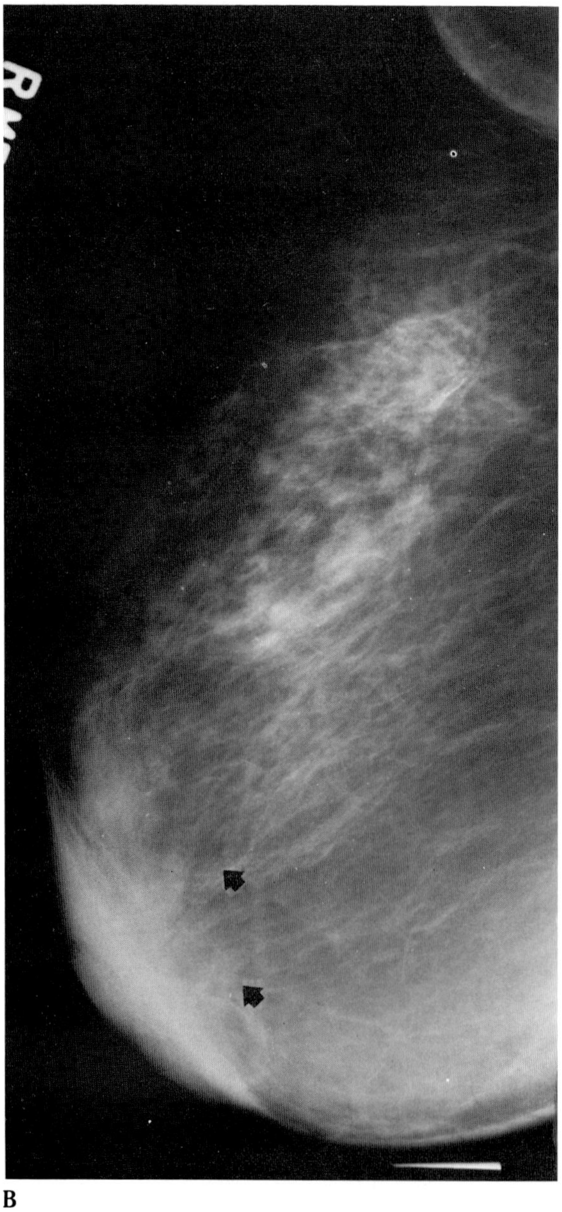

B

Fig. 21-17 **A:** Mammogram, right CC view. **B:** Mammogram, right lateral view. Note the markedly thickened area of the nipple. Spicules arising from the nipple area extend into the breast (arrows).

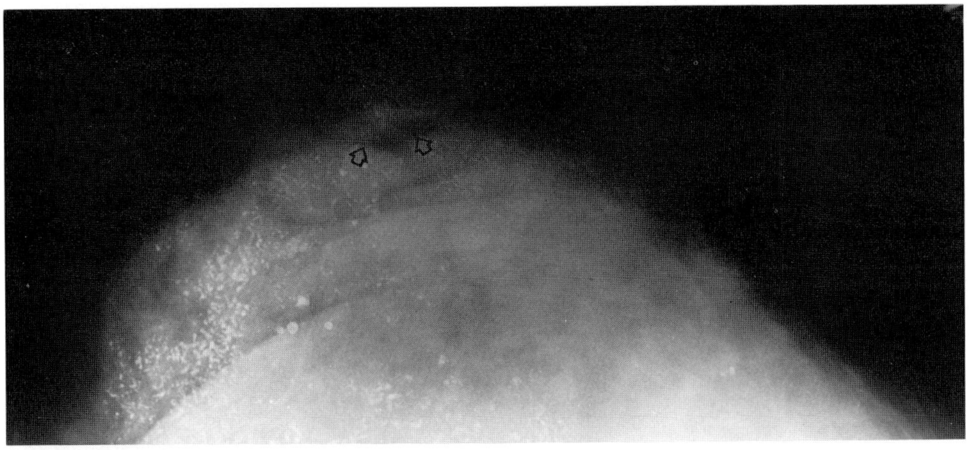

A

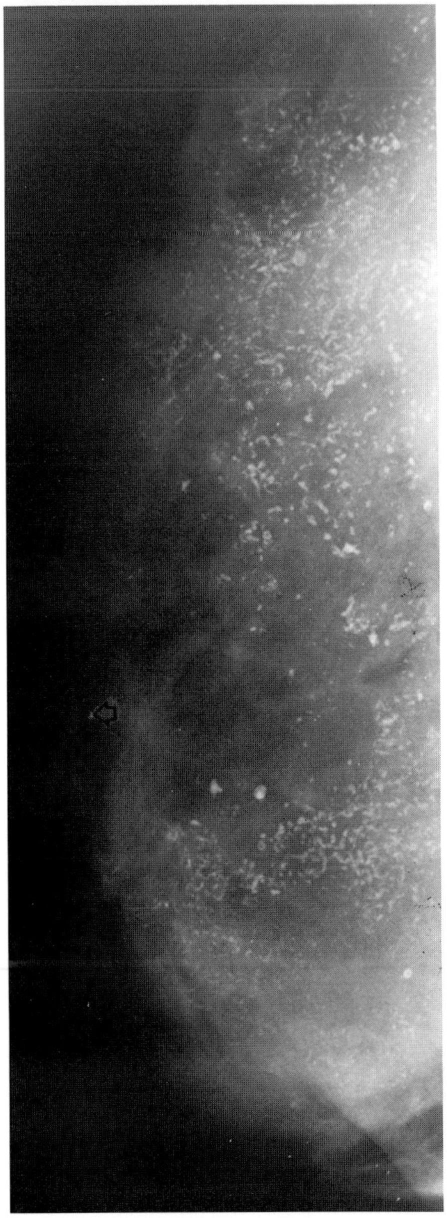

B

Fig. 21-18 A: Mammogram, right CC view. **B:** Mammogram, right lateral view. Diffuse malignant calcifications occupy more than half of the breast. The nipple is markedly swollen. Calcifications extend into the nipple (open arrow).

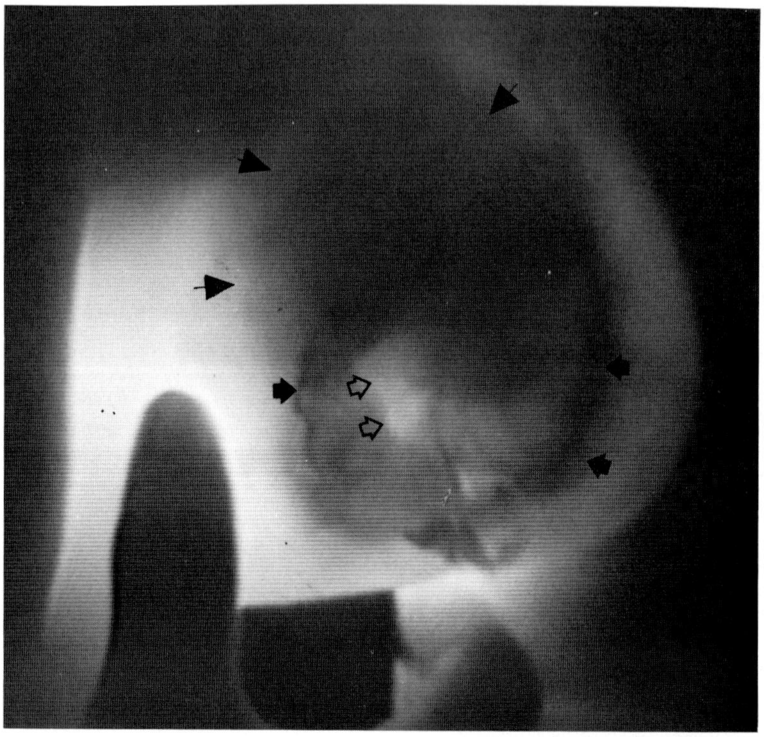

A

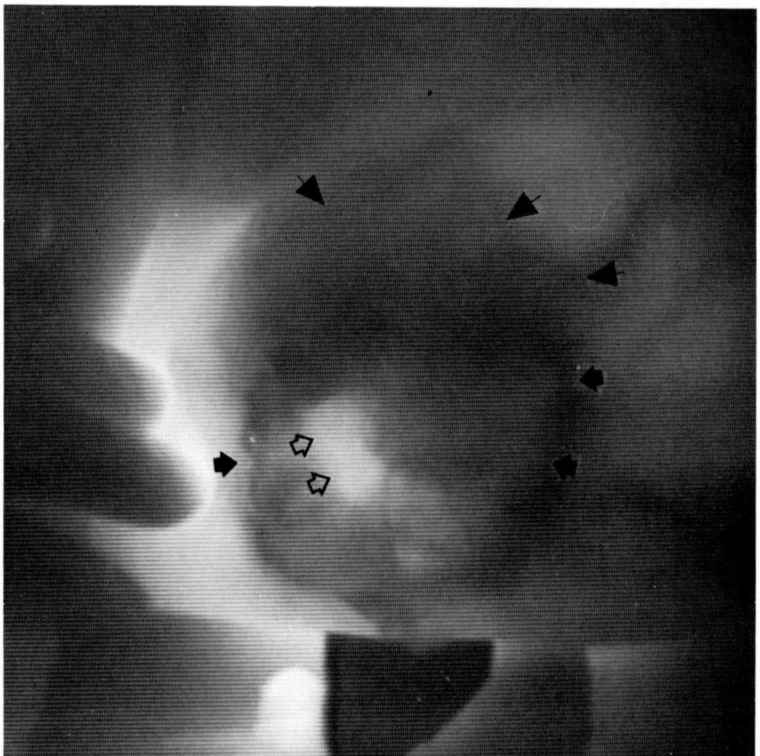

B

Fig. 21-19 A, B: Diaphanography. The ulceration is dark-edged, representing a rolled tumor edge (arrows) with a relative lucent center (open arrows). The tumor mass is the darkened area extending toward the axilla (arrowheads).

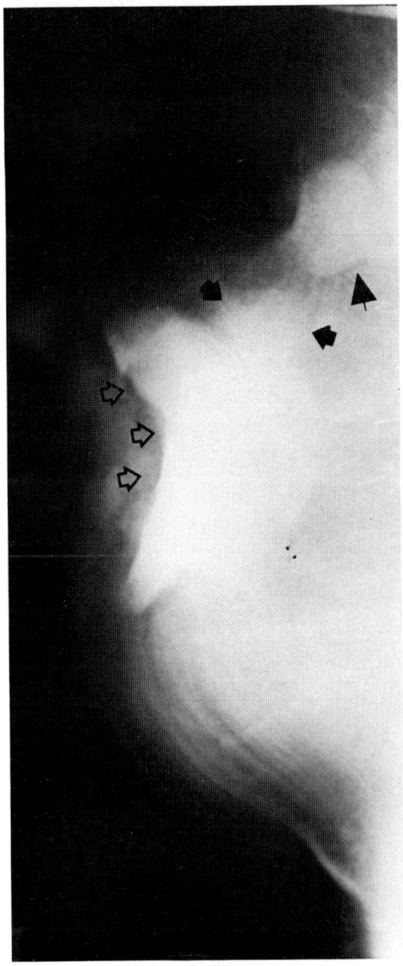

C

Fig. 21-19 C: Mammogram, lateral view. The mass with anterior ulceration (arrow) extends toward the axilla (open arrows), with a lymph node mass in the lower axilla (arrowhead).

Thermograms showed a marked increase in heat over the breast (Color Fig. 21). Diaphanography demonstrated the mass extending to the axilla, with a marked decrease in light transmission (Figs. 21-19A, B). Mammograms showed the large retracted mass on the right and the lymph node mass (Fig. 21-19C). There was moderate glandularity on the left with a dilated duct.

The patient underwent a modified radical mastectomy. A skin graft was necessary. All of 15 nodes were positive. Estrogen and progesterone receptors were both positive. After a course of radiation therapy to the chest wall, the patient refused to undergo chemotherapy. She also refused to be followed on a close basis but did return at 18 months, at which time the chest wall on the right was clear of metastasis, with the skin graft in good apposition. Radiation changes were present to the skin. The left breast was unchanged on mammography.

Case 22

A.H. is a 57-year-old woman who claimed that 2 weeks prior to being seen she fell from a chair against a hot stove, burning her breast, and her breast subsequently "opened up." On physical examination there was a large ulcerating mass on the lateral aspect of the left breast. The opening of the mass measured 8 cm across by 5 cm deep. There were firm, thick edges surrounding the cavity (Color Fig. 22).

Mammograms showed the presence of a large irregular mass with air in a central cavity open to the skin. The remaining areas of the breasts were normal (Fig. 21-20). A work-up for metastasis was negative.

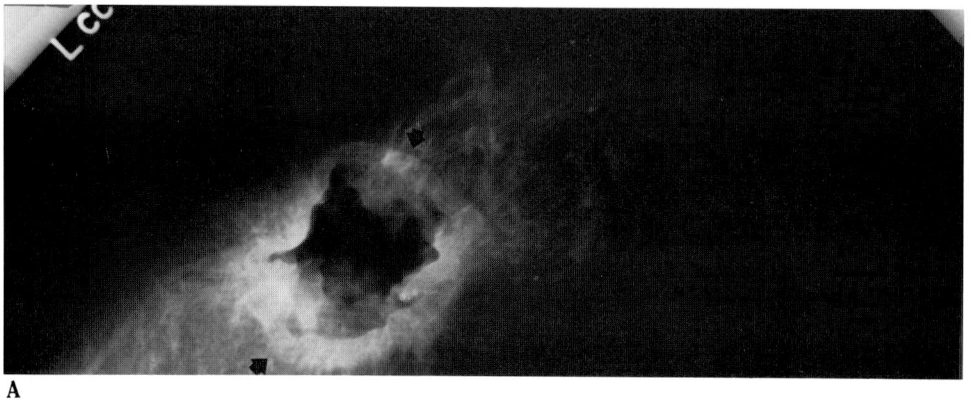

A

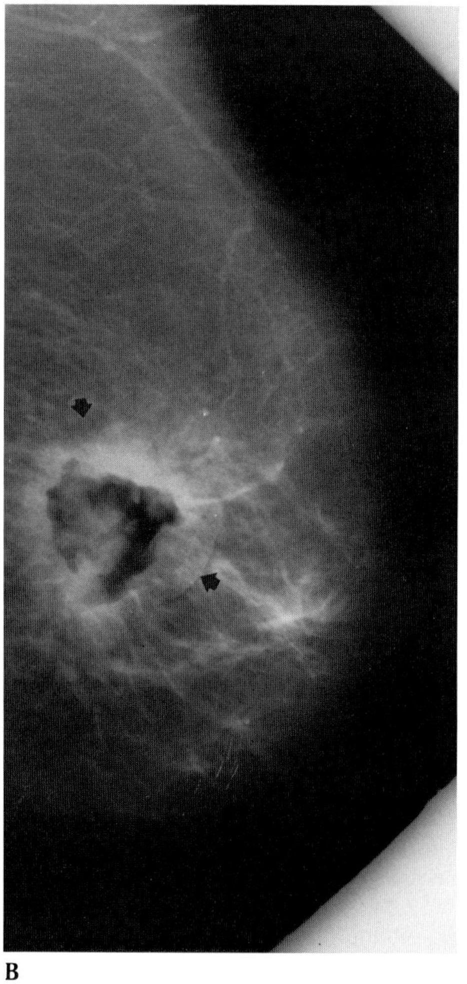

B

Fig. 21-20 A, B: Mammogram, left C.C. view. Mammograms, left lateral view. Note the rolled edges of a carcinoma (arrows), with the dark central area representing air in the cavity. Note the irregular walls extending into the central cavity outlined by the air.

The patient underwent a simple mastectomy and lymph node sampling. The diagnosis was infiltrating ductal carcinoma, with seven nodes negative. She refused radiation therapy or chemotherapy and has not been willing to be followed. At 1 year after surgery her son related that she was doing well.

Case 23

A.F. was a 42-year-old woman who related that she noticed a small lump on the inner lower aspect of the left breast 6 years prior to her appearance at the Woman's Breast Center. She presented with a fixed, fluctuant 10 cm mass occupying the entire medial lower aspect of the left breast. There was an ulcerating area at the skinfold of the under portion of the breast (Color Fig. 23). There was an additional 3 cm mass adjacent to the larger mass. Both axillary and left supraclavicular nodes were present.

Liquid crystal thermograms showed global hyperthermia of the left breast of more than 5°C, consistent with a Th V thermogram (Color Fig. 24). There was an inability on light scanning to penetrate the mass. A dime-sized area of marked light absorption was noted on the right, thought to represent a bruise. Mammograms showed a very large mass in the inner aspect of the left breast (Fig. 21-21A) and diffuse skin thickening and lymphatic changes. The second mass felt clinically was not seen. The right breast was normal. On ultrasound there was a large fluid center to the mass with multiple areas of solid tissue extending into the fluid center (Fig. 21-21B, C).

Partial aspiration of the mass revealed 120 cc of dark brownish fluid that was reported cytologically as atypical cells of a papillary nature and old blood. A bone scan demonstrated many metastatic areas. A cervical node biopsy demonstrated metastatic breast cancer. The patient died 3 months later.

Discussion

It is always amazing to see patients with late cancer, e.g., cases 21 and 22, who do well and recover from their disease or at least appear to on short-term follow-up. It substantiates the belief that not all breast cancers act the same, and that postmenopausal cancers may be less aggressive.

Aspiration of necrotic tumors often leads to an inconclusive diagnosis, as in case 23, if only fluid is obtained and if tissue masses are not needled.

Case Studies: Inflammatory Carcinoma

Case 24

B.W. was a 31-year-old woman who presented to the Woman's Breast Center in November 1983 with a 6-month history of a left breast mass and nipple retraction. She claimed that she had been seen at the time the mass was discovered by a physician who told her she had a duct inflammation that was causing the nipple retraction. This visit could not be documented, and it is probable that the patient lied about it.

On physical examination there was a 5 cm hard mass behind and medial to the nipple, with left nipple retraction. There were marked skin changes in the anterior portion of the breast with a peau d'orange effect. A lymph node mass was present in the axilla. The patient was wearing a neck collar, being treated by a chiropractor for neck pain of 2 months' duration.

Liquid crystal thermograms showed a marked temperature differential with a 6°C increase on the inner aspect of the left breast compared to the right. Diaphanography was unable to penetrate the mass. Mammograms showed a large mass measuring about 6 cm with spiculization. Marked skin thickening was noted with lymphatic enlargement (Figs. 21-22A, B). Ultrasound demonstrated a low-level echo mass with poor posterior borders (Fig. 21-22C).

A fine needle aspiration biopsy revealed highly atypical cells consistent with the clinical impression of inflammatory carcinoma. A bone scan was positive in the cervical area, and x-ray films showed metastasis to the cervical spine. The patient was put on a chemotherapy regimen. She expired in November 1984.

Case 25

S.W. is a 40-year-old woman who noticed a thickening on the medial aspect of the right breast in May 1983. A mammogram on 6/27/83 showed punctate calcifications and skin changes. A biopsy the next day demonstrated infiltrating carcinoma of the

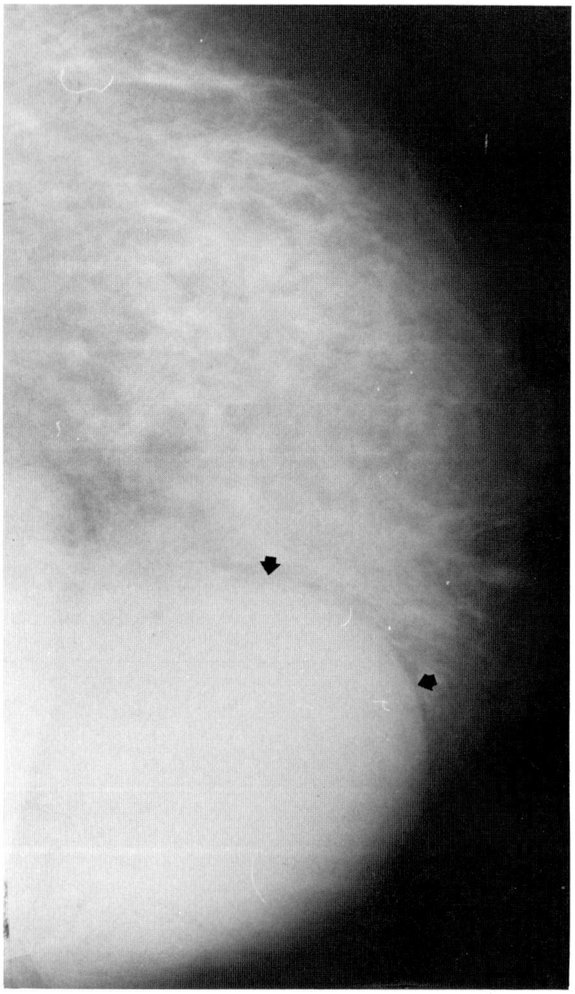

A

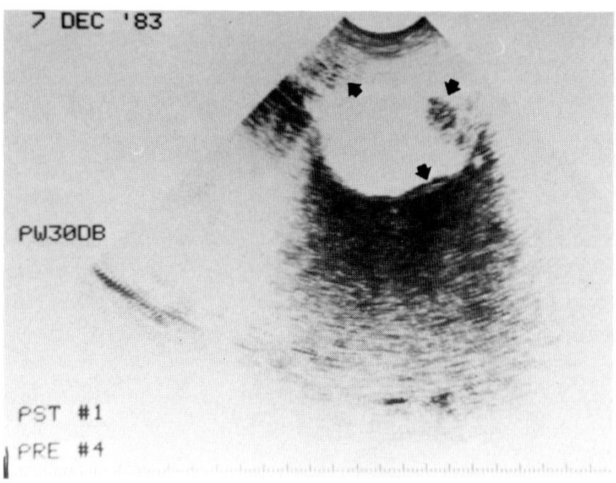

B

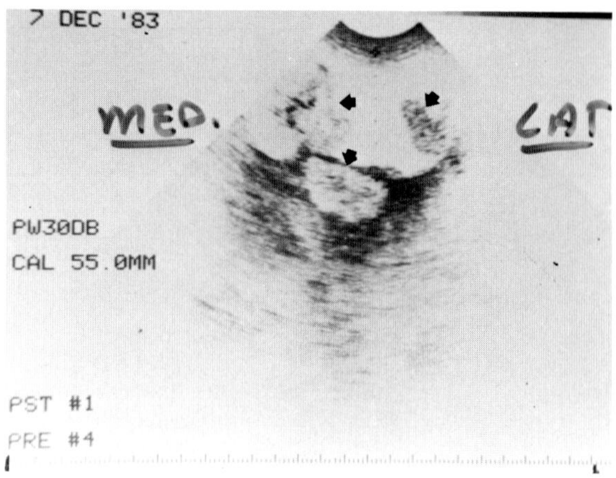

C

Fig. 21-21 **A:** Mammogram, lateral view. A large, well defined mass (arrows) occupies the inferior portion of the breast. Skin thickening is not apparent. **B, C:** Ultrasound. Extending into the fluid center of the mass are multiple solid areas (arrows). Note how much less tissue is seen in **B.** Care must be taken in cystic lesions to scan the entire lesion lest small areas of solid tissue are missed.

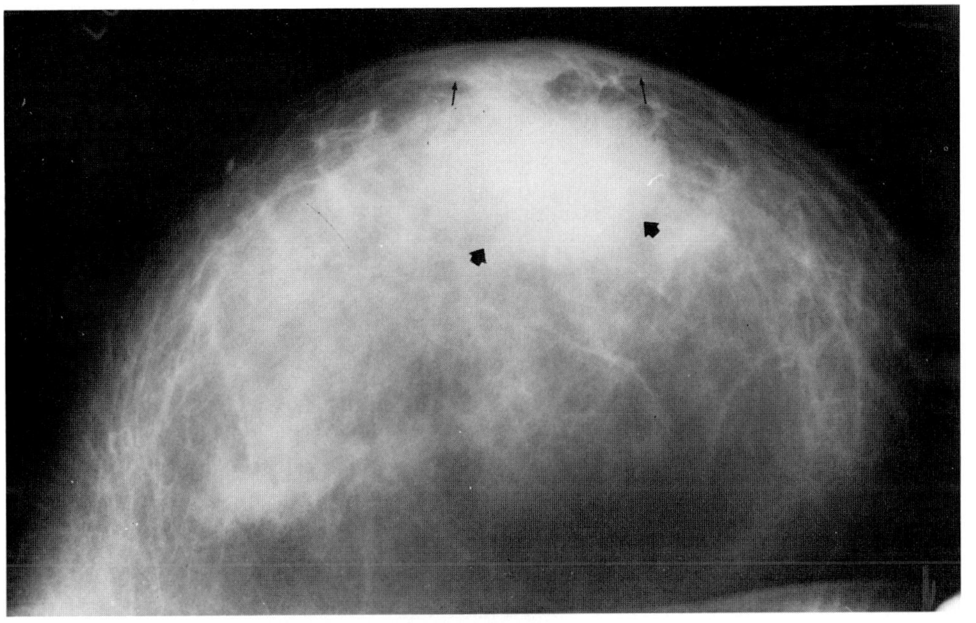

A

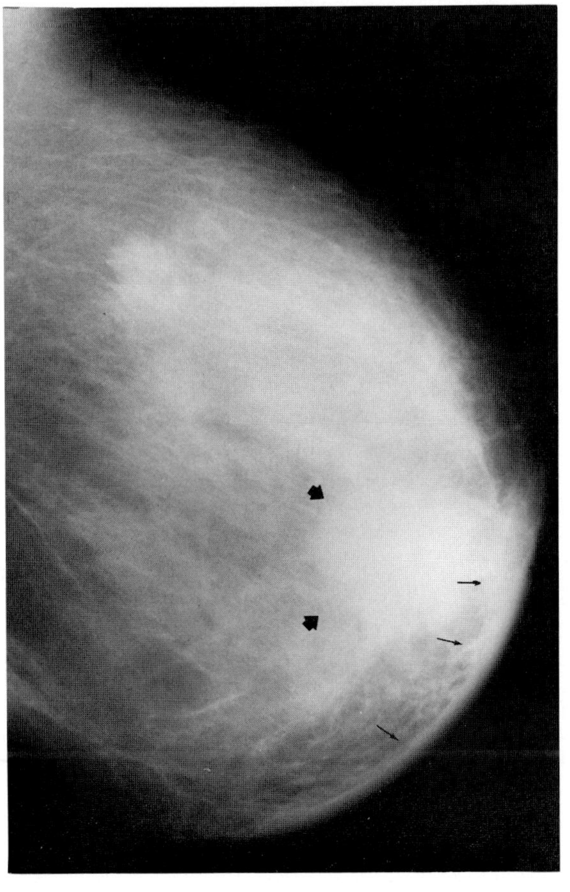

B

Fig. 21-22 Mammograms, left CC view **(A)** and left lateral view **(B)**. Note the large spiculated mass (thick arrows) behind the nipple with slight flattening of the nipple area. Note the marked skin thickening (thin arrows) and lymphatic engorgement consistent with inflammatory carcinoma. *(Figure continues.)*

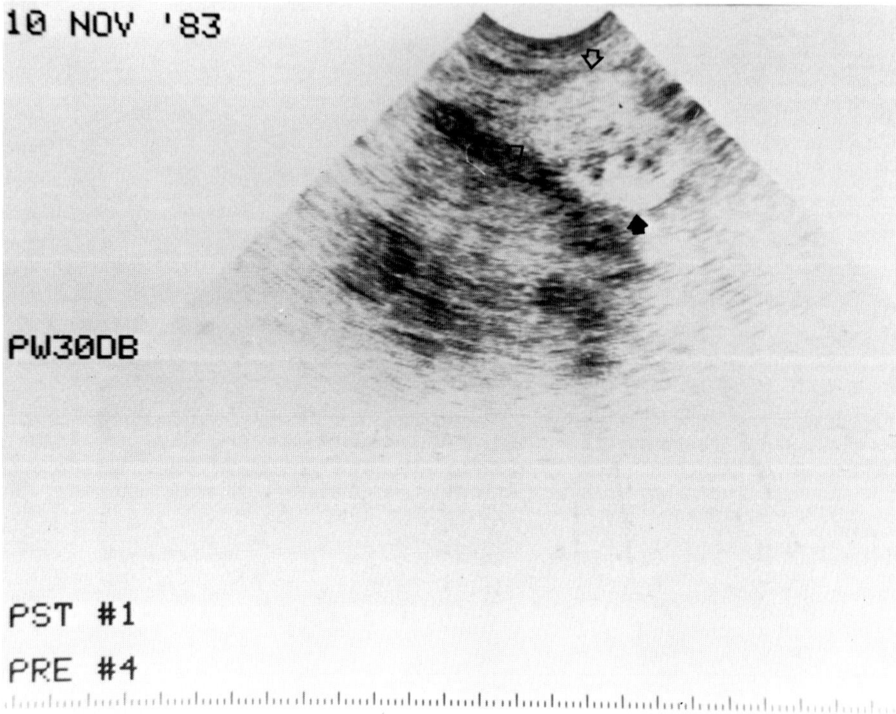

Fig. 21-22 C: Ultrasound. The large low-level echogenic mass (open arrows) with anechoic area posteriorly (arrow) represents a necrotic area.

breast with extensive lymphatic invasion consistent with an inflammatory carcinoma of the breast. Estrogen and progesterone receptors were positive.

The patient decided that since her prognosis with conventional medical therapy was so bad she would try unconventional therapy. She started megavitamin therapy and went on ADS, a plant derivative. There was an increasing size to the right breast.

She presented to the Woman's Breast Center on 8/4/83. On physical examination there was a large scar involving the inner aspect of the right breast and marked induration adjacent to the scar. Skin changes consistent with inflammation were noted in the inner aspect of the breast. There was no discrete mass. Marked nodularity was noted elsewhere in the right breast. The left breast was moderately glandular to palpation, without the degree of nodularity noted on the right.

Liquid crystal thermograms demonstrated markedly increased temperature in the nipple, periareolar area, and inner aspect of the right breast compared to the left (Th IV thermogram). There was decreased light transmission in the inner aspect of the right breast as well. Punctate calcifications were demonstrated in the inner right breast on mammography, less than preoperatively (Fig. 21-23A). In addition there was a conglomerate 2 cm nodal mass in the lower right axilla.

The patient has been followed for an additional 32 months at this time. She had a single course of 1 month's duration of tamoxifen but has otherwise been on a number of nonconventional therapies. In August 1984 there were two areas of redness noted on the left breast, thought to be areas of inflammatory carcinoma on the opposite breast; however, dermal biopsies were normal, and the redness subsided on cortisone cream. Chest x-ray films and liver function tests in October 1984 were normal. Physical examination of the breast on 10/30/84 showed the right breast to be slightly smaller than the left although during the interim the right breast had gotten larger and then regressed in size. The thermogram and diaphanography were essentially unchanged

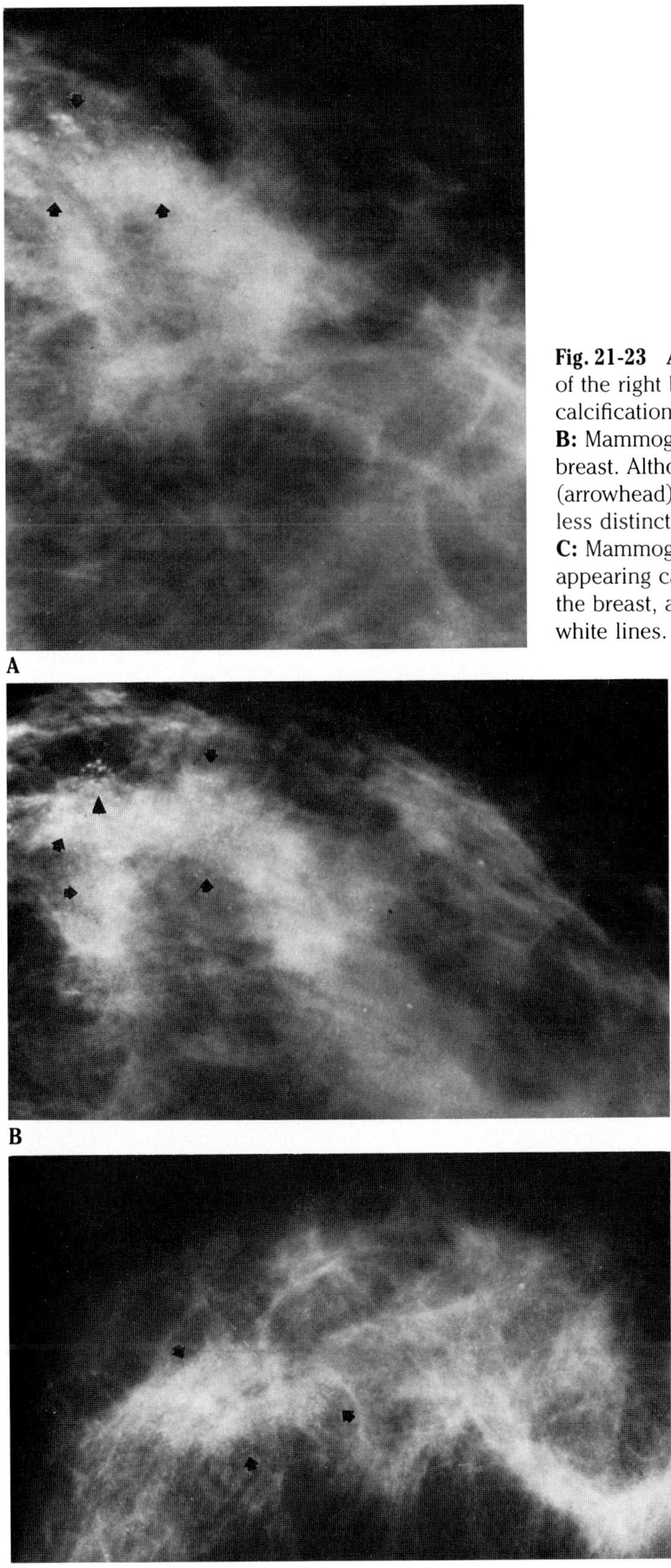

A

B

C

Fig. 21-23 **A:** Mammogram, magnified, inner aspect of the right breast. August 1983. Diffuse punctate calcifications remain postoperatively (arrows). **B:** Mammogram, magnified, inner aspect of the right breast. Although some of the calcifications (arrowhead) are as distinct as in **A,** most are less distinct and appear smudgy (arrows). **C:** Mammogram, magnified. Diffuse, smudgy-appearing calcifications (arrow) occur over half of the breast, appearing as indistinct, short, wavey white lines.

from the initial visit. Mammograms again demonstrated skin thickening and lymphatic changes. The calcifications were less distinct than on any subsequent examination although unchanged in number or distribution (Fig. 21-23B). The axillary nodal masses which became larger in December 1983 were unchanged. The patient had gained weight during the interim and "felt great."

In April 1985 the size of the right breast had decreased, with marked skin changes and hardening of the glandular tissue. Multiple skin nodules were seen in the inner aspect of the right breast. The lymph node masses in the right axilla were unchanged. Lymph nodes were felt in the left axilla. There were red streaks on the skin in the inner aspect of the left breast.

The thermogram was very positive, with an edge sign from the breast retraction. Diaphanography could not penetrate the right breast. On mammography there were groups of punctate calcifications, some of which corresponded to the skin nodules (Fig. 21-23C). The left breast was normal on mammography.

It is thought that there was a cross invasion of the skin on the left, with positive lymph nodes present in the left axilla. It is apparent that the inflammatory cancer on the right, which had been relatively stable, had exploded, with rapid growth over a 5-month period.

When seen in April, 1986 she had a contracted right breast, obvious cross spread to the left breast, massive bilateral axillary lymph nodes, and large bilateral pleural expressions on chest x-ray films.

Discussion

Case 25 is presented as a demonstration of inflammatory carcinoma, not to advocate nonconventional therapy. This case points out the need for the imager and the physician to accept that the patient is the ultimate decision maker in her own care, and that even if she elects to follow a course that is not of our choosing she still deserves to be followed.

The thermogram is the most *sensitive* test in inflammatory carcinoma, with diaphanography close behind. Neither is as *specific* as the mammogram. Ultrasound can also demonstrate the changes.

Case Studies: Carcinoma and Cysts

Case 26

S.M. is a 73-year-old woman who claimed to have had a firm mass adjacent to the right nipple for 30 years. She thought that the mass has gotten slightly larger over the past year. On physical examination there was a firm 1.5 cm mass just behind the right nipple and immediately medial to this a 3.5 cm softer, almost fluctuant mass. The masses could not be separated. There was no pain or tenderness.

Liquid crystal thermograms show a marked increase in periareolar and nipple heat on the right compared to the left (TH IV thermogram). Diaphanography showed marked light absorption in the smaller mass and marked light absorption in the rim of the larger mass with increased light transmission in the center of this mass (Fig. 21-24A).

Mammography demonstrated relative atrophy of the glandular tissue (Wolfe N1 pattern). On the right, adjacent to the nipple, was a bilobed mass. The smaller portion of the mass was just behind the nipple and contained multiple gross calcifications highly suggestive of a fibroadenoma. The larger portion of the bilobed mass measured slightly more than 3 cm and had smooth borders, except in the posterior portion where the two masses joined (Fig. 21-24B). In this area, seen best on magnification views, was a slight irregularity and minimal spiculization.

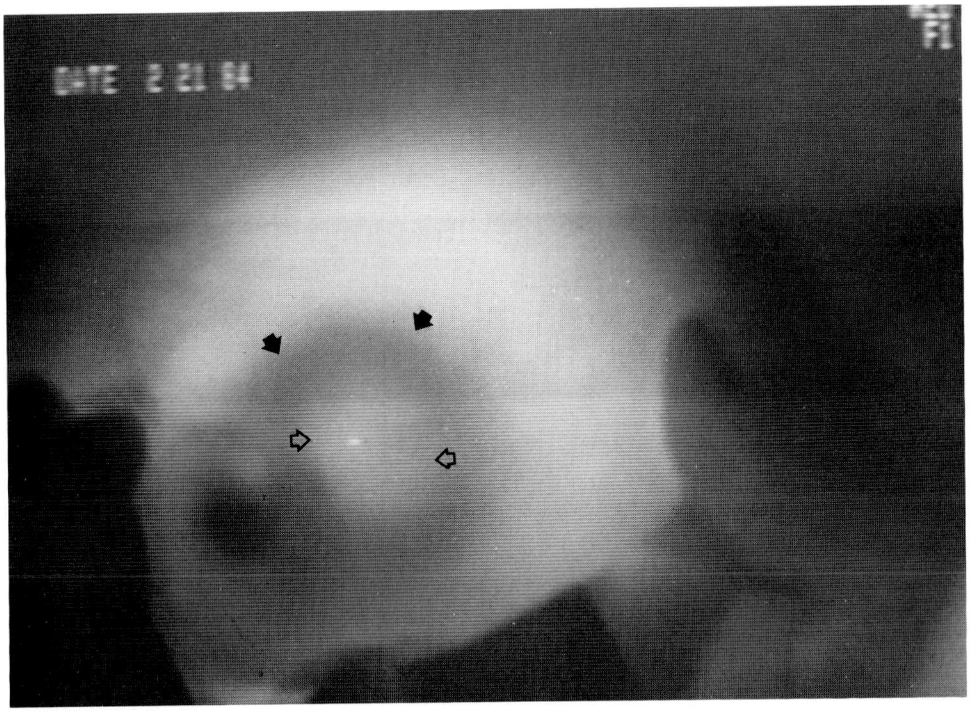

A

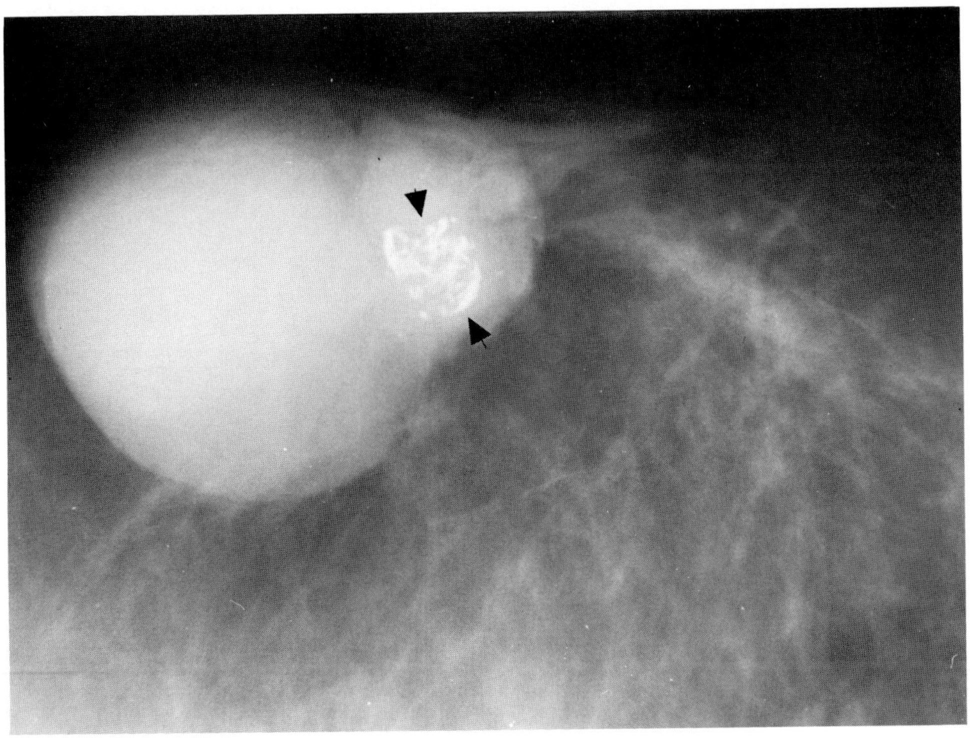

B

Fig. 21-24 A: Diaphanography. There is marked light absorption with a dark rim (arrows) from the edges of the lesion with increased light through the center (open arrows) representing fluid. **B:** Mammogram, magnified. The calcifications (arrows) in the smaller portion of this bilobed mass suggest a fibroadenoma. The larger mass has smooth borders.

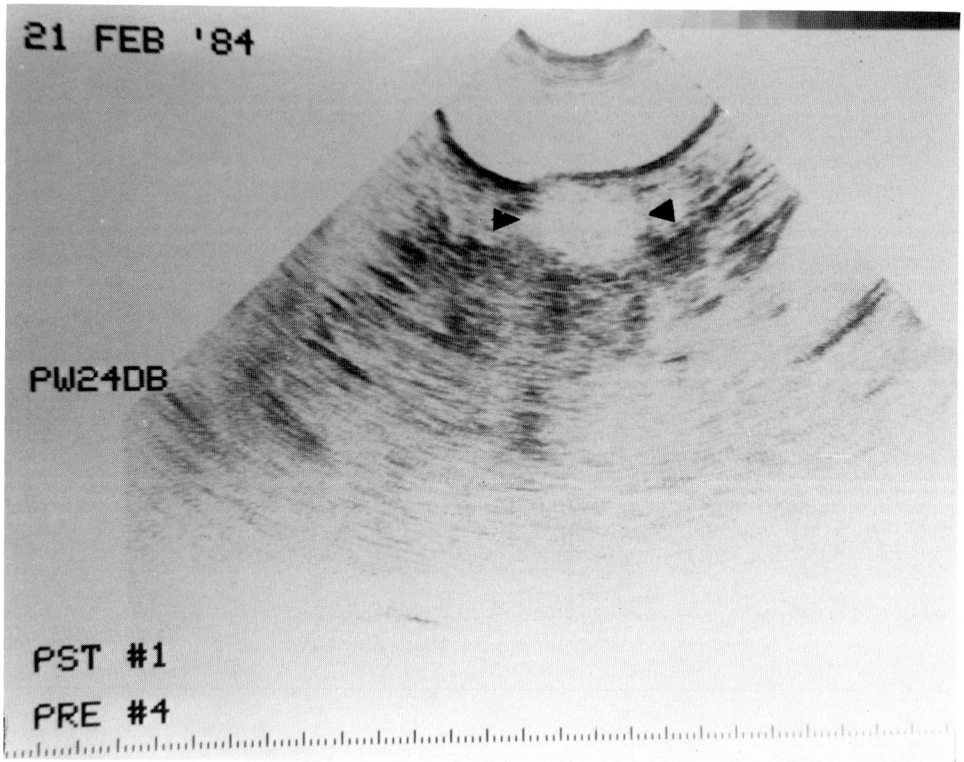

C

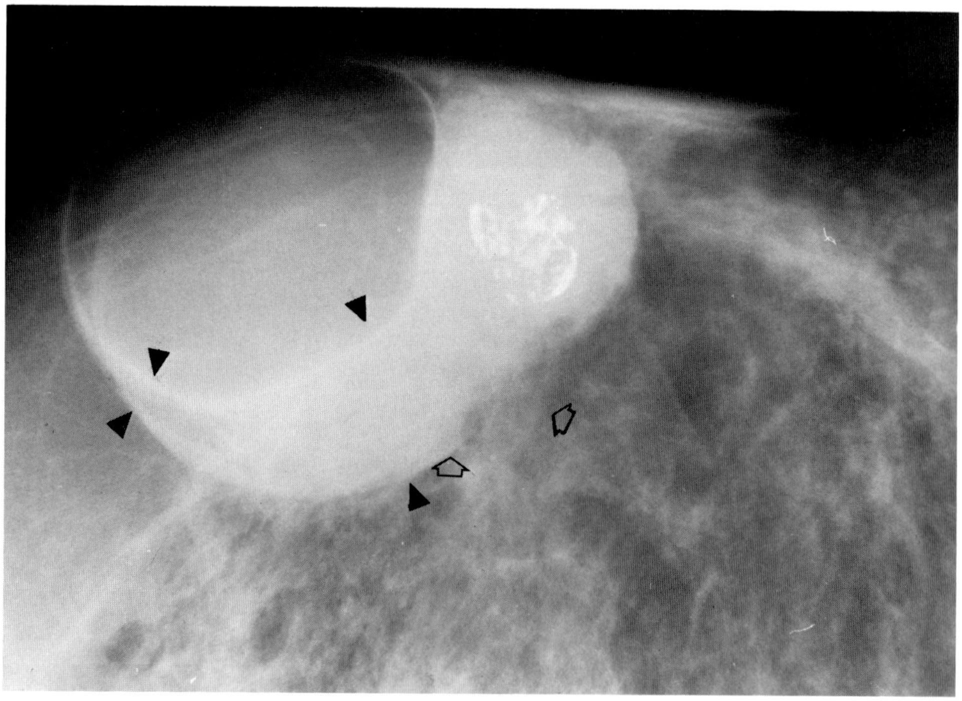

D

Fig. 21-24 **C:** Ultrasound through the smaller mass. The fluid area anteriorly is the water bag. The mass (arrows) is almost anechoic. The borders are poorly defined, and there is no increased through transmission. **D:** Pneumocystogram, magnified. Air partially fills the larger mass. Note the thick wall between the arrowheads. Note also the loss of detail (open arrows) at the junction of the masses not defined in **B.**

Ultrasound showed the larger mass to be echo-free and the smaller mass to be solid with diffuse low-level echoes; there was some shadowing from the posterior margin (Fig. 21-24C).

Cyst aspiration obtained 5 cc of dark brownish fluid. Air was then injected and a pneumocystogram obtained. A small amount of air escaped into the tissues. The air in the cystic lesion was noted not to fill the entire volume of the mass, especially posteriorly, suggesting a large posterior rim in this area (Fig. 21-24D). The cyst fluid was negative for malignant cells.

It was thought that these lesions represented a fibroadenoma, probably the mass present for 30 years, a cyst, and a carcinoma. At surgery an infiltrating ductal carcinoma 1.9 cm in greatest dimension, a cyst, and calcification consistent with a fibroadenoma were found. The carcinoma surrounded the calcification and invaded the posterior margin of the cyst wall. Ten axillary nodes were negative. A modified radical mastectomy was performed.

Case 27

T.G. is a 44-year-old woman who a month prior to this consultation had had a work-up elsewhere. At that time a well defined mass was seen on xeromammograms. There were two attempts at aspiration at which 2 cc of fluid was removed, and a pneumocystogram showed incomplete filling by the air of the mass.

On physical examination now there was a well defined lobulated 2.5 cm mass in the lower aspect of the left breast. Thermograms and diaphanography were normal. On mammography there was a well defined lobulated mass in the lower aspect of the left breast. In addition, there was a group of punctate calcifications in the outer left breast. On ultrasound the mass in the lower left breast was seen to be of two parts. The anterior portion was a well defined cyst, and the posterior part was well defined with internal echoes (Fig. 21-25). Although it was thought that it could be hemorrhage in the posterior portion, the possibility of a carcinoma was raised and biopsy recommended.

At surgery a ductal carcinoma in the posterior portion of a bilobed mass was found. The punctate calcifications were not found in the mastectomy specimen, but they were not looked for by use of specimen radiography. The patient underwent a modified radical mastectomy.

Discussion

In a patient the age of S.M. (Case 26) the occurrence of a cyst is suspect. She was not on replacement estrogens and had taken no medication that would be responsible for the cyst formation. The presence of a cyst adjacent to or in the same breast as a carcinoma has been commented on in the literature and is thought to be due to a stimulatory effect of the cancer, possibly a biochemical effect.

It is probable that the patient did indeed have a mass for 30 years, most likely a fibroadenoma that calcified. The ductal carcinoma either grew adjacent to the fibroadenoma or originated in tissue within the fibroadenoma, eventually replacing all the tissue of the original fibroadenoma except for the calcification.

The negative cytology of the cyst fluid is not unusual. In cysts with a wall malignancy or in necrotic tumors, there may be a relative lack of malignant cells in the fluid (see case 23, above).

On pneumocystography the air should fill the entire volume of the mass with a clear, well defined internal border, and a thin cyst wall should be noted. In this case the inability of the air to fully occupy the mass suggested a thick wall posteriorly, consistent with carcinoma (see Fig. 21-24D). Diaphanography identified the cystic nature of the internal portion of the larger mass and the thick wall with the cancer.

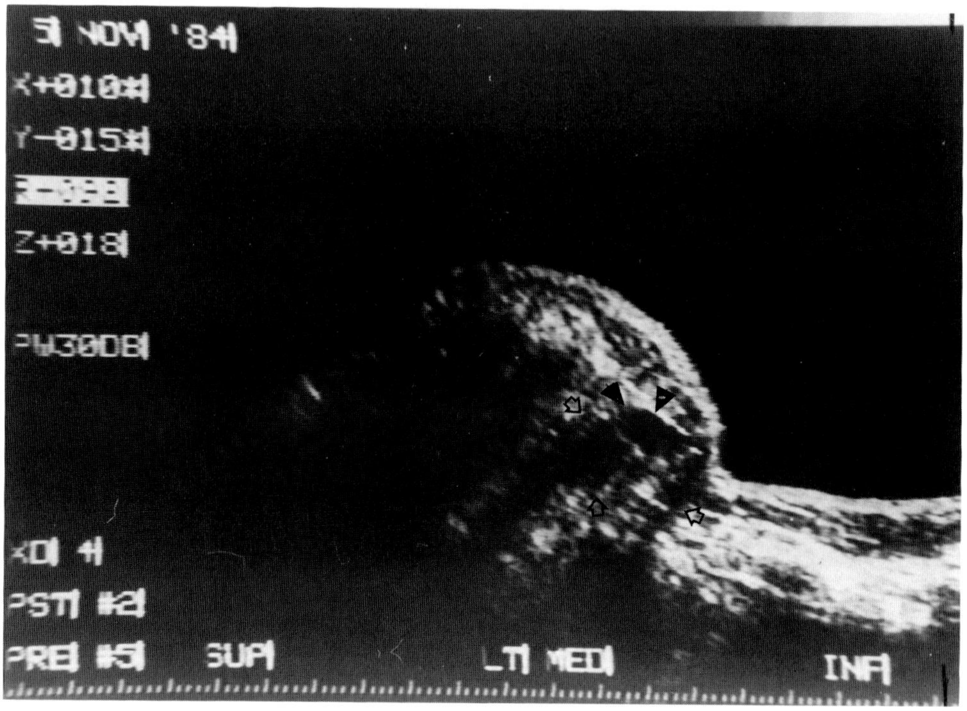

Fig. 21-25 Ultrasound, single transducer. The anechoic area anteriorly represents a cyst (arrowheads). There is a posterior mass with low-level echoes and irregular borders (open arrows). The normal increased through transmission seen with cysts is obscured by the posterior solid mass.

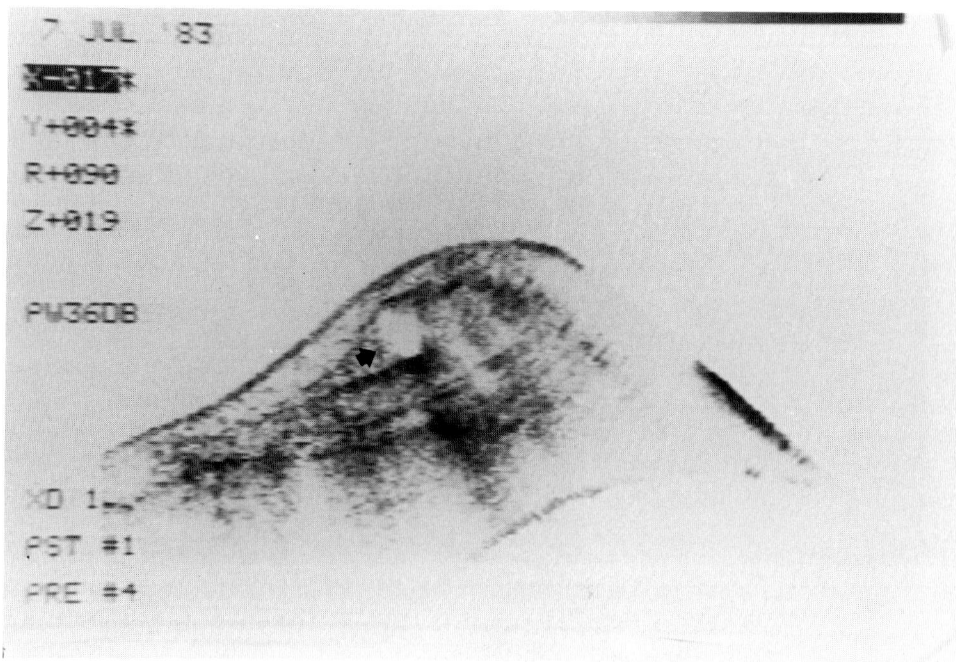

Fig. 21-26 Ultrasound. Note the anechoic area (arrow) with slightly increased through transmission.

In case 27 the presence of a mass after drainage of a cyst and the pneumocystogram that demonstrated a mass unfilled with air necessitated biopsy. This unfilled area represented the posterior portion of the mass seen on ultrasound to be echogenic, the area of cancer on biopsy. The lack of a search for the punctate calcifications on the mastectomy specimen is an error, because if there is a second tumor it is important to know the cell type for future therapy.

Case Study: False-Negative Needle Biopsies and Hemorrhage Masking a Cancer

Case 28

E.L. is a 47-year-old woman who saw a surgeon in August 1982 with thickening in the inner aspect of the right breast. A needle biopsy did not demonstrate malignancy. The area was unchanged when she was again seen in November 1982. Mammograms demonstrated diffuse glandular tissue, with no lesion noted. A true-cut needle biopsy did not demonstrate malignancy. There was a massive hemorrhage following the biopsy, and the surgeon drained blood from the area on three occasions during the following month.

The patient presented at the Woman's Breast Center on 4/27/83 with a hard mass occupying the entire inner upper portion of the right breast. Thermograms demonstrated increased nipple heat bilaterally and a marked increase in heat and vascularity in the inner aspect of the right breast (Th III on the left and Th V on the right) (Color Fig. 25). There was a marked decrease in light transmission over the inner right breast, with increased vascularity. Ultrasound showed small cysts on the left and markedly increased tissue density on the right with multiple fluid collections (Fig. 21-26). The patient refused mammography.

Aspiration of the fluid collections on the right yielded a small amount of blood, which on cytologic examination showed no malignancy. The patient was told that there may be a carcinoma present, but she declined formal biopsy. She was treated over the next 3 months with enzymes and warm packs. The area in question decreased to about one-half its original size.

Reevaluation on 7/7/83 showed decreased temperature on thermography, although it was still positive on the right. Diaphanography showed less light absorption over the area and a diminution in the size of the area by about one-half when compared to the initial study. A right mammogram demonstrated grossly increased glandular tissue on the right without a mass or calcifications. Ultrasound again demonstrated fluid areas. A needle aspiration of the fluid demonstrated malignant cells on cytology.

The patient underwent a modified radical mastectomy and partial muscle resection, as at the time of surgery tumor was found to be invading the underlying muscle. Ductal carcinoma invading the pectoralis muscle was found, with 11 of 20 nodes positive. After a course of radiation therapy to the chest wall she was placed on chemotherapy. She has had three episodes of chest wall metastasis, treated by surgery and repeat irradiation, while continuing on the chemotherapy. In January 1985 laser surgery was done to the chest wall metastasis. As of September 1985 she had en plaque metastasis of the right chest wall and bilateral pleural effusions. She expired in December, 1985.

Discussion

This case is a vivid example of the fact that needle biopsies are adequate only when they are positive; otherwise formal biopsy is indicated in any suspicious area. On this patient a thin needle biopsy, a true-cut needle biopsy, and multiple fluid aspirations were all negative despite a diffusely invasive cancer. The massive hemorrhage masked evaluation of the cancer as evidenced by the decreased size of the mass on enzyme therapy.

The invasion of the muscle increases the probability of chest wall recurrence, as happened in this patient. The growth of the recurrence despite continuing chemotherapy and radiation therapy is a bad prognostic sign. It is probable that the inability to control these chest wall recurrences will eventually lead to disseminated metastatic disease and death in patients who so present.

Case Studies: Carcinoma in Patients with Implants

Case 29

T.G. is a 56-year-old woman who presented with a 1.5 cm nodule on the lateral aspect of the left breast. The patient had bilateral silicone implants. Liquid crystal thermograms showed increased heat over the left breast, especially laterally, and increased nipple heat. Diaphanography showed decreased light transmission over the area of the mass with an abnormal vein in the area as well. Mammography demonstrated bilateral silicone gel implants. There was some increase in glandular tissue in the area of the mass, but no mass was delineated (Fig. 21-27A). A single benign calcification was noted. Ultrasound showed some glandular tissue with decreased echogenicity in the center portion (Fig. 21-27B).

Biopsy revealed an infiltrating ductal carcinoma. The patient underwent a modified radical mastectomy; all nodes were negative. At 2 years she has diffuse lung metastasis.

Case 30

K.L. is a 39-year-old woman who has a marked pectus excavatum deformity. She had had silicone gel implants inserted 10 years ago. The implants hardened, necessitating removal and new implants. At the time of surgery, the plastic surgeon noted an area of marked firmness, thought to be a calcification within the fibrous capsule that surrounded the first implant. This area was biopsied and found to be intraductal carcinoma. The patient was referred for evaluation.

On physical examination there was a swelling from the recent implant replacement surgery. The breasts were tender, and there was nodularity in the upper midportion of the right breast, the area of biopsy. Thermography was positive, with increased nipple heat and vascularity on the right. Diaphanography demonstrated decreased light transmission through this area. On mammography there were multiple punctate calcifications in the area of nodularity, measuring 2 cm in extent, and bilateral silicone gel implants (Fig. 21-28A). Ultrasound showed the bilateral implants and an echo-free area in the location of the calcifications (Fig. 21-28B).

A review of the original pathology slides demonstrated areas of invasion, changing the diagnosis from intraductal carcinoma to invasive ductal carcinoma. The patient underwent lumpectomy, axillary node dissection, and radiation therapy.

Discussion

Although the presence of implants can make the diagnosis of a lesion more difficult, it is possible to visualize the entire breast and the lesions with currently available imaging procedures. The presence of implants does not increase the patient's risk of breast cancer.

Case 30 is a prime example of the need for preoperative mammograms prior to plastic surgery procedures. It is the author's belief that every patient over the age

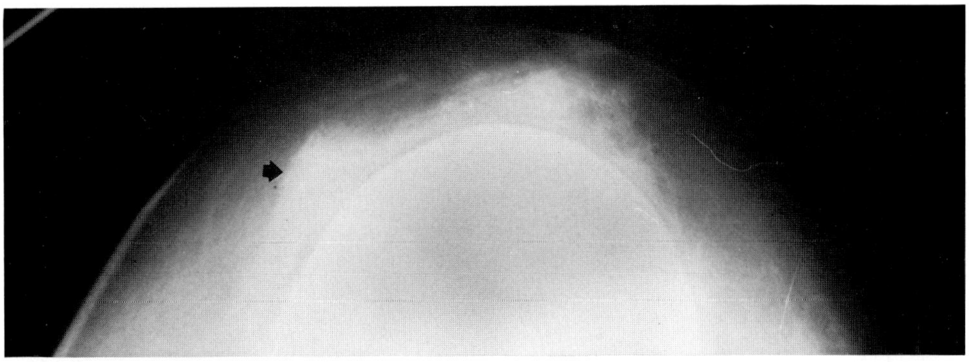

A

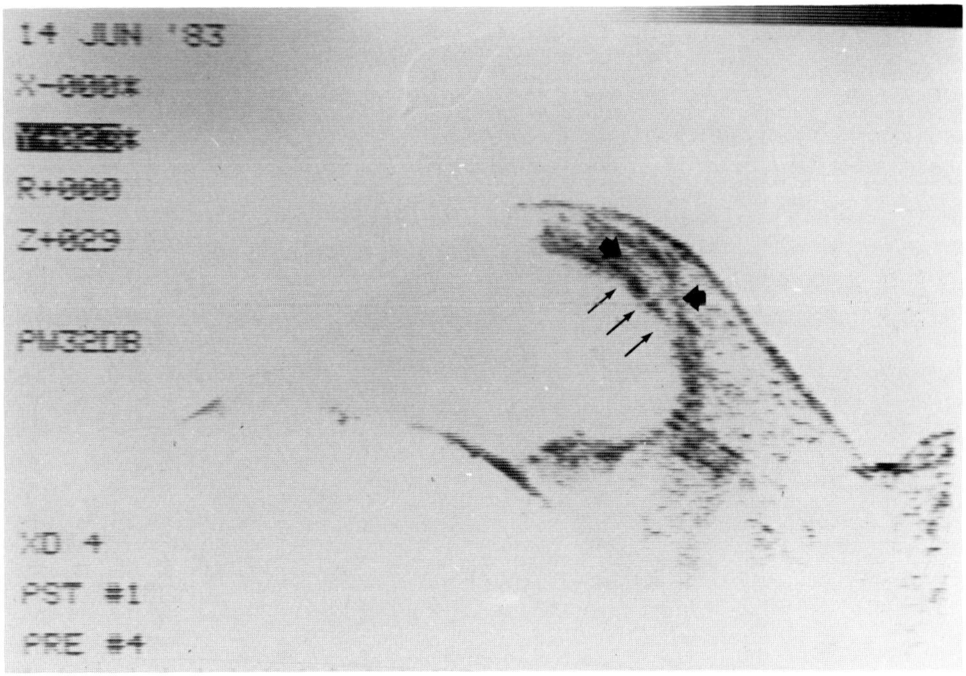

B

Fig. 21-27 A: Mammogram, CC view. There is a silicone gel implant with mild glandularity. Note the area of glandular density (arrow); no mass was identified.
B: Ultrasound, reverse image. A low-level echo area (thick arrows) is seen indenting the implant (thin arrows). Note how ultrasound helps identify the contents of the glandular area seen in **A.**

of 30 should have mammography prior to any breast surgery. The positive thermogram in this case was not due to the surgery, as both breasts had implant replacements, but was related to the cancer.

Case Studies: Lobular Carcinoma

Case 31

B.E. is a 68-year-old woman who presented with an ill-defined 2 cm lateral right breast mass. Liquid crystal thermograms demonstrated increased nipple heat and vascularity on the right (Th IV thermogram). Diaphanography was normal. Mammography showed

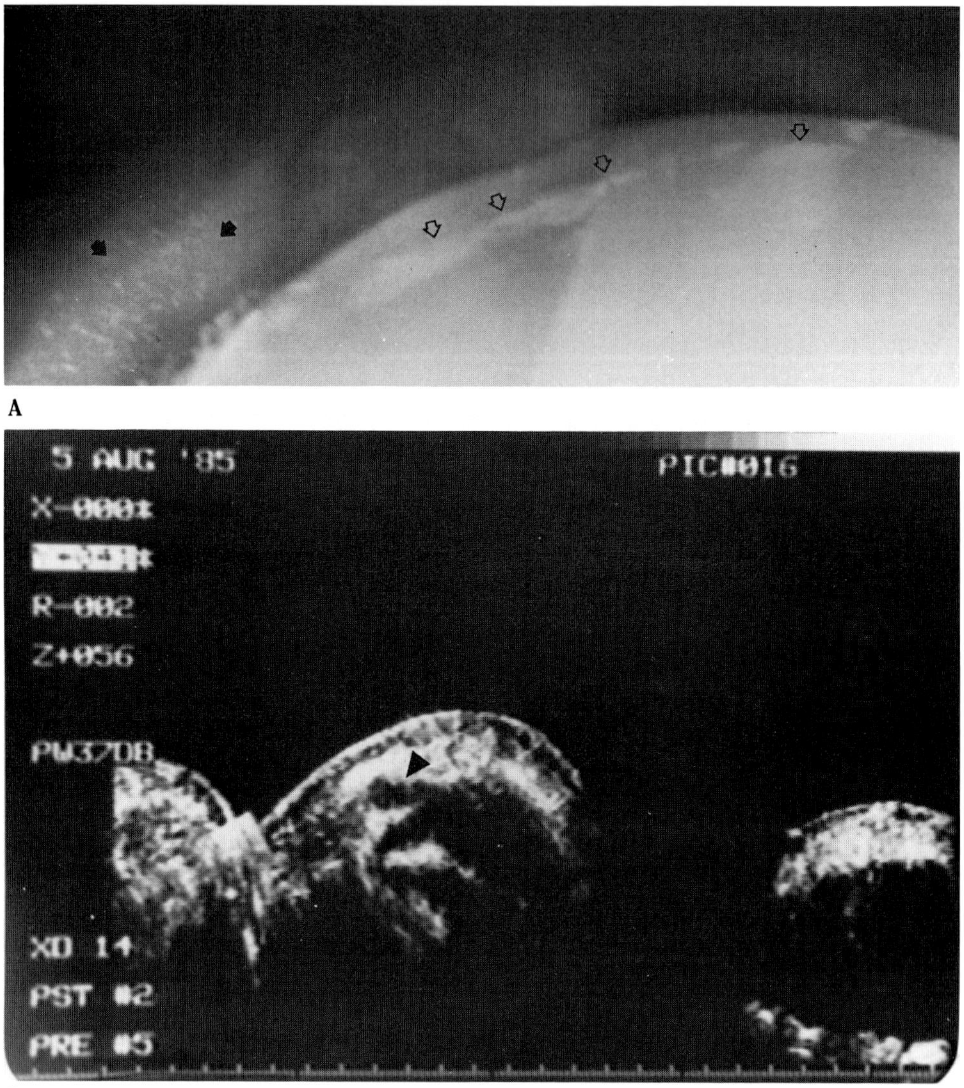

Fig. 21-28 **A:** Mammogram, magnified. Diffuse malignant calcifications (arrows) are seen adjacent to the implant. Gross calcifications (open arrows) are from calcification of the fibrous capsule around the old implant. **B:** Ultrasound. Note the low-level irregular mass (arrowhead) adjacent to the implant.

moderate glandularity (P2 pattern), more than expected for a patient of this age. There was a spiculated lesion with a dense center, the overall size measuring almost 3 cm (Fig. 21-29A). Ultrasound showed shadowing from the area of a low-level echo mass (Fig. 21-29B).

Review of prior mammograms showed no evidence of the lesion 18 months earlier; however, a mammogram 4 months prior to the examination was reported as a questionable spiculated lesion. On biopsy there was an infiltrating lobular carcinoma. The patient underwent a modified radical mastectomy.

Case 32

J.H. is a 36-year-old woman who presented with a 5 mm firm nodule of 1 month's duration in the upper outer right breast. Thermograms, diaphanography, mammography, and ultrasound were normal. It was assumed that this nodule was probably glan-

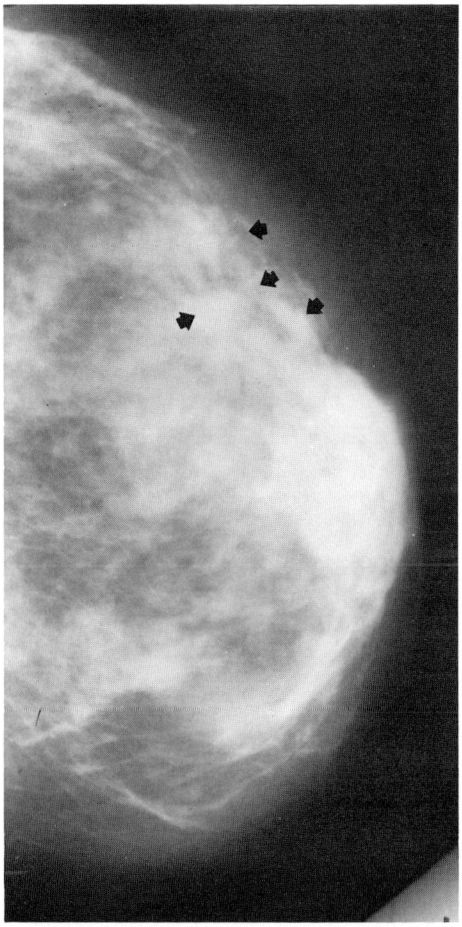

A

Fig. 21-29 **A:** Mammogram. Note the nodule with spicules (arrows). The center nodule is less than 1 cm whereas the spicules measure more than 3 cm overall. **B:** Ultrasound. There is a well defined low-level echo mass with slight posterior shadowing (arrows).

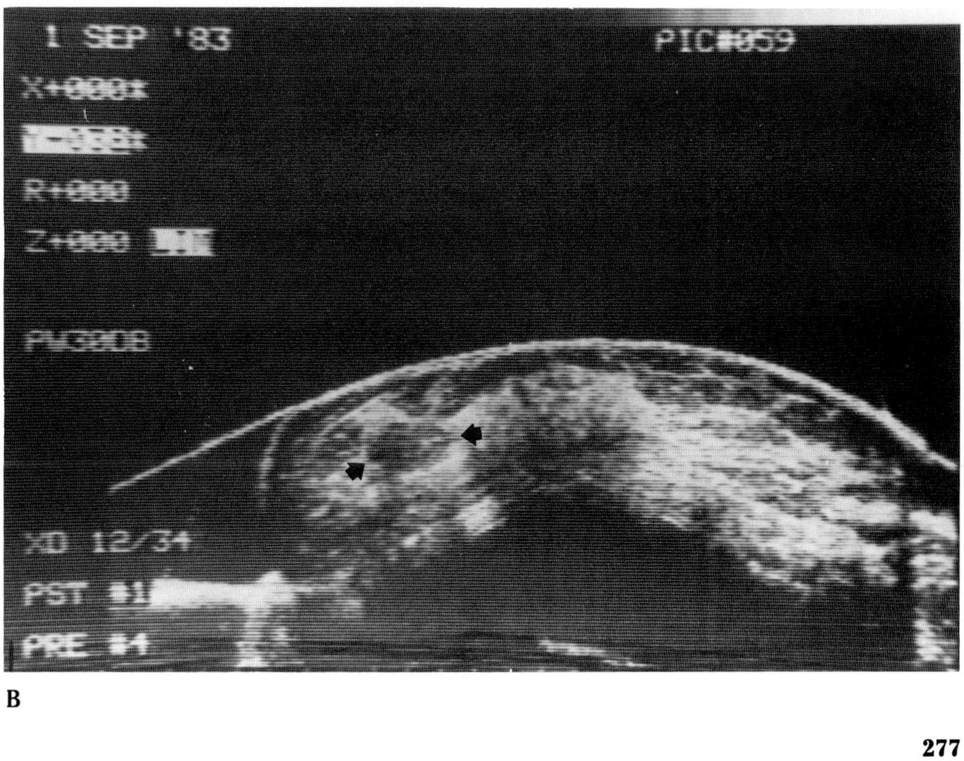

B

dular tissue and should change with the cycles. It did not change on two examinations by the primary physician at 6 and 12 months. On a repeat examination at 18 months the nodule was 6 mm in size. All tests were again normal. Excision was advised.

At biopsy there was an infiltrating lobular carcinoma as well as some foci of lobular carcinoma in situ. She has had a lumpectomy and radiation therapy.

Discussion

Lobular carcinoma can present in a myriad of ways, two of which are demonstrated here. In case 31 there was a mass and a spiculated lesion, and in case 32 there was a very small superficial nodule with no findings on the imaging examinations. Such variety of presentations can also be seen with ductal carcinoma. In case 31 there should have been a mammography report 4 months earlier that was more definite than questionable spiculization, as there was a mass with spiculization that was not present on the prior mammograms a year earlier. It is important to obtain and compare old mammograms whenever possible. Case 32 demonstrates the inability of our imaging procedures to visualize a 5 to 6 mm nodule.

(See case 10 in the section on multicentric carcinomas and case 14 in the section on bilateral breast cancers for additional case reports of lobular carcinoma.)

Case Study: Medullary Carcinoma

Case 33

M.R. is a 44-year-old woman who was evaluated by mammography at a local hospital for a left breast mass 4 cm in size. There was marked glandular tissue, with no mass identified. There was a disclaimer that because of the marked density of the breasts it was impossible to identify a mass, and therefore if a mass was present biopsy should be performed. Because of the persistence of the mass the patient was referred 4 months later.

On physical examination there was a movable 4 cm mass in the upper outer aspect of the left breast. Liquid crystal thermograms demonstrated diffuse increased vascularity over the left breast with an almost anarchic pattern over the area of the mass (Th IV thermogram) (Color Fig. 26). Diaphanography showed a marked decrease in light transmission over the mass. A magnification mammogram over the area showed marked glandularity (DY pattern), without a discrete mass or calcification. Ultrasound demonstrated a discrete low-level echo mass with increased through transmission (Fig. 21-30).

On the basis of these studies the diagnosis of a solid mass, either a fibroadenoma or carcinoma such as a medullary carcinoma, was offered. At biopsy a medullary carcinoma was found. The patient underwent lumpectomy and radiation therapy. At follow-up 2 years later there was no evidence of recurrence.

Discussion

This case illustrates a clinically evident mass which because of a negative mammogram did not have an appropriate biopsy. Unfortunately, this is not an isolated situation. In one report 165 patients were referred from a university surgical breast clinic to a university mammography department. All of the patients had a mass on

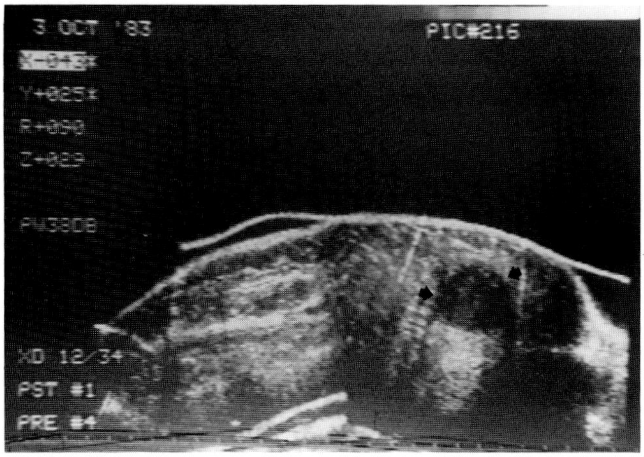

Fig. 21-30 Ultrasound. There is a moderately well defined low-level echo mass (arrows) with edge shadowing and some increased through transmission.

physical examination that was cancer on biopsy. The miss rate on mammography was 34.2 percent, and the miss rate in patients under the age of 45 was 52 percent. Because of the negative mammography report there was a delay of 2 to 24 months in the performance of biopsy. The thermograms, diaphanography, and ultrasound in this case all demonstrated an abnormality.

Case Studies: Lymphoma

Case 34

V.B. is a 73-year-old woman who was originally seen on 8/25/83 for a checkup. Physical examination and thermograms were normal. Diaphanography demonstrated slightly decreased light transmission adjacent to the nipples, thought to represent ductal changes. Mammograms were essentially normal.

The patient returned on 9/20/84 with a 3 cm mass in the left axilla. The breast was free of masses. Thermograms demonstrated increased vascularity on the left more prominent than previously seen. Diaphanography was essentially normal. Mammograms again showed a glandular pattern without lesion, unchanged since previous films, except that there were lymph node masses present in the left axilla (Fig. 21-31).

Left axillary lymph node biopsy revealed Hodgkin's lymphoma. The patient is undergoing chemotherapy.

Case 35

J.S. is a 56-year-old woman whose physical examination was normal. Telethermography demonstrated increased temperature of the left breast (Th III thermogram). Mammograms showed mild glandularity (P1 pattern). There was a trilobed 2 cm mass in the upper outer left breast and a smaller density elsewhere in the left breast (Fig. 21-32). The mass was solid on ultrasound, with a hypoechoic area and no increased through transmission.

The mass was localized preoperatively by mammography, and at biopsy a malignant lymphoma, of a well differentiated lymphocytic type, was found involving an intramammary lymph node. Bone marrow aspirate showed chronic lymphocytic leukemia. The patient is undergoing chemotherapy.

(This case was loaned by The Breast Center, Van Nuys, CA, courtesy of Drs. Silverstein and Gamigami.)

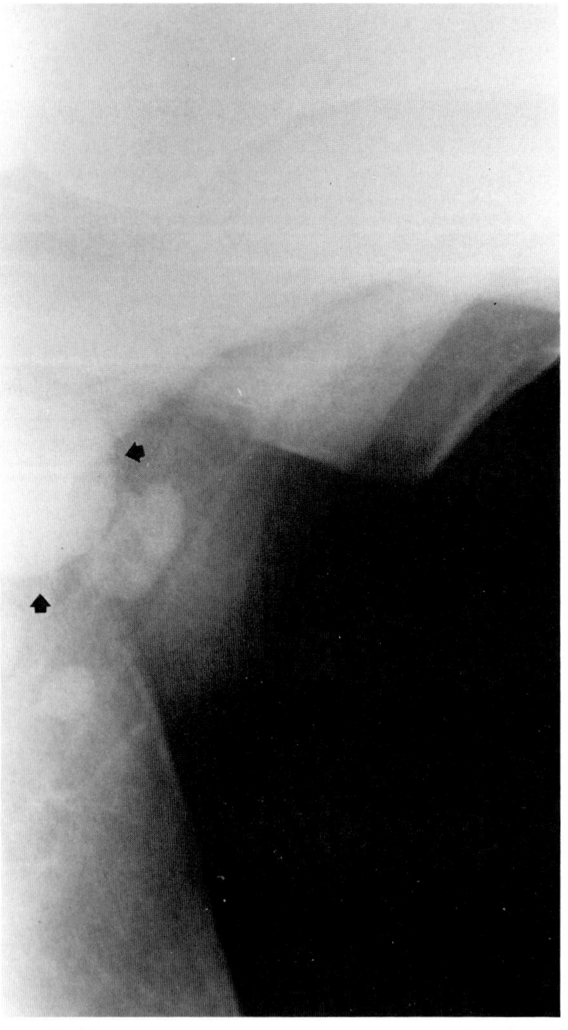

Fig. 21-31 Mammogram, magnified, left axilla. This large mass (arrows) represents a lymph node with lymphoma. Compare with the more normal size and shape of adjacent nodes.

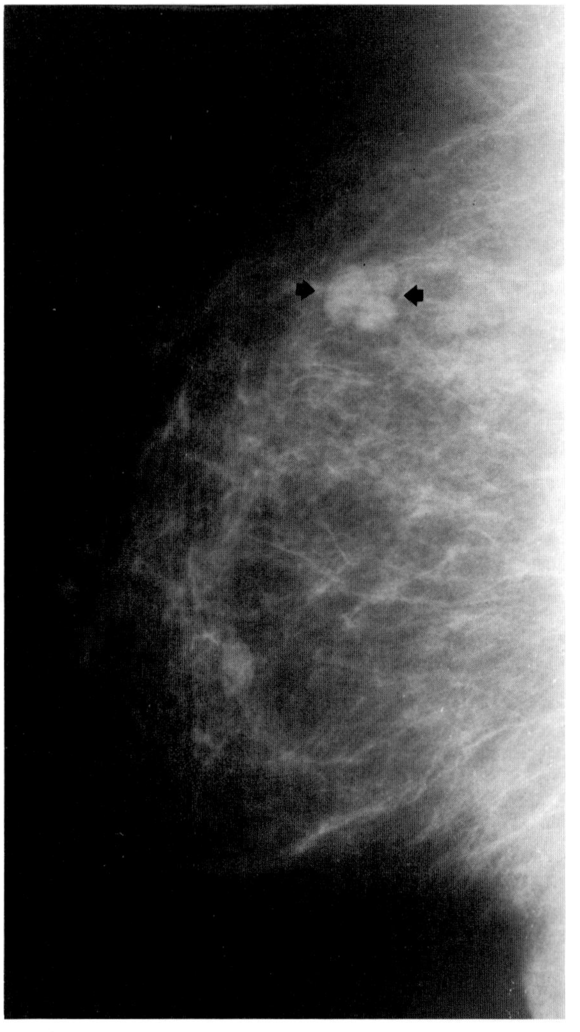

Fig. 21-32 Mammogram. There is a trilobed, well defined (arrows) mass with smooth borders.

Discussion

Lymphoma is usually found in the lymph nodes of the axilla or within the breasts, and occasionally there is a deposit within the glandular tissue itself. The treatment is usually chemotherapy, often in combination with radiation therapy.

Case Study: Metastatic Breast Lesions

Case 36

R.C. was a 70-year-old woman who presented with a hard area directly over the sternum barely extending into the inner aspect of both breasts. There was some ecchymosis in the area where her primary care physician had attempted an aspiration.

Thermograms and diaphanography were normal. Mammograms demonstrated three well defined, smooth densities—two on the left, one on the right—with a slight ovoid configuration in an otherwise fatty breast. The densities were thought to be intramammary lymph nodes. The lesion over the sternum could not be demonstrated on mammography, even with special films over the area.

A biopsy of the area revealed a metastatic papillary adenocarcinoma of either lung, ovary, or breast origin. The patient died of a coronary 2 weeks later. The site of the primary was never established. The family refused an autopsy.

Discussion

Nodules in the medial folds are very difficult to visualize on mammography, especially when they extend over the sternum, rather than into the breast. The best success comes from placing both breasts on the plate at the same time, although it was not successful in this case. In the differential diagnosis of any solid, well defined nodule of the breast the possibility of metastasis should be considered.

Bibliography

General

Amalric R, Giraud D, Altschuler C, et al: The contribution of infra-red thermography to the integrated diagnosis of early breast cancer, in Gautherie M, Albert E, Keigh L (eds): *Thermal Assessment of Breast Health*. Boston, MTP Press, 1984, pp 150–155.

Baker LH: Breast cancer detection demonstration project: 5-Year summary report. *CA* 1982;32:194.

Carlsen E: Transillumination light scanning. *Diagn Imaging* April 1982, pp 28–34.

Carlsen E: Transmission spectroscopy: An improvement in light scanning. *RNM Images* February 1983, pp 23–25.

Carter D: *Interpretation of Breast Biopsies, Biopsy Interpretation Series*. New York, Raven Press, 1984.

Cole-Beuglet C, Soriano R, Pasto M, et al: Solid breast mass lesions: Can ultrasound differentiate benign and malignant? in Jellins J, Kobayashi T (eds): *Ultrasonic Examination of the Breast*. London, Wiley, 1983, pp 45–55.

Croll J: Ultrasonic diagnosis of malignant tumors of the breast, in Kossoff G, Fukuda M (eds): *Ultrasonic Differential Diagnosis of Tumors*. New York, Igaku-Shoin, 1984, pp 90–107.

Cutler M: Transillumination as an aid in the diagnosis of breast lesions. *Surg Gynecol Obstet* 1929;48:721.

Dempsen PJ, Wilson PC: The use of automated sonography in total clinical breast evaluation, in Leopold G (ed): *Ultrasound in Breast and Endocrine Disease, Clinics in Diagnostic Ultrasound*. New York, Churchill Livingstone, 1984, pp 57–81.

DiMaggio C, Muzzio P, DiBello A, et al: Transillumination of the breast. *Radiol Med (Torino)* 1976;62(6):401–413.

Egan RL, McSweeney MB: Breast sonography—interpretative criteria, in Jellins J, Kobayashi T (eds): *Ultrasonic Examination of the Breast*. London, Wiley, 1983, pp 307–318.

Feig SA, McLelland R (eds): *Breast Carcinoma, Current Diagnosis and Treatment*. New York, Masson, 1983.

Frank G, Ackerman M: Xeromammography and 1200 breast cancers. *Radiol Clin North Am* 1983;21(1):81–91.

Gallager HS: Problems in the classification of breast cancer. *Radiol Clin North Am* 1983;21(1):13–26.

Gautherie M, Cros Ch: Breast thermography and cancer risk prediction. *Cancer* 1980;45:51–56.

Gautherie M, Haehnel P, Walter JP, et al: Improved survival rate of breast cancer patients with an early diagnosis based on initial thermal assessment and subsequent follow-up, in

Gautherie M, Albert E, Keith L (eds): *Thermal Assessment of Breast Health*. Boston, MTP Press, 1984, pp 180–200.
Haagensen CD, Bodian D, Haagensen DE: *Breast Carcinoma: Risk and Detection*. Philadelphia, Saunders, 1981.
Isard HJ: Breast disease and correlation of images: Mammography-thermography-diaphanography, in Gauthers M, Albert E (eds): *Biomedical Thermology* New York, Alan R Liss, 1982, pp 321-328.
Kobayashi T: *Clinical Ultrasound of the Breast*. New York, Plenum Press, 1978.
Kobayashi T: Current status of interpretative criteria for breast tumor, in Jellins J, Kobayashi T (eds): *Ultrasonic Examination of the Breast*. London, Wiley, 1983, pp 57–64.
McSweeney MB, Egan RL: Automated breast sonography: Comparison with other imaging modalities, in Jellins J, Kobayashi T (eds): *Ultrasonic Examination of the Breast*. London, Wiley, 1983, pp 325–333.
Porrath S, Bernay T: The role of thermography in the multimodality approach to breast cancer diagnosis, in Gautherie M, Albert E, Keith L (eds): *Thermal Assessment of Breast Health*. Boston, MTP Press, 1984, pp 156–166.
Reuter K, D'Orsi CJ, Reale F: Intracystic carcinoma of the breast: The role of ultrasonography. *Radiology* 1984;153:233–234.
Sadowsky N, Kopans DB: Breast cancer: Symposium on mammography. *Radiol Clin North Am* 1983;21(1):51–65.
Spitalier JM, Ayme Y, Brandone H, et al: The importance of infra-red thermography in the early suspicion and detection of minimal breast cancer, in Gautherie M, Albert E, Keith L (eds): *Thermal Assessment of Breast Health*. Boston, MTP Press, 1984, pp 173–179.
Tabár L, Dean PB: *Teaching Atlas of Mammography*. New York, Thieme-Stratton, 1983.

Infiltrating Ductal Carcinoma

Carter D: *Interpretation of Breast Biopsies, Biopsy Interpretation Series*. New York, Raven Press, 1984.
Feig SA, McLelland R (eds): *Breast Carcinoma, Current Diagnosis and Treatment*. New York, Masson, 1983.
Haagensen CD, Bodian D, Haagensen DE: *Breast Carcinoma: Risk and Detection*. Philadelphia, Saunders, 1981.
Ozzello L, Gump FE: The management of patients with carcinomas in fibroadenomatous tumors of the breast. *Surgery* 1985;160(2):99–104.
Tabár L, Dean PB: *Teaching Atlas of Mammography*. New York, Thieme-Stratton, 1983.

Multicentric Carcinoma in the Same Breast

Egan RL: Multicentric breast carcinomas. *Cancer* 1982;49(6):1123–1130.
Lagios MD: Multicentricity of breast carcinoma demonstrated by routine correlated serial subgross and radiographic examination. *Cancer* 1977;40:1726–1734.
Morgenstern L, Kaufman PA, Friedman MB: The case against tylectomy for carcinoma of the breast: The factor of multicentricity. *Am J Surg* 1975; 130:251–258.
Qualheim RE, Gall EA: Breast carcinoma with multiple sites or origin. *Cancer* 1957;10:460–468.
Schwartz GF, Patchesfsky AS, Feig SA, et al: Multicentricity of nonpalpable breast cancer. *Cancer* 1980;45(12):2913–2916.

Bilateral Breast Cancer

Egan RL: Bilateral breast carcinomas, role of mammography. *Cancer* 1976;38:931–938.
Egan RL, McSweeney MB, Sewell CW: Intramammary calcifications without an associated mass in benign and malignant diseases. *Radiology* 1980;137:1–7.

Haagensen CD, Bodian C, Haagensen DW: *Breast Carcinoma: Risk and Detection*. Philadelphia, Saunders, 1981.
Leis HP, Cammarata A, La Raja R, et al: Bilateral breast cancer. *Breast* 1981;7(4):13–17.
Schenker JG, Levensky R, Ohel G: Multiple primary malignant neoplasms in breast cancer patients in Israel. *Cancer* 1984;54:145–150.

Paget's Disease of the Breast

Ashikari R, Park K, Huvos AG, et al: Paget's disease of the breast. *Cancer* 1970;26:680–685.
Barth V: *Atlas of Diseases of the Breast*. Chicago, Year Book, 1979.
Haagensen CD, Bodian C, Haagensen DW: *Breast Carcinoma: Risk and Detection*. Philadelphia, Saunders, 1981.
Lagios MD, Westdahl PR, Rose MR, et al: Paget's disease of the nipple. *Cancer* 1984;54:545–551.
Paget J: On disease of the mammary areola preceding cancer of the mammary gland. *St Bartholomews Hosp Rep* 1967;10:87–89.
Paone JF, Baker PR: Pathogenesis and treatment of Paget's disease of the breast. *Cancer* 1981;48:825–829.

Ulcerating and Necrotic Carcinomas

Barth V: *Atlas of Diseases of the Breast*. Chicago, Year Book, 1979.
Haagensen CD, Bodian C, Haagensen DE: *Breast Carcinoma: Risk and Detection*. Philadelphia, Saunders, 1981.

Inflammatory Carcinoma

Barker JL, Nelson AT, Montague ED: Inflammatory carcinoma of the breast. *Radiology* 1976;121:173–176.
Barth V: *Atlas of Diseases of the Breast*. Chicago, Year Book, 1979.
Buzdar AU, et al: Management of inflammatory carcinoma of breast with combination modality approach—an update. *Cancer* 1981;47:2537–2542.
Cammarata A, Georgiou J, Cruz E, et al: Inflammatory carcinoma in a patient with a breast implant. *Breast* 1984;10(3):24–26.
Haagensen CD, Bodian C, Haagensen DE: *Breast Carcinoma: Risk and Detection*. Philadelphia, Saunders, 1981.
Tabár L, Dean PB: *Teaching Atlas of Mammography*. New York, Thieme-Stratton, 1983.

Carcinoma and Cysts

Cooke CG, Grant EG, Cigtoy OS: Ultrasound demonstration of giant malignant breast cyst undetected by xeromammography. *J Clin Ultrasound* 1981;9:461–462.
Haagensen DC, Bodian C, Haagensen DE: *Breast Carcinoma: Risk and Detection*. Philadelphia, Saunders, 1981.
Kasumi F, Tanaka H: Diagnosis of intracystic tumors by ultrasound, in Jellins J, Kobayashi T (eds): *Ultrasonic Examination of the Breast*. New York, Wiley, 1983, pp 283–291.

False-Negative Needle Biopsies and Hemorrhage Masking a Cancer

Bell DA, Hajdu SI, Urban JA, et al: Role of aspiration cytology in the diagnosis and management of mammary lesions in office practice. 1983; *Cancer* 51:1182–1189.

Norton LW, David JR, Wiens LC, et al: Accuracy of aspiration cytology in detecting breast cancer. *Surgery* 1984; 96:806–814.
Sommers RG, Young GP, Kaplan MJ, et al: Fine-needle aspiration biopsy in the management of solid breast tumors. *Arch Surg* 1985;120:673–677.
Wanebo HJ, Feldman PS, Morton CW, et al: Fine-needle aspiration cytology in lieu of open biopsy in management of primary breast cancer. *Ann Surg* 1984;199:569–579.

Carcinoma in Patients with Implants

Cammarata A, Georgiou J, Cruz E, et al: Inflammatory carcinoma in a patient with a breast implant. *Breast* 1984;10(3):24–26.
Cole-Beuglet C, Schwartz G, Kurtz AB, et al: Ultrasound mammography for the augmented breast. *Radiology* 1980;136:505–507.
Frantz P, Herbst CA: Augmentation mammoplasty, irradiation, and breast cancer. *Cancer* 1975;36:1147–1150.
Holt RW, Spear SL: Cancer in the augmented breast: Diagnosis and treatment. *Breast* 1984;10(4):16–18.
Piontek RW, Kase KR: Radiation transmission study of silicone elastomer for mammary prosthesis. *Radiology* 1980;136:505–507.

Lobular Carcinoma

Ashikari R, Huvos AG, Urban JA, et al: Infiltrating lobular carcinoma of the breast. *Cancer* 1973;31:110–116.
Carter D: *Interpretation of Breast Biopsies*. New York, Raven Press 1984, pp 145–146.
Cole-Beuglet C, Soriano RZ, Kurtz AB, et al: Ultrasound analysis of 104 primary breast carcinomas classified according to histopathologic type. *Radiology* 1983;147:191–196.
Fechner RE: Infiltrating lobular carcinoma without lobular carcinoma-in-situ. *Cancer* 1972;29:1539–1545.

Medullary Carcinoma

Barth V: *Atlas of Diseases of the Breast*. Chicago, Year Book, 1979.
Carter D: *Interpretation of Breast Biopsies*, New York, Raven Press, 1984, pp 112–119.
Cole-Beuglet C, Soriano RZ, Kurtz AB, et al: Ultrasound analysis of 104 primary breast carcinomas classified according to histopathologic type. *Radiology* 1983;147:191–196.
Kalisher L: Factors influencing false negative rates in xeromammography. *Radiology* 1979;133:297–301.
Mann BD, Giuliano AE, Bassett LW, et al: Delayed diagnosis of breast cancer as a result of normal mammograms. *Arch Surg* 1983;118:224.

Lymphoma

D'Orsi CJ, Feldhaus L, Sonnenfeld M: Unusual lesions of the breast. *Radiol Clin North Am* 1983;21(1):76–78.
Fisher MG, Chideckel NJ: "Primary" lymphoma of the breast. *Breast* 1984;10(3):7–12.
Kushner LN: Hodgkin's disease simulating inflammatory breast carcinoma on mammography: A case report. *Radiology* 1969;92:350.
Mambo NC, Burke JS, Butler JJ: Primary malignant lymphomas of the breast. *Cancer* 1977;39:2033–2040.
Meyer JE, Kopans DB, Long JC: Mammographic appearance of malignant lymphoma of the breast. *Radiology* 1980;135:623–626.
Tabár L, Dean PB: *Teaching Atlas of Mammography*. New York Thieme-Stratton, 1983.
Wiseman C, Liao KT: Primary lymphoma of the breast. *Cancer* 1977;39:2033–2040.

Metastatic Breast Lesions

Bohman LG, Bassett LW, Gold RH, et al: Breast metastases from extramammary malignancies. *Radiology* 1982;144:309–312.

D'Orsi CJ, Feldhaus L, Sonnenfeld M: Unusual lesions of the breast. *Radiol Clin North Am* 1983;21(1):78–80.

Hadju SI, Urban SA: Cancers metastatic to the breast. *Cancer* 1972;29:1691–1696.

Martin JE: *Atlas of Mammography*. Baltimore, Williams & Wilkins, 1982.

McIntosh IH, Hooper AA, Mills RR, et al: Metastatic carcinoma within the breast. *Clin Oncol* 1976;2:393-401.

Tabár L, Dean PB: *Teaching Atlas of Mammography*. New York, Thieme-Stratton, 1983.

22

Carcinoma In Situ

Saar Porrath

In situ carcinoma implies a noninvasive process. The cancer has not broken through the basal membrane of the lobule or duct. As the entity is microscopic, it is often an incidental finding at surgery done for another reason. A mass is seldom present, and there are usually no signs and symptoms except for the occasional presentation of malignant calcifications seen more commonly with intraductal carcinoma.

There are two basic types of carcinoma in situ: lobular carcinoma in situ and carcinoma in situ. Carcinoma in situ is also called intraductal carcinoma.

Being microscopic in its presentation, thermography, diaphanography, and ultrasound usually play no role, although they may be positive in individual cases. Mammography may show a group of malignant calcifications, either punctate or rodlike.

For purposes of the discussion of incidence and treatment, carcinoma in situ here implies intraductal, but not lobular, carcinoma in situ. Most carcinomas in situ are seen in premenopausal women, although they can occur postmenopausally. They are usually in a single focus, although they may be multifocal. The presentation is almost always unilateral. If careful inspection shows no infiltrating portion, the treatment varies from wide excision and careful follow-up to lumpectomy, axillary node dissection, and radiation therapy. There is a question if axillary node dissection is really necessary when a single small focus of carcinoma in situ is found, as the nodes are almost always negative. Some surgeons advocate modified radical mastectomy. If there is an area of invasion, the lesion is a ductal carcinoma and treatment is directed.

Lobular carcinoma in situ, when it occurs alone without coexisting carcinoma, has been defined by Haagensen et al. as a benign pathologic-clinical entity. They coined the term lobular neoplasia, reflecting the view that this lesion is a premalignant condition, not a true cancer.

Most cases are in premenopausal women (89 percent in Haagensen et al.'s study, the remaining 11 percent postmenopausally). The disorder constituted 3.8 percent of all their benign epithelial lesions. It was present in the left breast 51.9 percent of the time and in the right breast in 41 percent of patients; 26 percent of the time it occurred bilaterally.

The subsequent development of carcinoma in the same breast has been reported as from 4 to 22 percent. (In Haagensen et al.'s large series the figure was 10.5 percent). Carcinoma of the opposite breast was found in 10.5 to 20 percent of the cases, the lower number in Haagensen et al.'s study. The total number of patients developing invasive breast cancer who had a diagnosis of lobular neoplasia is reported to be 17.1 to 36.9 percent. (In Haagensen et al.'s study it was 18 percent.)

It is this incidence of subsequent development of carcinoma and its frequency of bilaterality that has led to a diversion of opinions as to the proper therapy. Whereas many surgeons recommend unilateral mastectomy and a blind mirror biopsy of the opposite breast, others recommend bilateral mastectomy. (These recommendations more closely follow those given with a diagnosis of invasive lobular carcinoma.) Haagensen et al. recommended following the patient closely, without mastectomy.

It is interesting to note that when carcinoma in situ becomes invasive it is almost always ductal carcinoma. This is also the case for the invasive carcinoma which follows lobular carcinoma in situ; it is small cell or ductal carcinoma in 90 percent of the cases, seldom lobular carcinoma.

Case Studies: Intraductal Carcinoma

Case 1

J.K. is a 56-year-old woman who was referred for breast screening. On physical examination there was mild glandularity in the breast without a mass. Thermograms and diaphanography were normal. On mammography there was moderate glandularity (P2 pattern), with a group of punctate calcifications over a 1 cm area without a mass (Fig. 22-1). Ultrasound failed to demonstrate any abnormality.

After preoperative localization, a biopsy demonstrated an area of intraductal carcinoma 1.5 cm in length, without invasion. The patient underwent a modified radical mastectomy, and all nodes were negative.

Case 2

R.C. is a 61-year-old woman who was referred for screening. Physical examination was normal. Thermograms and diaphanography were also normal. On mammography there was marked glandularity and a group of punctate calcifications (Fig. 22-2). Ultrasound demonstrated nonspecific shadowing from the outer aspects of both breasts.

After mammographic localization, a 3 mm comedocarcinoma (intraductal) was found at surgery. It was elected not to do an axillary node dissection. The patient underwent radiation therapy to the left breast. At 36 months there has been no recurrence.

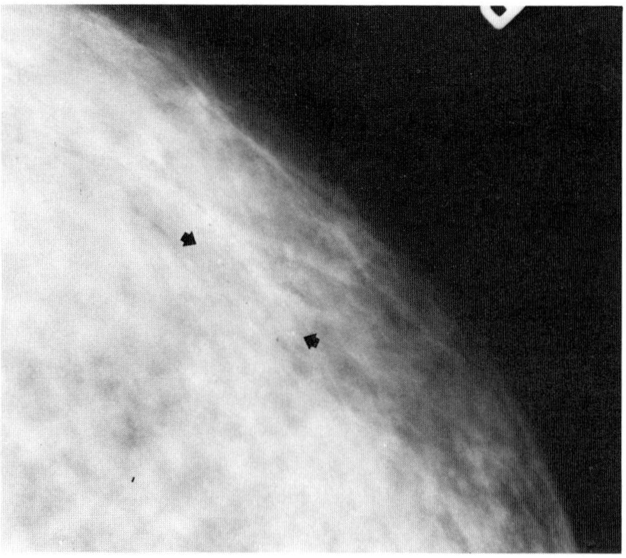

Fig. 22-1 Mammogram. Note the small group of faint punctate calcifications (arrows) along the duct. Further photographic magnification was attempted, but all detail was lost because of the small size and lack of contrast of the calcific areas.

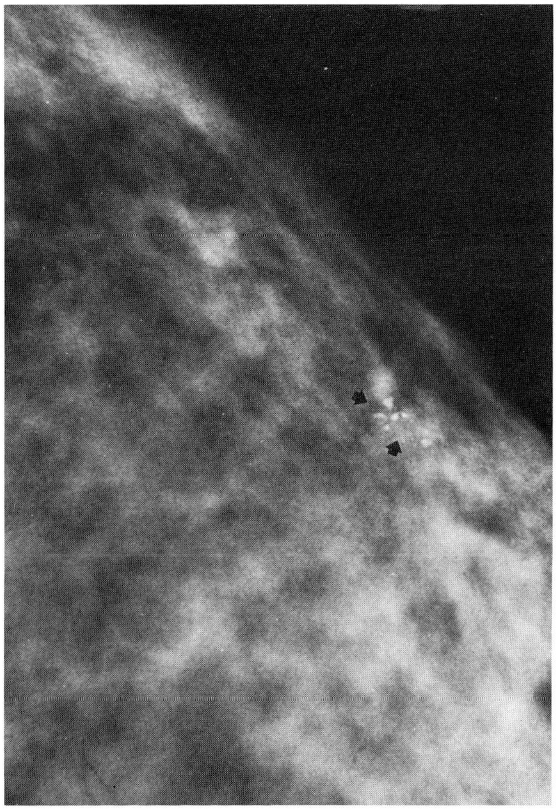

Fig. 22-2 Mammogram, magnified. Note the group of irregular small and punctate calcifications (arrows).

Case 3

B.S. is a 45-year-old woman referred for evaluation because of breast lumpiness and nipple discharge. On physical examination there was diffuse glandularity in the breasts, no discrete mass, and a bilateral whitish discharge.

Thermograms and diaphanography were normal. On mammography there was moderate glandularity (P1 pattern). There were diffuse calcifications noted along the extent of a duct, the calcifications being irregular, some rod-shaped or Y shaped (Fig. 22-3).

A biopsy was recommended. The initial surgeon claimed he could feel nothing and wanted to reevaluate the patient in 3 months. The primary physician urged a second surgical opinion. At surgery a multifocal intraductal carcinoma with a predominantly comedocarcinomatous pattern was found. In addition, there was extensive fibrocystic disease with sclerosing adenosis, microcysts, focal apocrine metaplasia, and intermediate and terminal duct dilatation with considerable stromal fibrosis.

Discussion

The finding of an intraductal carcinoma is what screening is all about. It would be wonderful if all cancers could be found before there was invasion or if they were not palpable. Any group of punctate calcifications should be biopsied. Most of these are not cancer, but if the imager tries to be too selective there will be misses, an unacceptable situation.

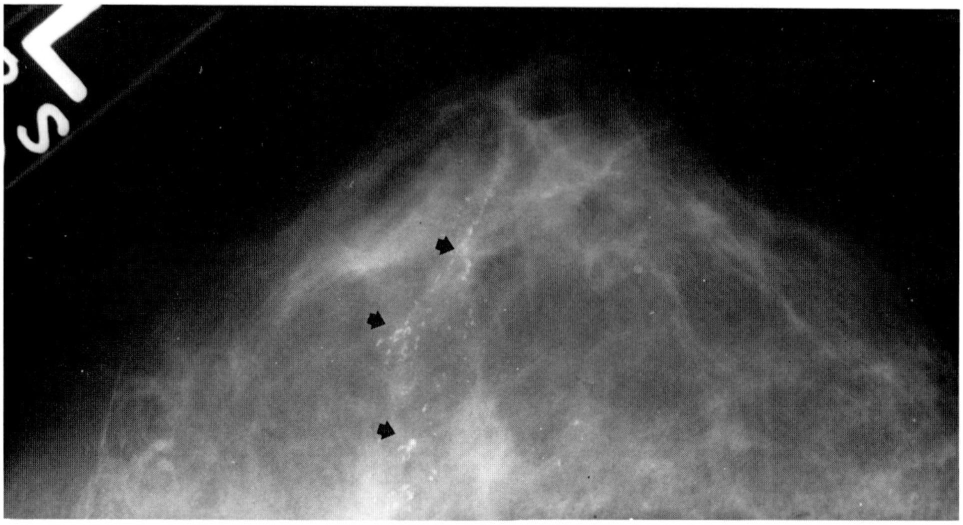

A

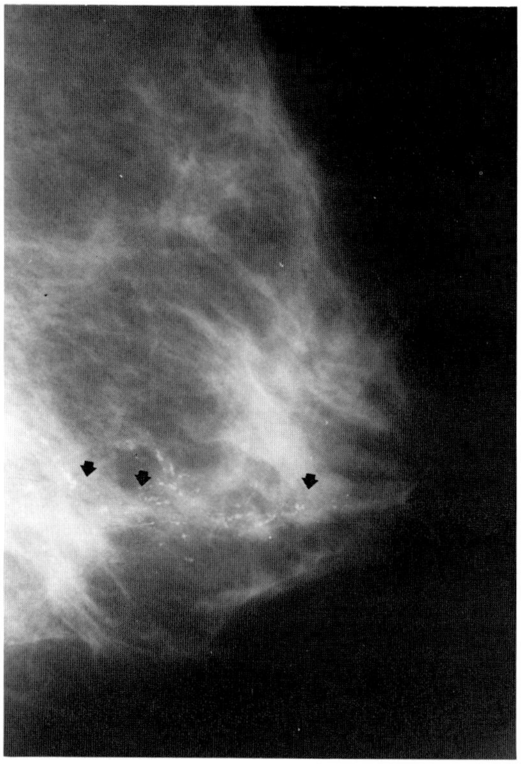

B

Fig. 22-3 Mammograms, CC view (**A**) and lateral veiw (**B**). There are diffuse calcifications along the duct (arrows) that are punctate, irregular, rod- and Y-shaped.

There is controversy about the proper therapy for an intraductal carcinoma. Cases 1 and 2 illustrate the alternatives. Most patients with intraductal carcinoma undergo mastectomy because of the relative lack of information concerning the results of radiation therapy. Hopefully in the future there will be more breast-saving procedures in these cases, which present the best prognosis.

In case 3 the initial surgeon did not feel any mass and therefore was unwilling to operate. It is important that when these types of calcification are found at mammography the patient undergoes biopsy. It has been proved too many times that they can signify cancer. The opinion of "wait until it is palpable" is outdated and must not be allowed delay the necessary surgery.

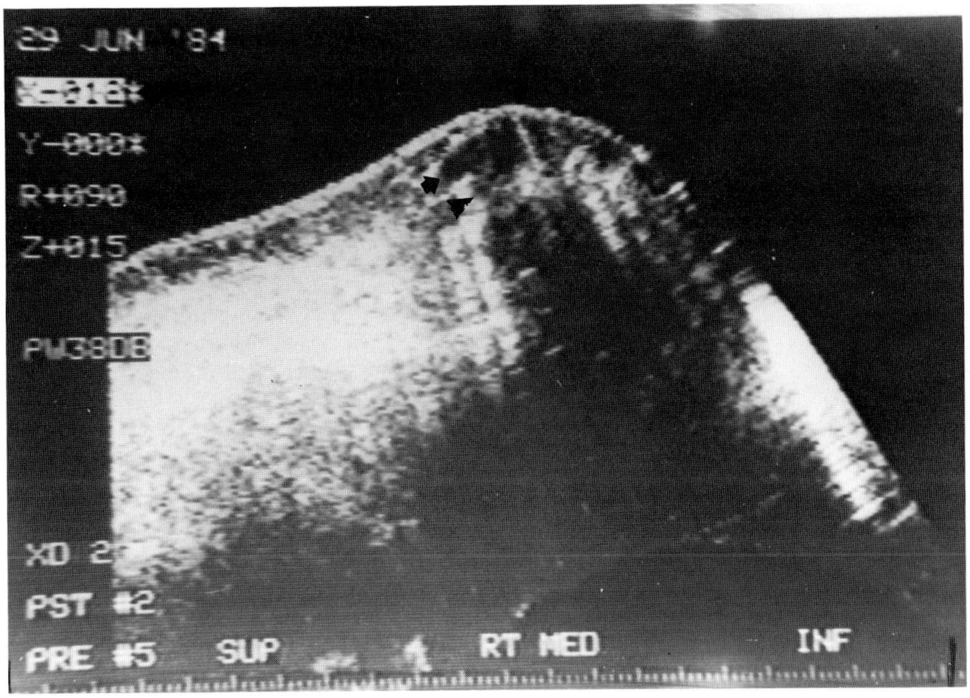

Fig. 22-4 Ultrasound. Note the cyst (arrow) and adjacent low-level echo area (arrowhead).

Case Studies: Lobular Carcinoma In Situ (Lobular Neoplasia)

Case 4

B.C. is a 40-year-old woman referred because of breast lumps of 1 week's duration. On physical examination there was marked glandularity to the breasts with multiple densities felt throughout both breasts. In particular, there were firm, moderately well defined, 1 cm nodules at 12 o'clock in each breast. There was no pain or tenderness.

The thermographic pattern was slightly abnormal with increased heat and vascularity above the right nipple. Diaphanography was normal. Mammography showed marked glandular tissue (Wolfe DY pattern). No lesion was identified, and no calcifications were seen. Whole breast water-bath ultrasound showed a well defined 1 cm cyst in the location of the mass on the left. An additional cyst was seen deep on the left. On the right there was a 0.5 cm cyst and immediately below it an area of decreased echogenicity with slightly increased sound through transmission. This area was poorly defined (Fig. 22-4). An attempt at aspiration obtained no fluid. Biopsy was advised.

Pathologic study revealed several foci of lobular carcinoma in situ, without an invasive component, occurring in a background of fibrosis, cystic dilatation, apocrine metaplasia, and adenosis. After lengthy consultations with the patient it has been elected to follow her with physical examination every 3 months and breast imaging procedures every 6 months, at least for the first 3 years.

Case 5

H.D. is a 40-year-old woman who at age 34 was discovered to have bilateral lobular carcinoma in situ in the upper outer aspects of the breasts. She underwent lumpectomy and radiation therapy at M. D. Anderson Hospital, receiving 5000 rads to each breast.

On physical examination scars were noted in the upper outer portions of the breasts. The skin was soft and supple with no evident radiation changes except over the sternum where there was slight telangiectasia. No masses were present. Thermograms and diaphanography were normal. Mammograms showed moderate glandularity (P2 pattern). Ultrasound demonstrated minimal skin thickening but no other abnormality.

Case 6

D.S. is a 49-year-old woman who had bilateral breast biopsies for lumps. The tissue showed a lobular carcinoma in situ on the left and atypical lobular hyperplasia on the right. She was referred for consultation. On physical examination three scars were noted on the right and one on the left. There were no masses.

Thermograms and diaphanography were normal. On mammography there was marked glandularity (DY pattern). Diffuse, benign-appearing calcifications were seen scattered throughout both breasts consistent with sclerosing adenosis. There was a conglomeration of glandular tissue in multiple areas without discrete masses. Ultrasound showed cysts bilaterally (Fig. 22-5).

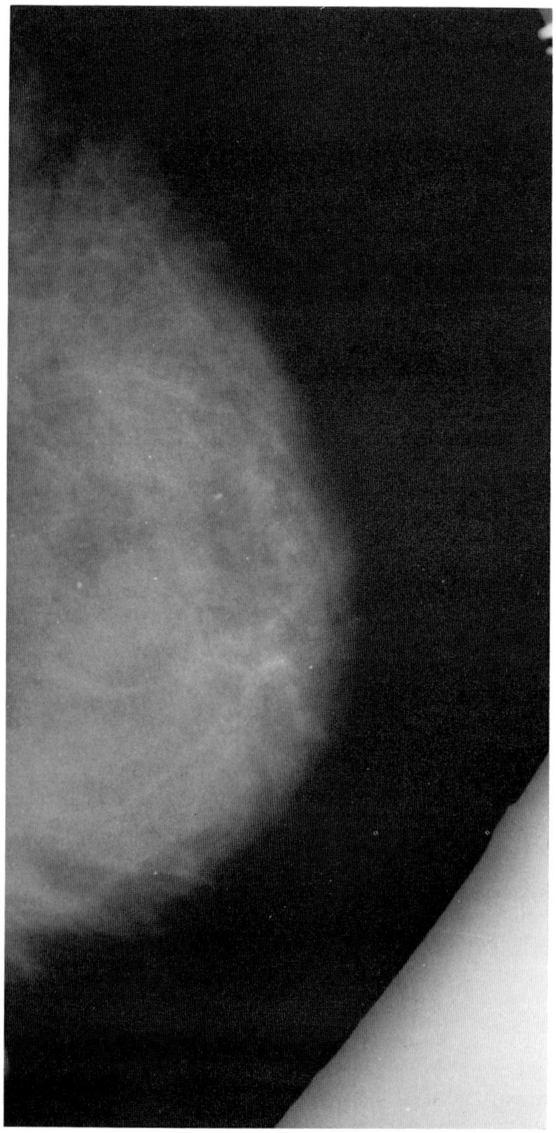

A

Fig. 22-5 A: Mammogram. The diffuse small calcifications probably represent sclerosing adenosis superimposed on dense glandularity.

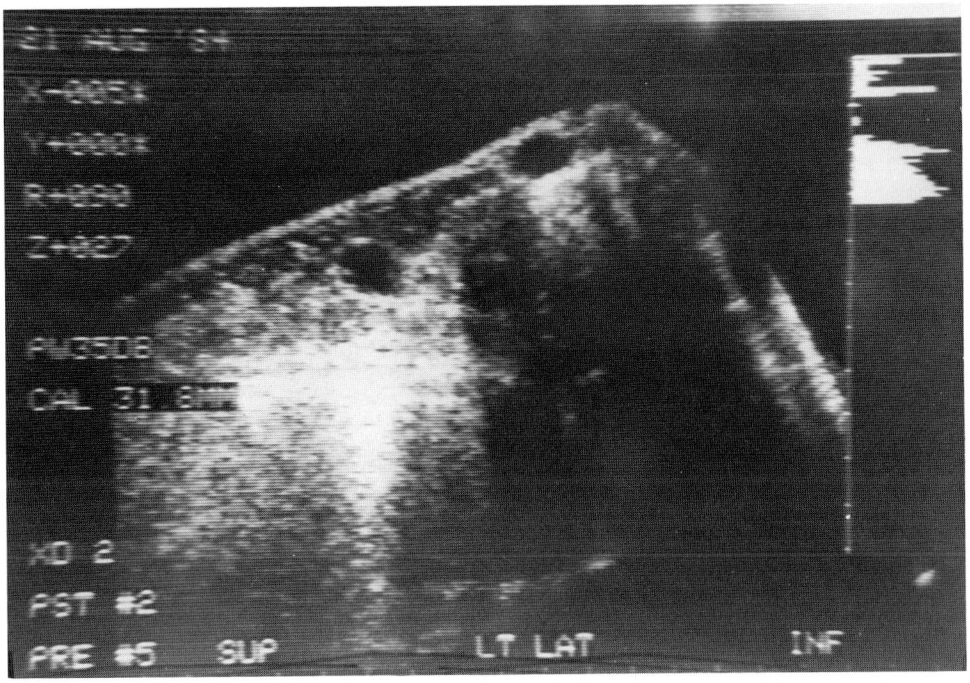

B

Fig. 22-5 B: Ultrasound. There are two well defined cysts and glandular tissue with marked shadowing.

This patient presents a marked quandry. Following the recommendations of Haagensen et al., this patient should be followed very carefully, without mastectomy. The marked calcifications and glandularity seen on mammography make follow-up difficult. The presence of cysts on ultrasound can be documented. It is wondered if this patient would not be better served with a bilateral subcutaneous mastectomy, with careful evaluation of all the tissue and, if normal, a second-stage implant insertion.

Discussion

It is doubtful if the lobular carcinoma in situ in case 4 would have been identified if there was not accompanying cystic dilatation that caused a small mass. Most cases are seen because of a biopsy for other reasons, as lobular carcinoma in situ (termed lobular neoplasia by Haagensen et al.) almost never causes a mass unless it becomes invasive.

Case 5 is a demonstration of a bilateral lobular carcinoma in situ. There had been a nodule on the left. The biopsy on the right was a blind mirror-image biopsy.

Bibliography

Carter D: Intraductal lesions of the breast, in *Interpretation of Breast Biopsies, Biopsy Interpretation Series.* New York, Raven Press, 1984, pp 25–75.

Carter D: Lobular lesions, in *Interpretation of Breast Biopsies, Biopsy Interpretation Series* New York, Raven Press, 1984, pp 76–94.

Cole-Beuglet C, Soriano RZ, Kurtz AB, et al: Ultrasound analysis of 104 primary breast carcinomas classified according to histopathologic type. *Radiology* 1983;147:191–196.

Egan RL, McSweeney MB, Sewell CW: Intramammary calcifications without an associated mass in benign and malignant diseases. *Radiology* 1980;137:1–7.

Fisher B, Bauer M, Margolese R, et al: Five-year results of a randomized clinical trial comparing total mastectomy and segmental mastectomy with or without radiation in the treatment of breast cancer. *N Engl J Med* 1985;312:665–673.

Gautherie M, Haehnel P, Walter JP, et al: Improved survival rate of breast cancer patients with an early diagnosis based on initial thermal assessment and subsequent follow-up, in Gautherie M, Albert E, Keith L (eds): *Thermal Assessment of Breast Health*. Boston, MTP Press, 1984, pp 180–200.

Haagensen CD, Bodian C, Haagensen DE: *Breast Carcinoma: Risk and Detection.* Philadelphia, Saunders, 1981.

Haagensen CD, Bodian C, Haagensen DE: Lobular neoplasia (lobular carcinoma in situ), in *Breast Carcinoma: Risk and Detection.* Philadelphia, Saunders, 1981, pp 238–291.

Kopans DB: "Early" breast cancer detection using techniques other than mammography. *AJR* 1984;143:465–468.

Moskowitz M: Mammographic screening: Significance of minimal breast cancers. *AJR* 1981;136:735–738.

Porrath S, Bernay T: The role of thermography in the multimodality approach to breast cancer diagnosis, in Gautherie M, Albert E, Keith L (eds): Thermal *Assessment of Breast Health.* Boston, MTP Press, 1984, pp 156–166.

Sickles EA: Mammographic detectability of breast microcalcifications. *AJR* 1982;139:913–918.

Sickles EA: Mammographic features of "early" breast cancer. *AJR* 1984;143:461–464.

Silverstein MJ, Rosser RJ, Gamagami P, et al: Axillary lymph node dissection for intraductal breast carcinoma. Proceedings American College of Surgeons and Obstetricians, Houston, 1985.

Unzeitig GW, Frankl G, Ackerman M, et al: Analysis of the prognosis of minimal and occult breast cancers. *Arch Surg* 1983;118:1403–1404.

Section IV

Male Breast Disease

23

Male Breast Disease

Saar Porrath

Virtually all the disorders, anomalies, and diseases that are present in the female breast can be found in the male breast, although to a much lesser degree of frequency.[1–5]

The male breast consists of fat with a minimal amount of stromal tissue. It does possess the ability to become a glandular organ if stimulated. Male infants at or soon after birth may have a small amount of milky discharge, stimulated by intrauterine female hormones. This discharge also occurs in female infants. Nipple discharge in the adult man may be secondary to medication such as antidepressives and antihypertensives, continued use of marijuana, or hormonal stimulation such as estrogen therapy for prostatic cancer.

Normal Male Breast

The normal male breast is fatty, with a few strands of stromal tissue. On physical examination the fat may feel nodular but seldom masslike. The thermogram varies depending on the amount of fat but is usually normal and symmetrical. The light scan shows increased light transmission. The mammogram is fatty with occasional stromal streaks. Ultrasound findings are typical of the normal fatty female breast.

Gynecomastia

The most common disorder of the male breast is gynecomastia. The term means "woman's breast" and is descriptive of the entity. Many men at some time during their lives have gynecomastia, although it varies greatly in degree. It usually occurs in the adolescent, primarily during the late teens. It may be unilateral or bilateral. It usually resolves by the early twenties, although persistent gynecomastia may be present throughout adult life. This type of gynecomastia is hormonal, responding to the normal variation of both male and female hormones in men. Not infrequently, because of psychological reasons there is a need for surgical removal of the glandular tissue.

Gynecomastia secondary to medications, hormones, cirrhosis of the liver, chronic renal disease, chronic congestive heart failure with digitalis therapy, starvation, and metabolic disorders secondary to chronic infection may occur in later life. This type is more persistent and may not resolve after the disorder has been corrected. Gynecomastia secondary to estrogen therapy for prostatic cancer has become very common. It can be very painful, and prehormonal radiation therapy has been advocated to prevent the pain.[6]

There are two presentations of gynecomastia.[4,6–8,9] The first mimics the female breast and is ductal hyperplasia and glandular hypertrophy in a lobular fashion. The second is primarily hypertrophy of the connective tissue with fewer glandular elements. There can be a mixture of the types.

On physical examination there is a varying-sized unilateral or bilateral nodularity in the breast, almost always centered on the nipple. It may be tender or even painful. Nipple discharge, although uncommon, may be present, and the nipple may be more prominent on the side of the involvement.

Thermography shows an increase in heat and occasionally vascularity if the man is moderate-sized or especially if he is obese. The normal or increased fat of the noninvolved breast acts as insulation on the thermogram. If the man is slender, the involved side may actually be cooler on thermography as the glandular tissue may act as a buffer to the normally transmitted heat of the chest wall. The light scan shows some diminution in light transmission, which increases as the amount of tissue increases.

The mammographic appearance varies[4,6–8] depending on the amount of tissue present and the predominant type of tissue, glandular or connective. When there are ductal and glandular elements the mammographic pattern is one of increased density spreading from the nipple area with the greatest radiographic density immediately beneath the nipple. As the amount of connective tissue or stromal elements increases, there is a greater density seen on mammography, with a more button-type appearance seen. Obviously there can be mixed presentations. The radiographic density is usually spread throughout the tissue, whereas masses, if also present, show as an area of localized increased density.

Ultrasound demonstrates the increased tissue as echogenic,[10–13] differentiated from the low echogenicity of the surrounding fat. On occasion, though rarely, a dilated duct is seen. The appearance is not unlike that of the early adolescent female breast.

Benign Lesions

True cysts are uncommon in men. The cysts that are seen are usually inclusion cysts or of epidermoid nature.

Benign lesions such as adenomas are very rare. Their presentation is similar to that in the female breast. Because of the predominantly fatty nature of the male breast, lipomas are somewhat more common but are also unusual.

Accessory nipples are not uncommonly present in the milk line, which extends in mammals from the axilla to the groin. Rashes and skin lesions such as dermatitis are common, and their presentation is similar to that in women.

Cancer

Male breast cancer, although similar in presentation to that in the female breast, is in many other ways a dissimilar disease.[4,6–11,12,14,15] There has been little change in the incidence of male breast cancer over the past 50 years, whereas the incidence of female breast cancer has reached almost epidemic proportions. There is little hormonal influence, as seen with female breast cancer. Diet may not be a factor, and family history may not be influential. Whereas breast cancer in female paternal relatives increases the risk to women, there are no large studies to show the risk of a male relative with breast cancer on either the male or female offspring.

Almost all male breast cancers are discovered because of a lump, which may vary in size. It is usually hard and well defined but may be soft and poorly defined. Nipple discharge secondary to cancer is unusual. Occasionally there is unilateral gynecomastia stimulated by the cancer.

The thermogram may be positive, but the results depend on the size of the breasts, as explained previously. Light scanning may show an area of decreased transmission and increased vascularity, depending on the size of the lesion. Mammography varies. The usual presentation is that of a mass of increased density, either well or poorly defined. Malignant calcification may be present, and spiculization may be seen. Ultrasound often shows a mass. The presentation is not unlike that of cancer in the fatty female breast, with an area of diminished density with shadowing noted. Because of the relative rarity of male breast cancer there are few large reports of imaging examinations other than mammography.

Most male breast cancers are ductal in origin. The usual treatment is mastectomy. Because they are often found late, metastatic disease is not infrequent.

Case Study: Male Breast Cancer

Case 1

J.B. is a 44-year-old man who presented with left nipple retraction (Fig. 23-1) and a 2 cm left breast mass of 1 year's duration. Telethermography demonstrated a hot spot of 2.5°C increase over the right side (Th III thermogram on the left). On mammography

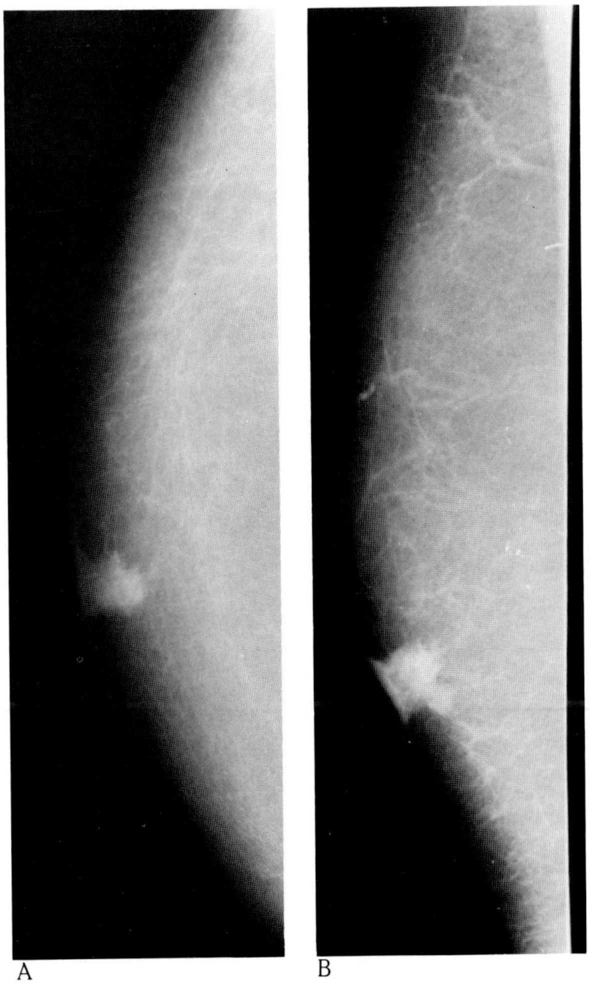

A B

Fig. 23-1 Mammograms, CC view **(A)** and lateral view **(B)**. There is a dense mass behind the nipple with slight nipple retraction. The posterior aspect of the mass is irregular, suggesting spiculization.

there was an irregular 2 cm mass density behind the left nipple, with skin thickening and dimpling (Fig. 23-1).

A needle biopsy was class II, raising the question of gynecomastia. At surgery a ductal carcinoma was noted. At mastectomy 12 nodes were negative. Six months later a metastatic nodule was biopsied in the lung. The patient is on chemotherapy.

(This case was loaned by The Breast Center, Van Nuys, CA, courtesy of Drs. Silverstein and Gamagami.)

Case Study: Benign Male Breast Disease

Case 2

G.R. is a 60-year-old man who was referred because of a right breast nodule of unknown duration. On physical examination there was a 1 cm firm, movable nodule at 9 o'clock in the right breast. The right nipple was very prominent with slight skin thickening of the surrounding areola.

Thermograms were normal. Diaphanography showed slightly decreased light transmission over the nodule (Fig 23-2A). Mammography demonstrated a fatty breast without a definite nodule (Fig. 23-2B). Ultrasound showed fatty tissue without a mass.

Although the patient had multiple lipomas elsewhere on his trunk, the firm feel and the positive diaphanography were against this lesion being a lipoma, although the mammogram showed just fatty tissue.

It was thought that the nodule represented a hematoma or a peculiarly firm lipoma. It was elected to follow the patient. On follow-up 3 months later there was no change clinically in the nodule. Biopsy was suggested. At surgery a nodular density visually resembling a fibroadenoma was found, but on pathologic slides it proved to be a lipoma.

The patient was seen 3 months later because of right nipple tenderness. He related that approximately 1 year earlier he had had a small pustule on the nipple which he squeezed. The nipple remained slightly prominent and tender since then. On physical examination the right nipple was three times as large as the left, a finding not seen on either of the earlier two visits, although the nipple had been prominent. There was a scar at the site of the previously described nodule, with the nodule now absent. There was a small mass effect behind the right nipple. Thermograms were normal. Diaphanography showed slightly decreased light transmission over the scar and markedly diminished light transmission over the nipple. A single-view mammogram failed to reveal a mass behind the nipple. Ultrasound did not show a mass but did demonstrate nipple enlargement with thickened walls.

The mass effect was thought to be conglomerate fatty tissue. The nipple change was probably postinflammatory without active infection. Hydrocortisone cream was prescribed. A pustule developed 1 week later on the right nipple, which the patient squeezed. The tenderness and nipple prominence diminished. Three months later there was no pain or tenderness; the nipple is no longer reddened, although it remains about twice the size of the left nipple.

Discussion

The presentation of the lipoma in this case was peculiar on palpation and diaphanography. It even appeared different at surgery. The reason is not known. The nipple changes on the right with recurrent pustules a year apart is also unusual in men. Breast infections in men are rare. It is probable that a small nidus of infection was present in a duct, resulting in a recurrence of the nipple pustule. (See also cases 4 and 5 under Breast Abscesses, Chapter 15.)

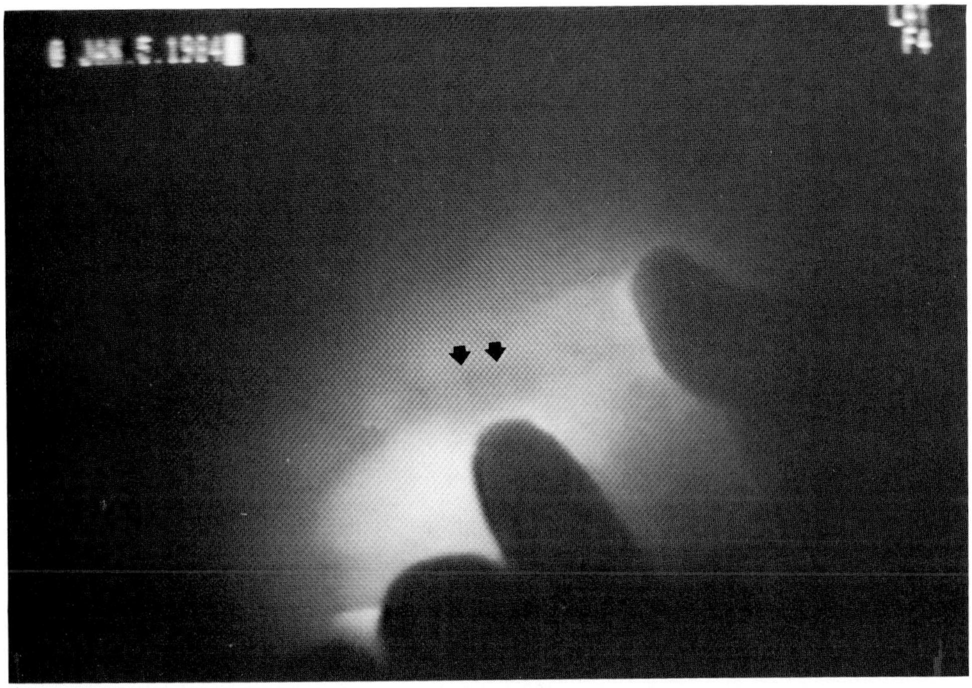

A

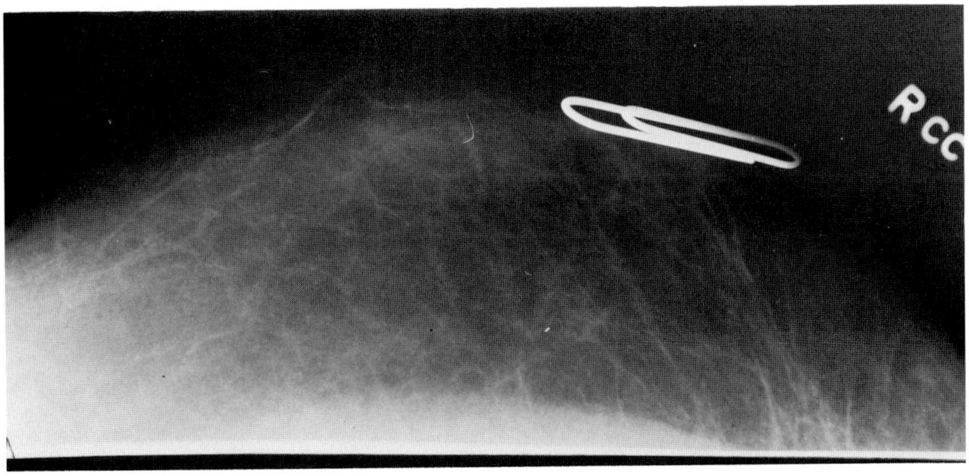

B

Fig. 23-2 A: Diaphanography. Note the slight decrease in light transmission (arrows) over the area of the mass. **B:** Mammography. Fatty breast normally seen in men. The paperclip overlies the areas of the mass. Nothing is seen on the mammogram.

Case Studies: Gynecomastia

Case 3

Z.D. is a 17-year-old boy who presented with a 3-year history of a right breast mass. There had been no essential change during that time period. There was no pain or tenderness.

On physical examination there was a fairly large breast present on the right, especially so for a boy. There was firmness with a glandular mass behind the right nipple. The left breast was normal, and there was no nipple discharge.

Liquid crystal thermography showed markedly increased heat diffusely over the right breast compared to the left (Color Fig. 27). Diaphanography showed slightly decreased light transmission on the right (Fig. 23-3A). Mammography demonstrated a small amount of glandular tissue on the left behind the nipple and a large amount of glandular tissue on the right distributed over the entire breast (Figs. 23-3B, C). Ultrasound demonstrated the glandular tissue bilaterally without other masses (Fig. 23-3D).

The modular density on the right was thought to represent a glandular area. Because of the large differential in size and the fact that there had been no change for 3 years, surgery was advised for cosmetic and psychological reasons. Surgery on the right breast removed 66 g of tissue, a significant amount. The pathologic diagnosis was gynecomastia.

Case 4

J.C. is a 37-year-old man who has had a mild gynecomastia since his teenage years. There was a strong family history of breast cancer: his mother and both maternal and paternal grandmothers. He presented with a soft, movable 1 by 1.5 cm nodule at 3 o'clock in the left breast.

Thermography and diaphanography were normal. Mammography showed marked glandular tissue bilaterally without a mass. Ultrasound demonstrated glandularity without a mass (Fig. 23-4).

The nodule was thought to be glandular. The patient was seen 2 months later. In the interim his internist had given him two injections of testosterone. A prolactin level was normal. On reexamination the nodule was absent. The glandular tissue on the left was more prominent and somewhat more diffuse.

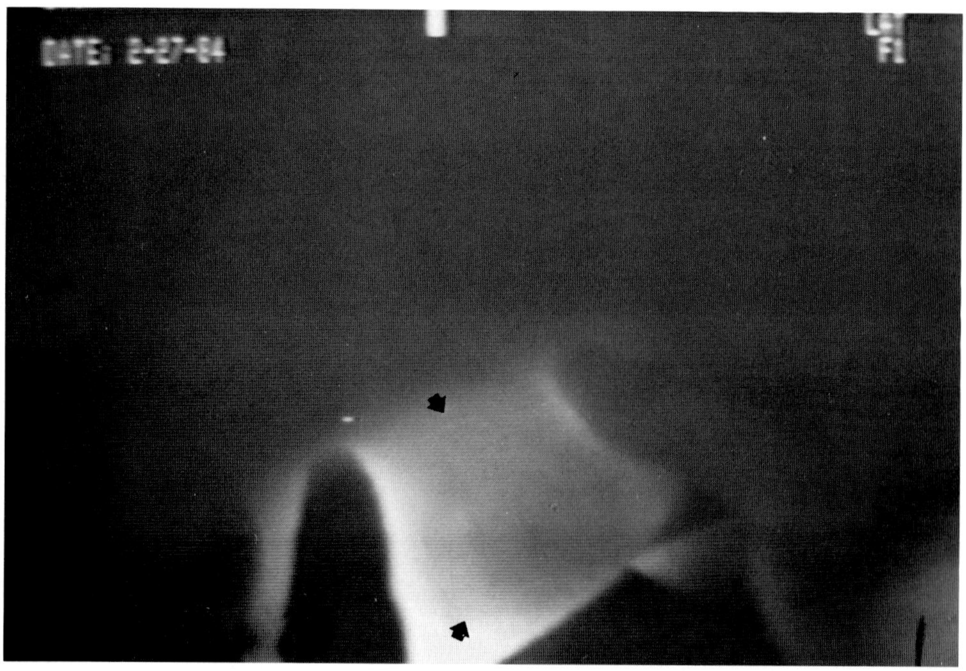

A

Fig. 23-3 A: Diaphanography. Note the decreased light transmission over the right breast (arrows).

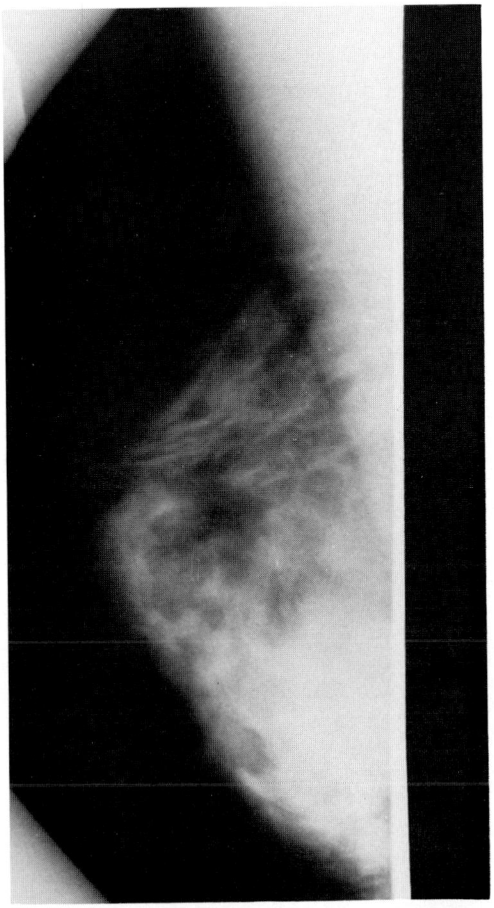

B

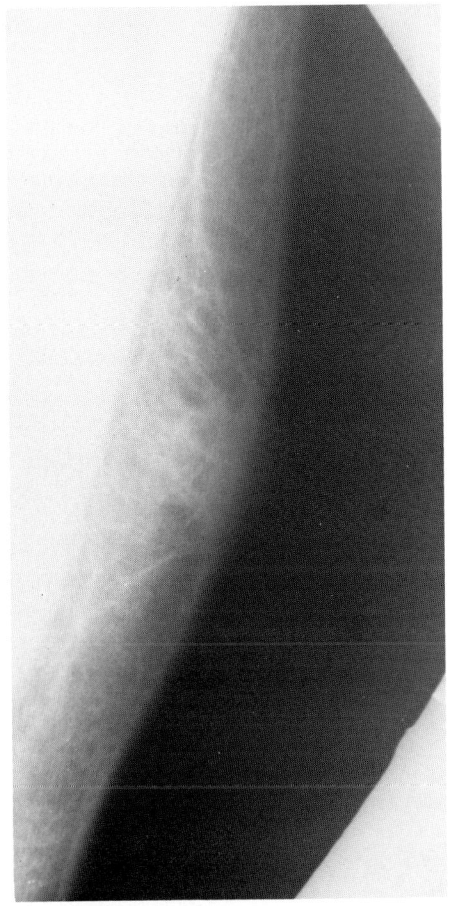

C

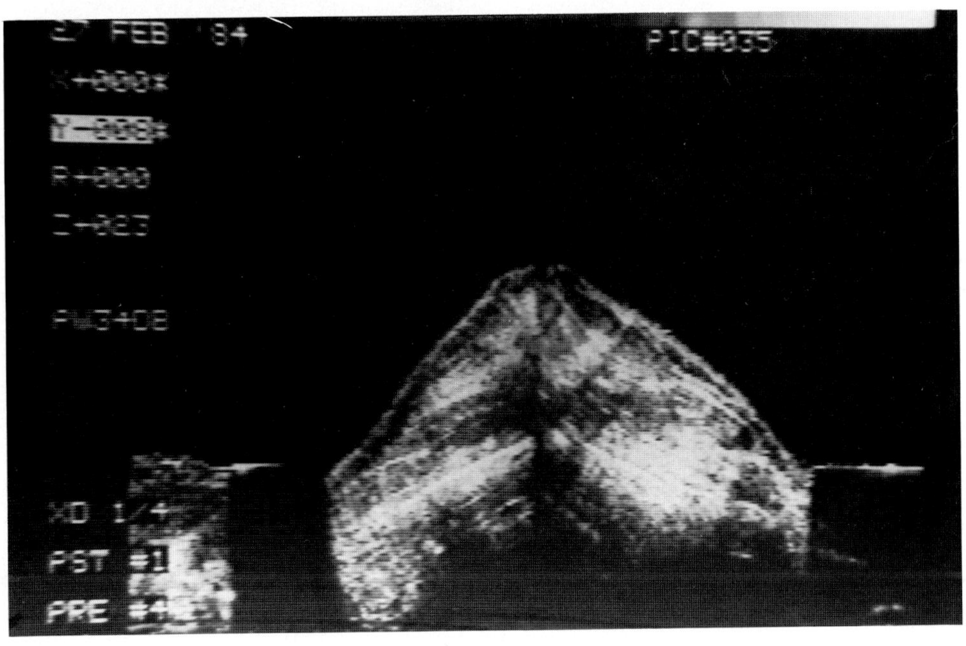

D

Fig. 23-3 **B:** Mammogram, right lateral view. There is marked glandularity with a grossly enlarged right breast. **C:** Mammogram, left lateral view. Mild glandularity extends from the nipple. Compare with **B** (marked glandularity) and Fig. 23-2B (benign male breast disease). **D:** Ultrasound, right transverse view. Note the marked glandularity and increased size of the right breast. Compare with the mammogram in **B.**

Case 5

T.R. is a 64-year-old man referred because of left breast pain and a left nipple discharge. On physical examination there was a small tender mass behind the left nipple. No nipple discharge was seen at the time of the examination. The right breast was normal.

Liquid crystal thermograms demonstrated increased periareolar and nipple heat on the left (Th III thermogram). On diaphanography there was some decrease in light

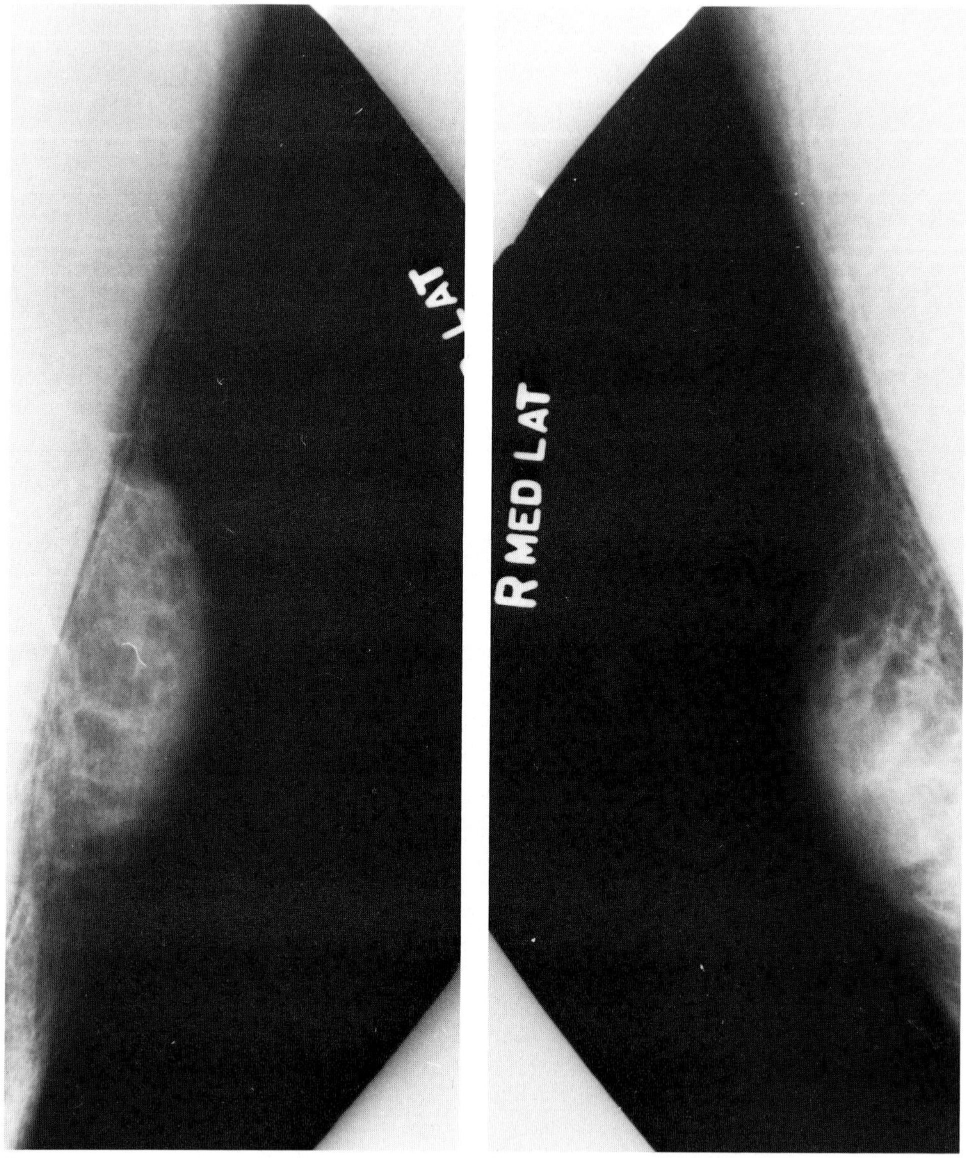

A B

Fig. 23-4 Mammograms, left lateral **(A)** and right lateral **(B)** views. Note the marked glandularity distributed over both breast areas consistent with gynecomastia. *(Figure continues.)*

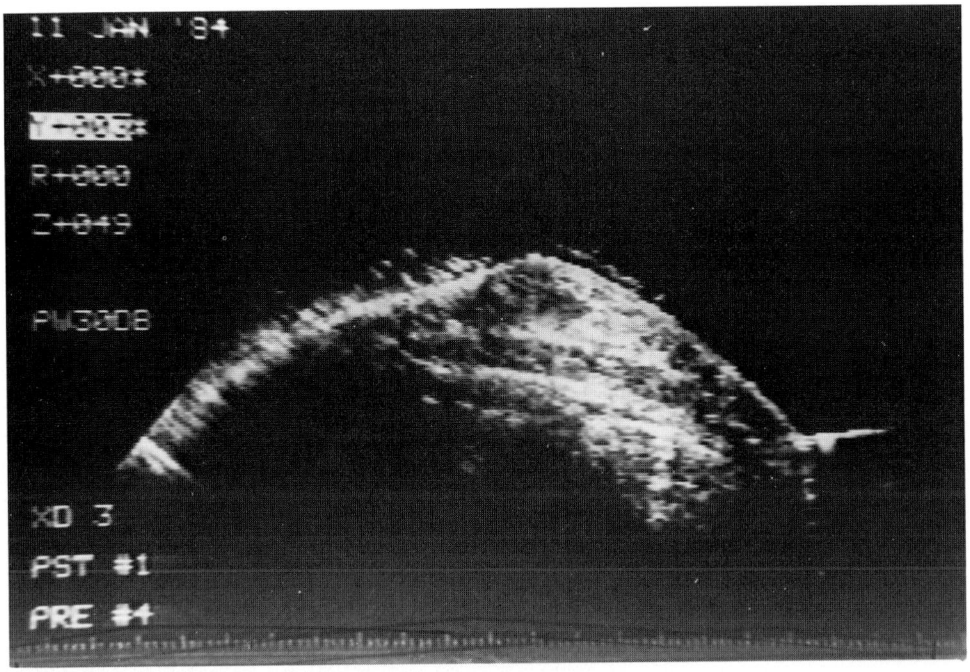

C

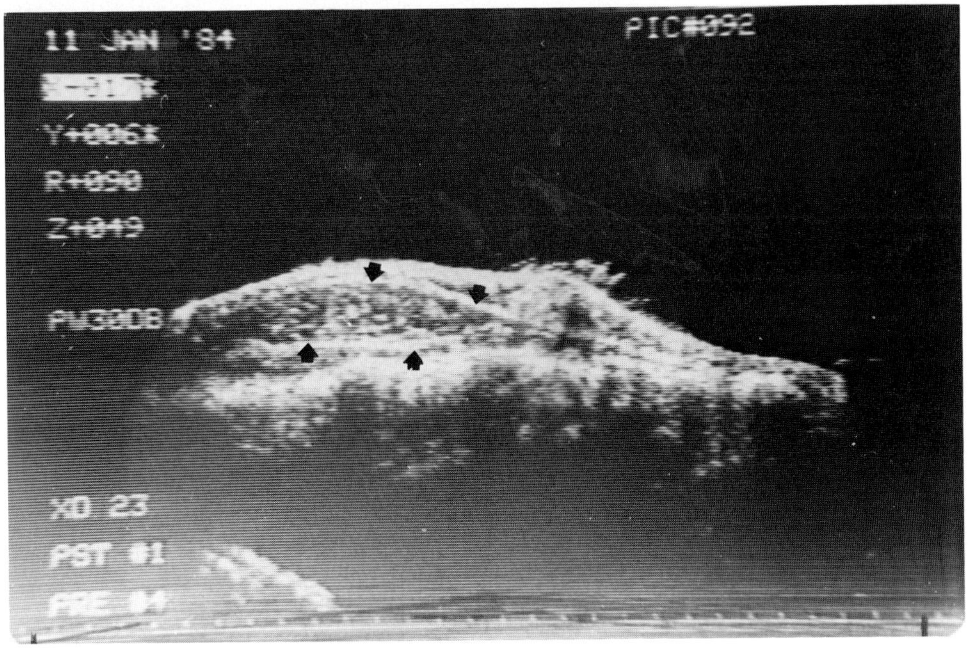

D

Fig. 23-4 **C:** Ultrasound, left transverse view. Diffuse echoes anterior to the skin represent hair on the chest. Note the diffuse glandular pattern with slight shadowing behind the nipple area. **D:** Ultrasound, left longitudinal view. Note the well defined pectoralis muscle (arrows), slight nipple shadowing, and diffuse glandular pattern.

transmission adjacent to the left nipple. Mammograms showed a fatty breast on the right and a small nubbin of glandular tissue behind the left nipple (Fig. 23-5).

The patient was thought to have unilateral gynecomastia secondary to antidepressant medications. There was also an elevation in the beta-hCG of 5100 m I.U. the normal level in men being up to 2500 m I.U. The small tender area disappeared when the patient's medication was discontinued.

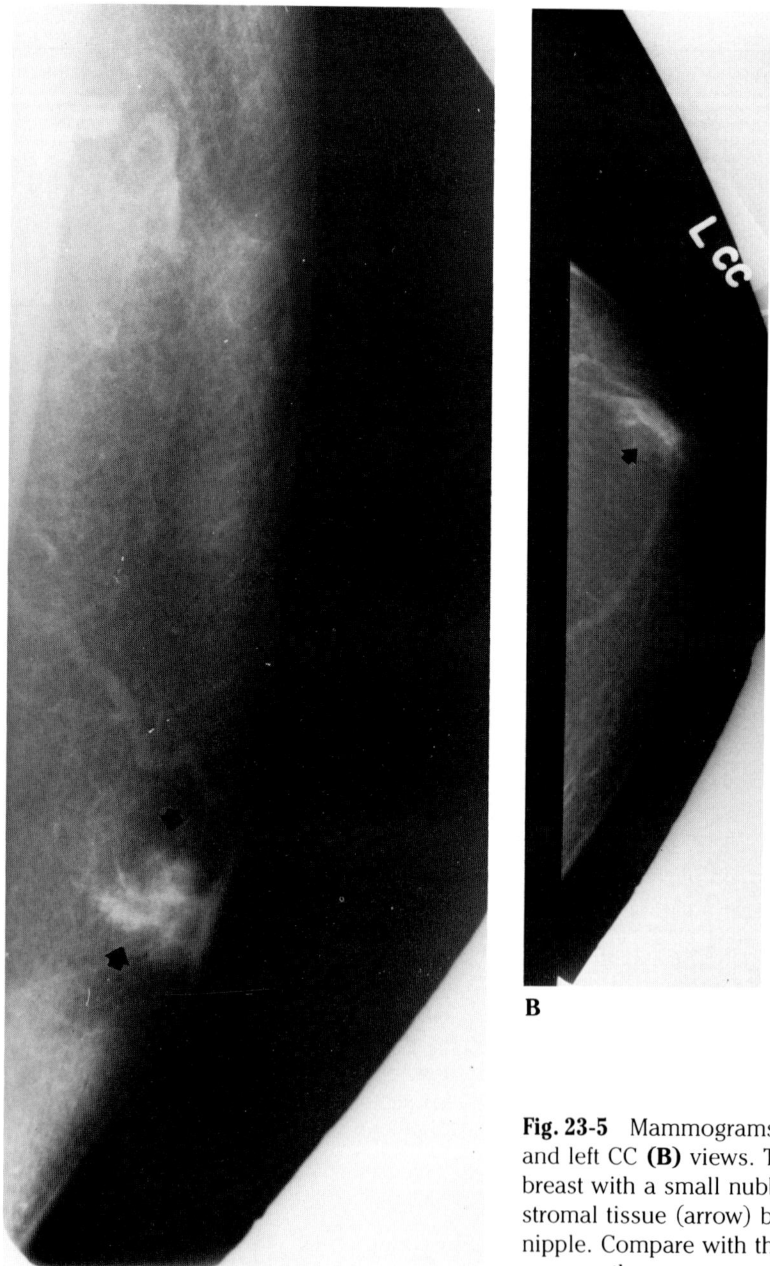

A

B

Fig. 23-5 Mammograms, left lateral **(A)** and left CC **(B)** views. This is a fatty breast with a small nubbin of primarily stromal tissue (arrow) behind the left nipple. Compare with the denser area seen on the mammogram of male breast cancer (Fig. 23-1).

Discussion

In most cases the diagnosis of gynecomastia can be made with a large degree of certainty. Surgery may be indicated for cosmetic or psychological reasons, as in case 3. In case 4 the nodule could not be demonstrated on any imaging examinations, increasing the suspicion that it was glandular. If it had not disappeared on follow-up, biopsy would have been indicated. In case 4 it is unsure at what risk the patient is for developing breast cancer with a strong family history of breast cancer in female relatives, as there seems to be no good study of male breast cancer outlining familial risk factors.

Case 5 is an example of iatrogenic gynecomastia caused by the patient's medication. Antidepressants are among many medications that have an effect on the breast, both male and female. A history is important to determine if there has been a change in medications or in the dosage, although as in this case it was the long-term administration of the drug that caused the effect without dosage alteration.

References

1. Bannayan GA, Hajdie SI: Gynecomastia: Clinico-pathologic study of 351 cases. *Am J Clin Pathol* 1972;57:431-437.
2. Carlson HE: Current concepts, gynecomastia. *N Engl J Med* 1980;303(14):795–799.
3. Cordiano C, Ninfo G, Gagni C: Gynecomastia: Statistical and clinical findings on 203 observations. *Int Surg* 1971;55:131–136.
4. Kapdi CC, Parekh NJ: The male breast. *Radiol Clin North Am* 1983;21(1):132–148.
5. Nuftall FQ: Gynecomastia as a physical finding in normal men. *J Clin Endocrinol Metab* 1979;48(2):338–340.
6. Michels LG, Gold RH, Arndt RD: Radiography of gynecomastia and other disorders of the male breast. *Radiology* 1977;122:117–122.
7. Kalisher L, Peyster RG: Xerographic manifestations of male breast disease. *AJR* 1975;125(3):656–660.
8. Martin JE: The male breast, in *Atlas of Mammography*. Baltimore, Williams & Wilkins, 1982, pp 341–352.
9. Gagnon JD, Moss WT, Stevens KR: Pre-estrogen breast irradiation for patients with carcinoma of the prostate: A critical review. *J Urol* 1979;121:182–184.
10. Cole-Beuglet C, Schwartz GF, Kurtz AB, et al: Ultrasound mammography for male breast enlargement. *J Ultrasound Med* 1982;1:301–305.
11. Jackson VP, Gilmor RL: Male breast carcinoma and gynecomastia. *Radiology* 1983;149:533–536.
12. Jellins J, Kossoff G, Reeve TS: The ultrasonic appearance of pathology in the male breast. *Ultrasound Med Biol* 1975;2:43–44.
13. Wigley KD, Thomas JL, Bernardino ME, et al: Sonography of gynecomastia. *AJR* 1981;136:927–930.
14. Ouimet-Oliva D, Herbert G, Ladouceur J: Radiographic characteristics of male breast cancer. *Radiology* 1978;129:37–40.
15. Vercoutere AL, O'Connell TX: Carcinoma of the male breast. *Arch Surg* 1984;119:1301–1304.

Section V

Postirradiated Breast

24

Postirradiated Breast

Saar Porrath

With the increased use of lumpectomy and radiation therapy[1,2] it behoves the imager to become acquainted with the appearance of the postirradiated breast. Patients at M. D. Anderson Hospital get a postlumpectomy mammogram, another following recovery from radiation therapy, and then every 6 months for the first 2 to 3 years. It is only by close follow-up that early recurrences are found.

The findings on physical examination and on the imaging procedures depend on the amount of time that has elapsed following the irradiation as well as the degree of deformity caused by the initial surgery. If there has been an extensive resection at the time of the original lumpectomy, these findings may become somewhat more exaggerated after irradiation.[3,4]

Immediately following irradiation the breast is reddened, with areas of rawness. The axillary area may be "weepy," and the breast may be tender and feel firm. These problems tend to decrease with time. By a year there may be only a slight increase in skin turgor and some telangiectasia. The skin may be slightly browned, and the skin over the surgery scar tends to be tense. Care is taken to document any deformity or dimpling, as they can increase with time owing to retraction of the surgical area but may also signal the onset of a recurrence. As in any postsurgical breast, there may be areas of increased density. There may also be edges of tissue formed by the previous resection. They should be well documented to discern any changes.

The thermogram initially is extremely hot. With time, however, there is a decrease in heat and vascularity. The thermographic pattern should have reached a "normal base" by a year. If the pattern remains hot, Gautherie[5] has shown that there may be a poorer prognosis and perhaps an early recurrence. A thermographic pattern that returns to normal and then reverts to one of increased heat may be a early signal of recurrence.

The light scan initially shows a marked decrease in light transmission that diminishes as the radiation reaction subsides. There may be slightly diminished light transmission, exaggerated in the area of the scar or where there is skin thickening. A change in the pattern with a decrease in light transmission may represent either further late scarring or a recurrence[6–9] (see also Chapter 4).

Ultrasound can be very sensitive to the postirradiation changes.[10,11] Initially there is marked skin thickening that returns to almost normal with time. In fact, the skin changes may be so slight as to be practically undetectable except in the area of the scar. The subcutaneous tissues show markedly increased echoes secondary to the irradiation, which may return to normal. While in the acute radiation phase, the glandular tissue may show an increased density and shadowing. Often some of the glandular areas remain ultrasonically dense with increased shadowing. The areas of the scars show marked shadowing. If, after a baseline is obtained, new areas of shadowing are seen, it may represent either delayed scarring or a recurrence. A recurrence may also present as an ill-defined mass with some shadowing.

Obtaining a baseline mammogram for comparison purposes following irradiation is important for the later recognition of subtle changes. The mammogram, like the other studies, reflects the radiation changes of increased skin thickening, increased glandular density, scar formation, and an increase in the subcutaneous tissues. Most of these changes resolve with time. Benign calcifications may occur. The baseline mammogram also allows recognition of any malignant calcifications not removed during the initial surgery. These remaining calcifications may partially resolve with time. If new malignant calcifications occur, a recurrence must be suspected. The same is true of any densities that develop.[12–14]

Case Studies

Case 1

D.H. is a 55-year-old woman who presented elsewhere for mammography in October 1982. She had a small mass in the lower area of the right breast, and a 2 cm mass was seen on mammography in the upper portion of the right breast at 11 o'clock. It was an infiltrating ductal carcinoma. She was treated with lumpectomy and radiation therapy. The mass in the lower portion of the breast was glandular tissue.

A follow-up mammogram on 5/20/83 showed minimal scarring in the upper right breast. A mammogram on 10/18/83 showed increasing spiculization without definite mass. On 6/26/84 there was further spiculization noted on mammography with an increasing, ill-defined density. She was referred to the Woman's Breast Center on 10/31/84 because of a lump of 3 months' duration at the site of the previous cancer.

On physical examination there was slight skin retraction at 11 o'clock, high on the chest wall, and just below this a 2 cm moderately defined, firm mass. Slight skin thickening and postirradiation changes were noted in the right breast. Liquid crystal thermography showed marked increased heat over the upper right breast and nipple area (Color Fig. 28). Diaphanography showed decreased light transmission through the mass and adjacent areas (Figs. 24-1A, B). Repeat mammograms again demonstrated spiculization and a poorly defined density, essentially unchanged from the mammograms of 10/31/84 (Fig. 24-1C). Ultrasound showed postirradiation changes with slight skin thickening and two areas of shadowing, one in the area of the previous biopsy and the other in the area of the density felt clinically (Fig. 24-1D). The differential between postirradiation changes and recurrent cancer could not be made, and needle biopsy was recommended. (In the postirradiated breast needle biopsy is preferable, as formal biopsy may not heal well owing to the damaged vascularity from irradiation.) Tru-cut needle biopsies of the area revealed mild chronic inflammation and radiation reaction. When seen 14 months later the mass had decreased in size. The mammogram and ultrasound were normal. The thermogram has remained persistently very positive, probably reflecting the radiation changes to the breast.

Case 2

R.W. is a 64-year-old woman who was seen at the Woman's Breast Center in June 1984. She reported a slight, clear nipple discharge from the left breast. At the age of 52 in 1972 she had had a lumpectomy and radiation therapy for an intraductal carcinoma of the left breast. Her radiation therapy was given on a cobalt-60 radiation therapy unit.

On physical examination the left breast was contracted, hard, and about 40 percent smaller than the right. No mass was felt. There was a raw edge to the left nipple and redness of the nipple and areola. There was no nipple discharge. On closer

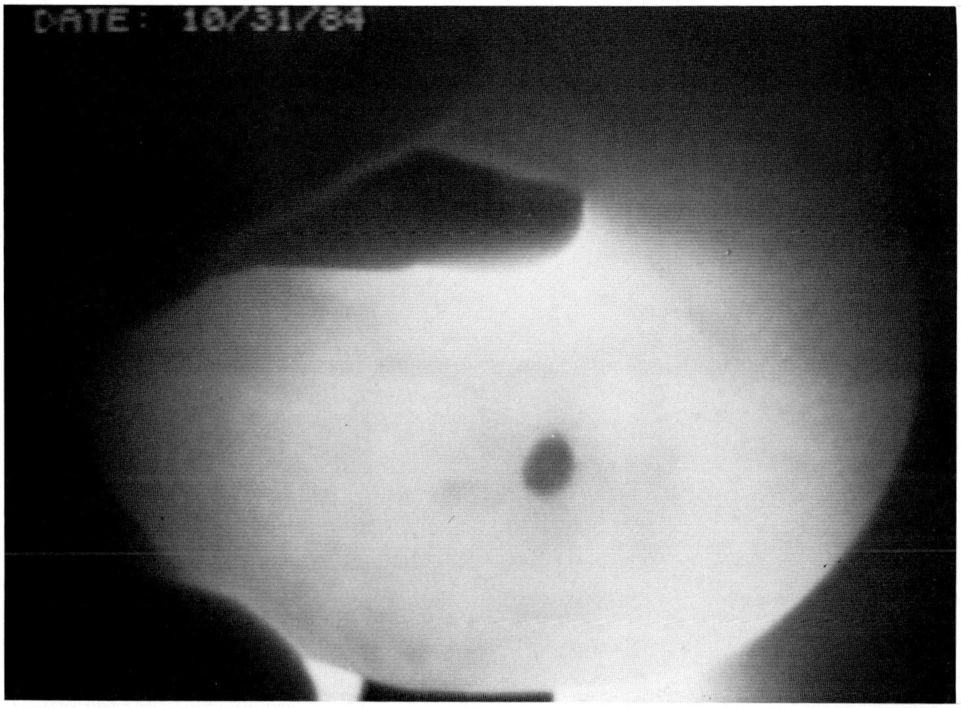

A

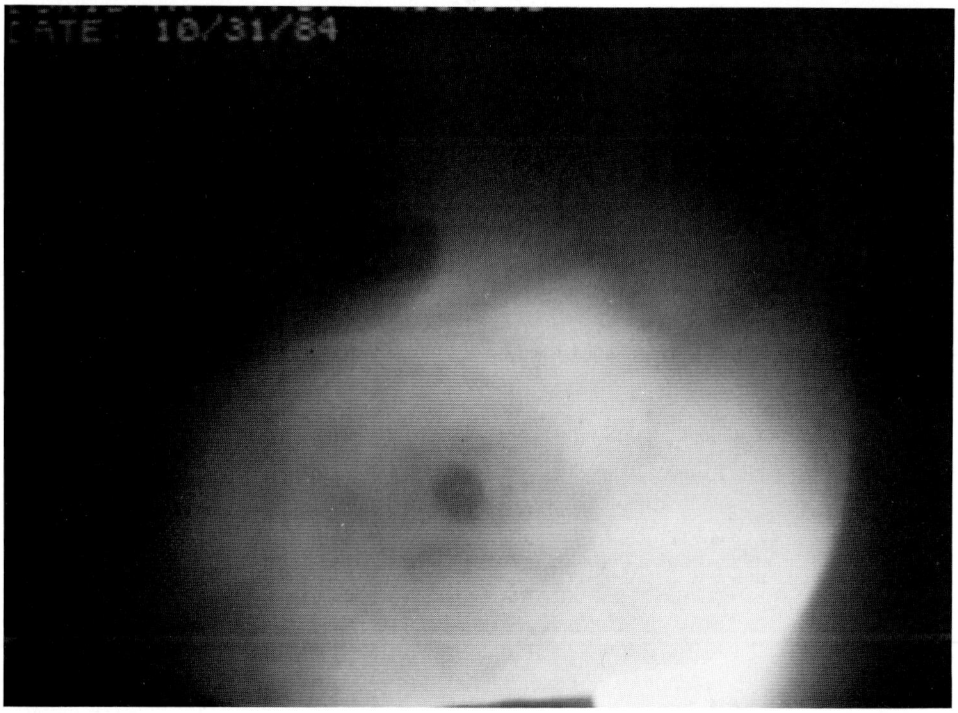

B

Fig. 24-1 **A:** Diaphanography, normal left breast. **B:** Diaphanography, irradiated right breast. Note the slight decrease in light transmission over the anterior right breast, the indistinctiveness of the right nipple, and the increased vascularity on the right. These findings represent mild radiation changes seen on light scanning.

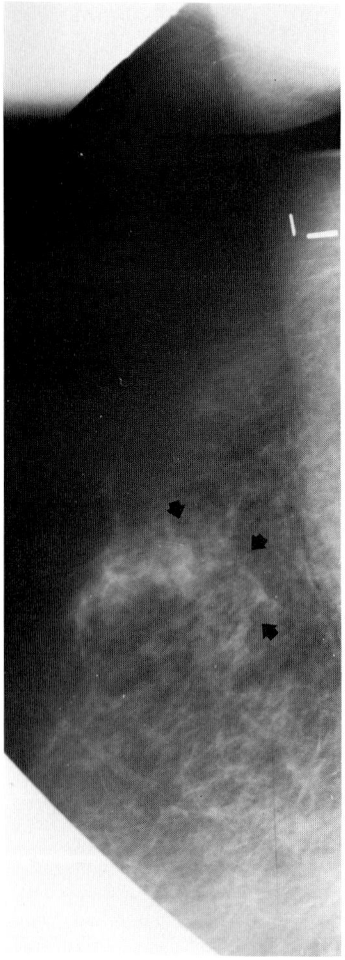

C

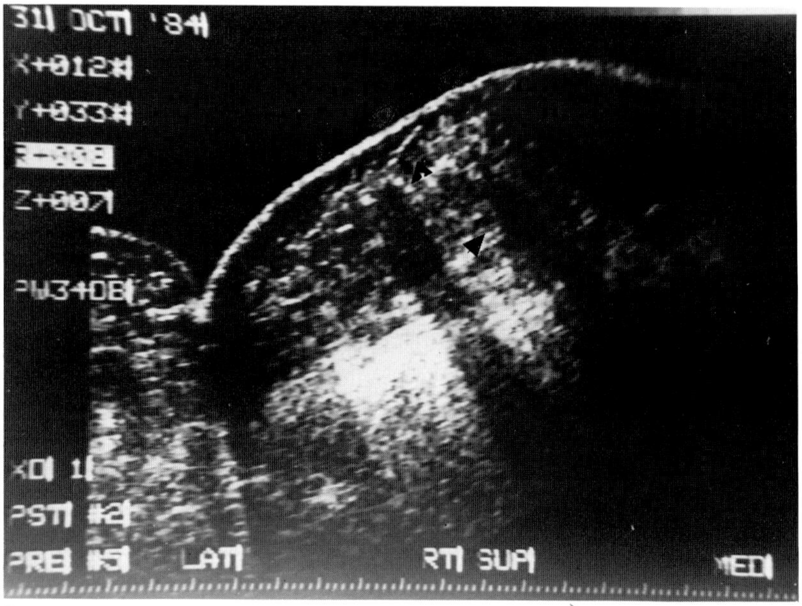

D

Fig. 24-1 **C:** Mammogram, magnified, upper right breast. Note the irregular density with slight spiculization (arrows). **D:** Ultrasound. Note the slight straightening of the skin contour (open arrows). The areas of marked shadowing (arrowheads) represent the irregular density seen on the mammogram in **C** and an area of previous biopsy.

questioning the patient related that what she thought was nipple discharge was really a serous fluid seen in the reddened area surrounding the nipple.

Liquid crystal thermograms revealed a left global hyperthermia of 4°C and increased nipple heat of 2°C compared to the right. Diaphanography showed a diffuse decrease in light transmission over the entire upper left breast. Chronic radiation changes with skin thickening, increased density of the glandular tissue, and increased markings throughout the subcutaneous tissues were evident on mammography. No mass or malignant calcifications were noted (Figs. 24-2A, B). Automated whole breast ultrasound also demonstrated these chronic radiation changes (Fig. 24-2C).

The reddened nipple edge was thought to be due to contact dermatitis caused by a new shampoo the patient was using and thought not be be related to the radiation changes. The patient was given cortisone cream, and the nipple edge was normal on a follow-up visit 1 month later. There has been no recurrence of the dermatitis 22 months later.

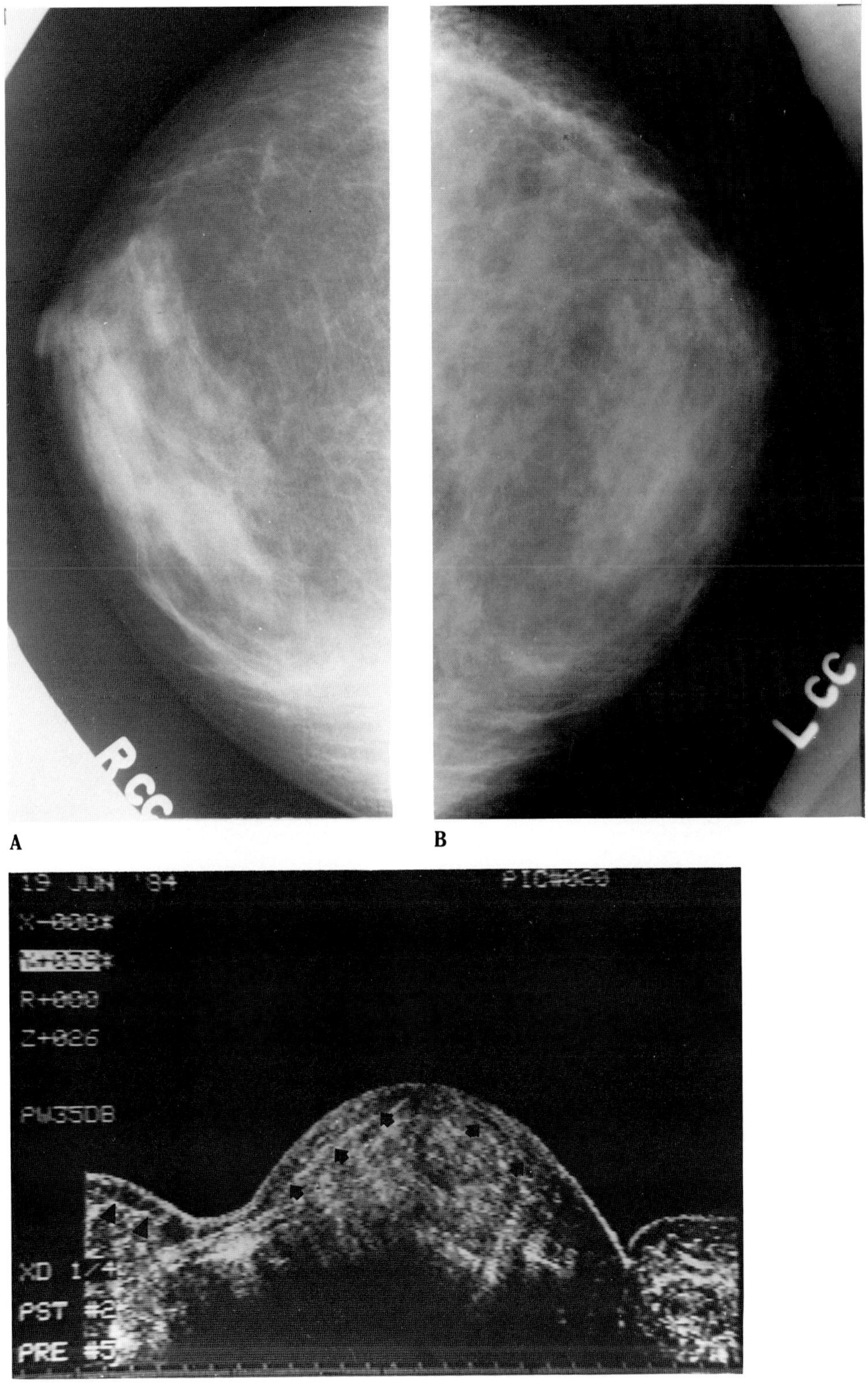

Fig. 24-2 **A:** Mammogram, right CC view, normal side. **B:** Mammogram, left CC view, irradiated breast. Note the diffuse increased markings throughout the left breast and increased subcutaneous markings. (The increased skin thickening is not visible here.) **C:** Ultrasound. Note the marked increase in echoes in the subcutaneous area (arrows) of the left breast. Compare with the medial aspect of the normal right breast with the normal fat–glandular interface and low-level echo area in the fatty layer (arrowheads).

Case 3

R.J. is a 52-year-old woman who was found to have a lump high on the chest wall on the right. Studies done on 4/28/82 revealed a 2 by 3 cm firm mass at 12 o'clock, where the breast met the chest wall. Thermography was markedly positive with a total right global hyperthermia of 5°C compared to the left (Color Fig. 29). Diaphanography was positive, with decreased light transmission. Mammograms showed an irregular 2 cm mass against the chest wall with some small calcifications. Ultrasound did not show the mass.

An infiltrating ductal carcinoma, scirrhous type, with three positive nodes were found on lumpectomy and lymphadenectomy. The patient was both estrogen-receptor and progesterone-receptor positive. She had radiation therapy with 4500 rads to the right breast and a boost of 2000 rads to the area of the tumor with an iridium implant. Chemotherapy was administered for a year.

She was seen at the Woman's Breast Center for follow-up on 5/24/84. On physical

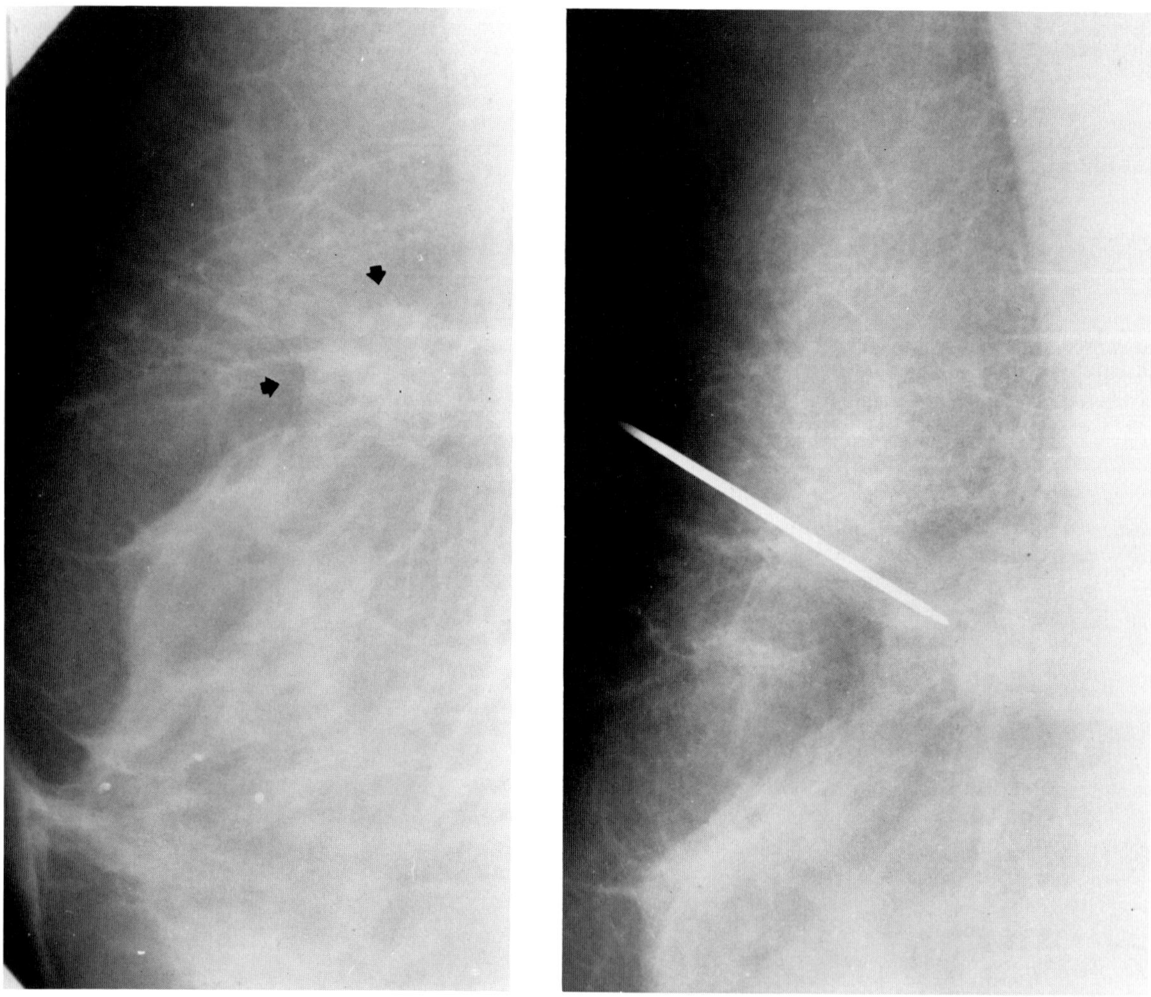

A B

Fig. 24-3 A: Mammogram, magnified, upper right breast. The benign-appearing calcifications were not present preoperatively and are presumed secondary to irradiation. Note the irregular mass of glandular density (arrows). **B:** Mammogram. There is a biopsy needle within the irregular area.

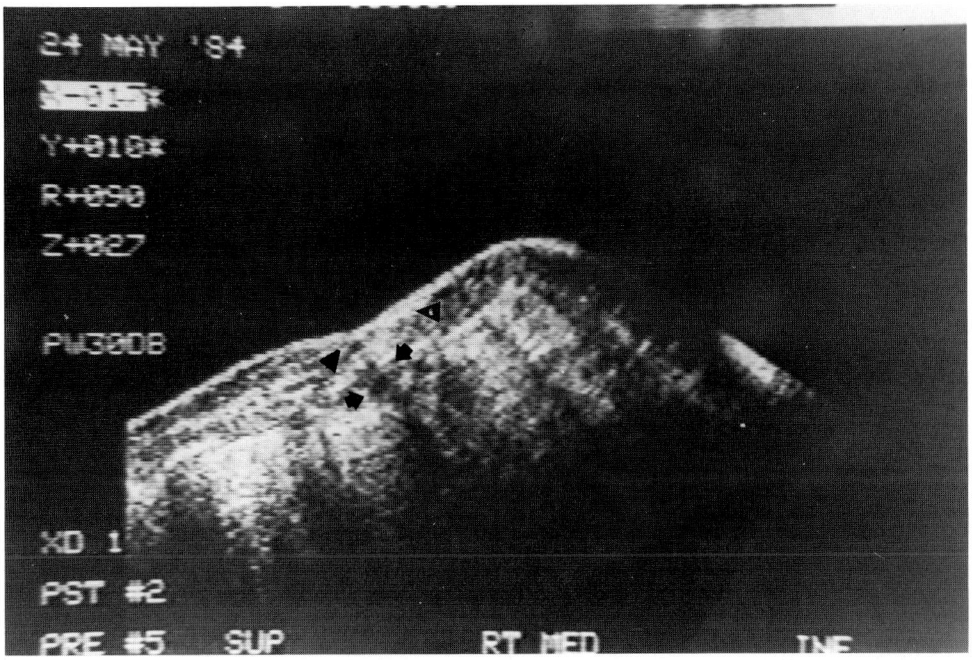

C

Fig. 24-3 C: Ultrasound. Note the slight skin thickening and retraction from postoperative and irradiation changes (arrowheads). An irregular mass of low-level echogenicity (arrows) with posterior shadowing is also noted.

examination there was retraction of the upper aspect of the right breast consistent with the surgery and irradiation. There was a firmness and hardness immediately below this area that the patient related had not been present previously. The remainder of the breast showed slight radiation changes. The left breast was normal.

Liquid crystal thermograms demonstrated increased right nipple heat and increased vascularity over the upper and inner aspect of the breast consistent with a slightly positive thermogram (Color Fig. 30). It was impossible to put the light wand behind the area in question because of the retraction on the right so that diaphanography could not be performed. Mammograms showed moderate glandular tissue (P2 pattern). There was a spiculated area at 12 o'clock on the right with small calcifications (Fig. 24-3A). The calcifications were grosser than those usually seen with malignancy. The spiculization could have been due to the previous surgery or could be new; unfortunately, no postoperative mammograms had been obtained. Ultrasound showed skin thickening and retraction in the upper right breast. There was a mass effect with slightly irregular borders, loss of echogenicity, and marked shadowing (Fig. 24-3C).

There was a high suspicion of recurrent malignancy. An initial needle biopsy did not obtain adequate material, so a repeat needle biopsy was done with a cutting needle under mammographic localization (Fig. 24-3B). The tissue obtained showed fibrinoid material and fat with radiation changes. There has been no change a year later.

Case 4

M.Q. is a 52-year-old woman who was seen on 11/17/83. Six years earlier in September 1977, she underwent lumpectomy and radiation therapy for a ductal carcinoma of the inner aspect of the right breast. She had follow-up for the first 2 years postirradiation and then declined further follow-up. She presented to us with a fixed mass in the inner aspect of the right breast measuring 3 by 6 cm, with retraction of the skin seen below this mass. The right breast was smaller on the medial side than the left breast. There were minor radiation changes noted to the right breast. No lymph nodes were palpated.

Liquid crystal thermograms showed markedly increased heat in the inner aspect of the right breast, as well as increased nipple heat thermogram Th IV (Color Fig. 31). There was an inability on diaphanography to penetrate the inner aspect of the right breast.

Mammograms showed marked skin thickening and lymphatic changes in the inner aspect of the right breast. There was an increased density with multiple calcifications, punctate and amorphous in character (Fig. 24-4A). On comparison with old mammograms, no calcification was seen in December 1977, minimal calcification in 1978, and more marked calcification in 1979, although less than in 1983. Ultrasound demonstrated shadowing in this area without a discrete mass, as well as marked skin thickening (Fig. 24-4B).

The patient has refused biopsy or further follow-up. It is presumed that she has a recurrence of her breast cancer.

Case 5

F.B is a 45-year-old woman who 7 years earlier had a BB-sized nodule at 12 o'clock in the left breast. A mammogram at the time was negative, and her physician told her that she had fibrocystic disease. When seen in December 1983 there was a hard 3 cm mass present in the same location. Although she knew that the mass had grown over the 7 year period, she had refused any work-up, clinging to the belief that the area was fibrocystic disease.

Liquid crystal thermograms showed increased nipple heat and diffuse increased vascularity on the left (Th IV thermogram (Color Fig. 32). There was a marked diminution in light transmission through the mass (Fig. 24-5A). Mammograms showed marked glandularity (DY pattern), with a poorly defined mass of about 2 cm with punctate calcifications. Immediately beneath this area was another group of punctate calcifications without a mass (Fig. 24-5B). Ultrasound demonstrated two masses adjacent to each other with poorly defined borders and shadowing (Fig. 24-5C).

A needle biopsy was inconclusive. A formal biopsy showed infiltrating ductal carcinoma. A lumpectomy and axillary node dissection was performed; all nodes were negative.

On physical examination prior to radiation therapy a fullness was noted in the upper outer left breast, with the sensation of fluid. This area persisted, and the patient was reevaluated after 2000 rads. The thermogram showed a marked heat increase in the left breast consistent with acute radiation changes (Color Fig. 33). Mammograms showed skin thickening and subcutaneous changes consistent with radiation changes; no mass was identified. Ultrasound demonstrated a 3 by 4 by 5 cm semifluid area with internal echoes (Figs. 24-5D, E). A needle aspiration revealed fresh and clotted blood consistent with a hematoma.

The radiation therapy continued, and 5000 rads was administered to the total left breast. At reevaluation the fluid collection was noted to have decreased in size to 3 by 3 by 3 cm (Fig. 24-5F). It was elected to do an external electron boost to the area of the original carcinoma rather than iridium implants so as not to run the remote risk of infection by transecting the area with needles; 1400 rads was administered.

Evaluation 6 months later showed radiation changes to the left breast, less than previously. The fullness in the upper outer area had diminished. The thermogram was again very hot, although less so than during the radiation therapy (Color Fig. 34). There was diminished light transmission. Mammograms showed postirradiation changes without a mass. Ultrasound also showed the changes, as well as a further decrease in the fluid collection to about a 2 cm area.

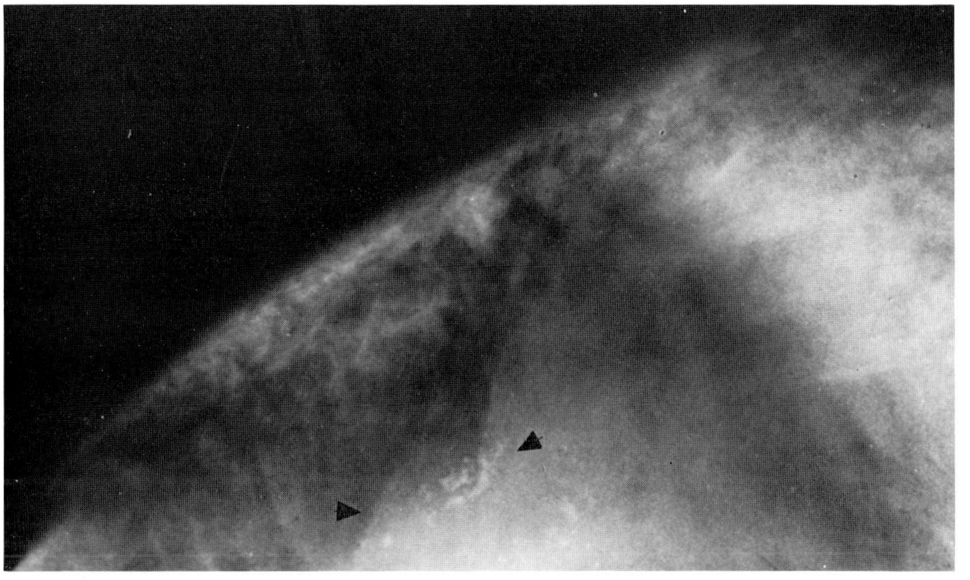

A

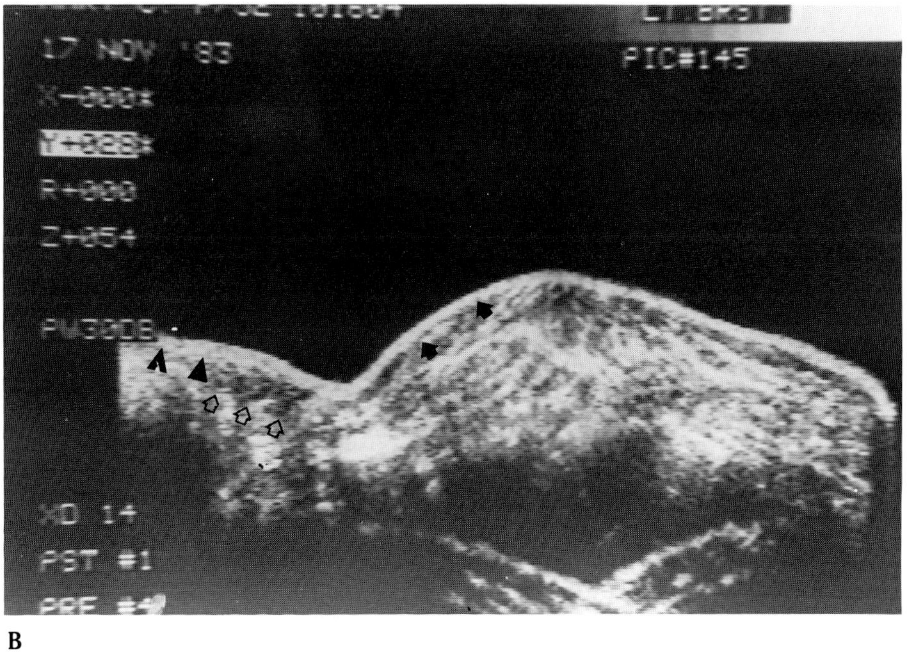

B

Fig. 24-4 **A:** Mammogram, magnified. There is diffuse skin thickening from radiation changes and malignant calcifications from recurrent tumor (arrowhead). **B:** Ultrasound. Compare the normal skin thickness on the left (arrows) with the thickened skin of the irradiated right breast (arrowheads). Note the abnormal irregular low-level echo area in the inner right breast (open arrows).

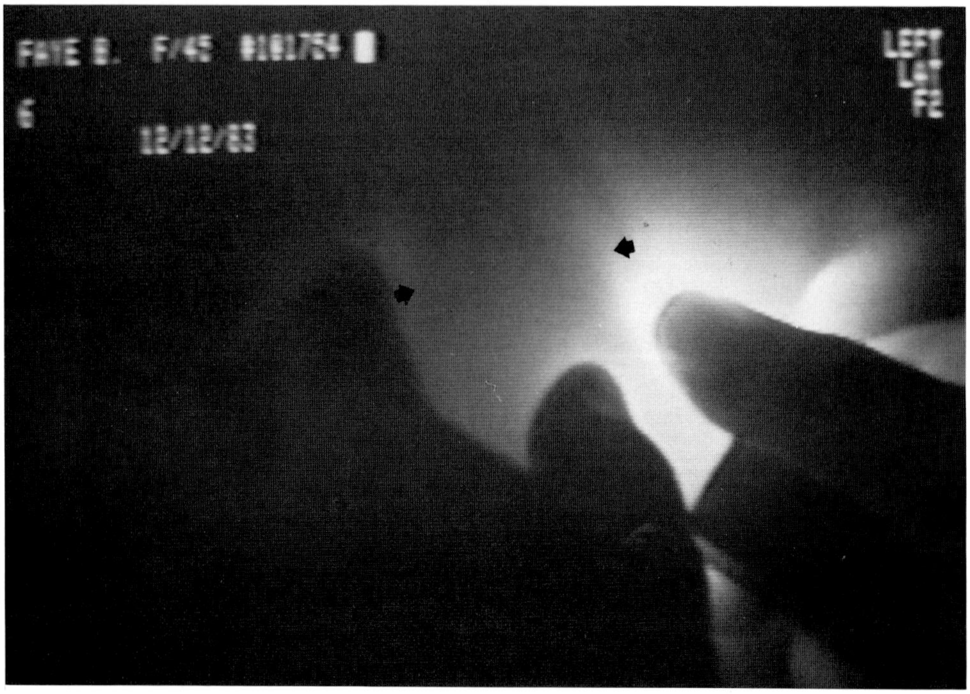

A

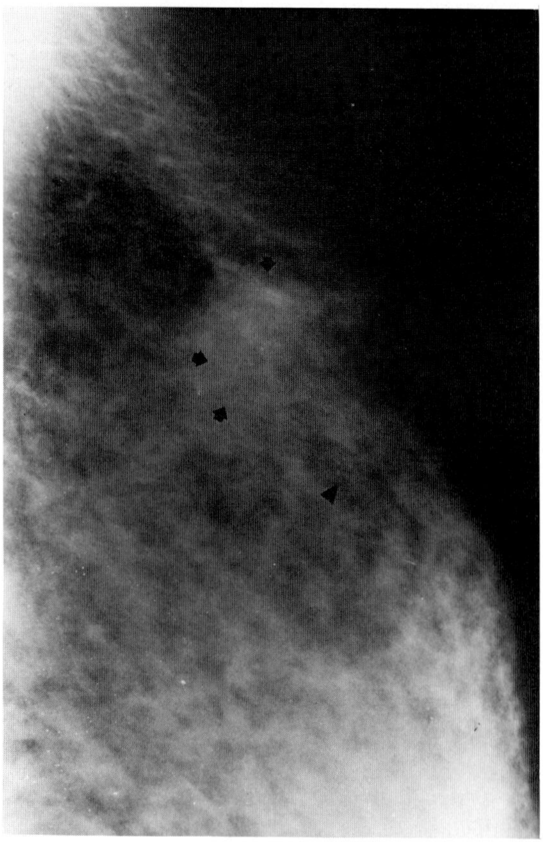

B

Fig. 24-5 **A:** Diaphanography. Note the area of decreased light transmission in the upper left breast (arrow). **B:** Mammogram, magnified, upper left. There are a mass with malignant calcifications (arrows) and an adjacent area of malignant calcifications without a mass (arrowhead).

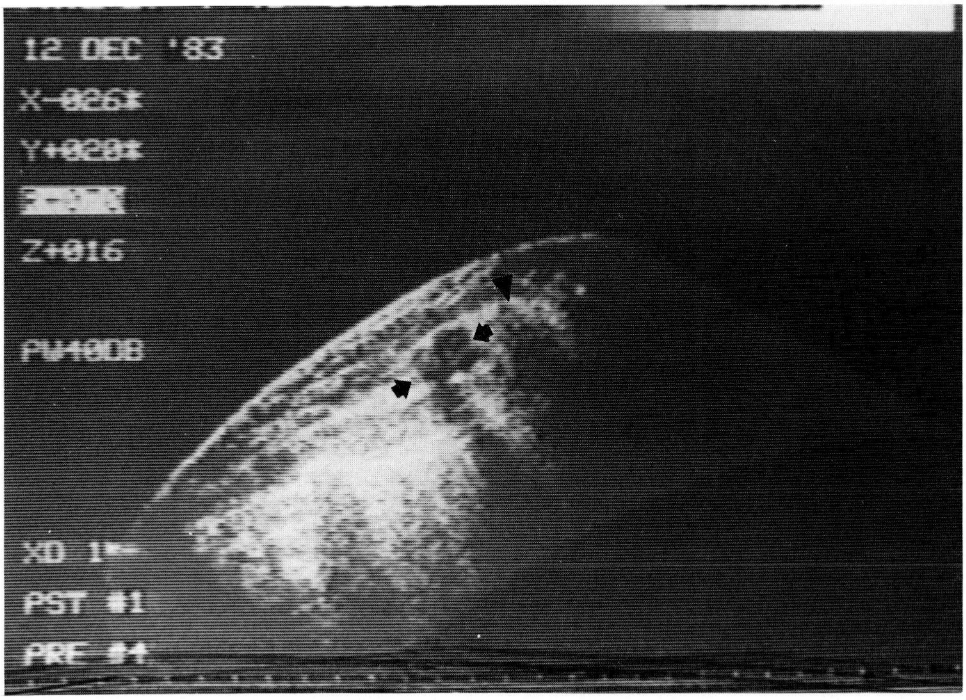

C

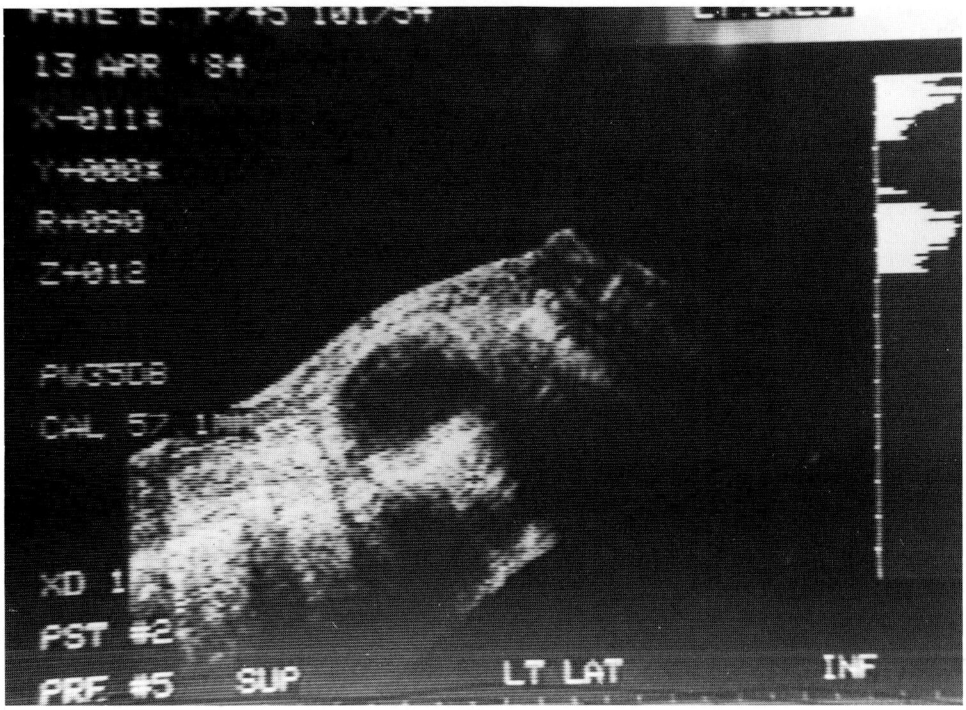

D

Fig. 24-5 **C:** Ultrasound. Note the irregular low-level echo mass (arrows) with posterior shadowing. The adjacent area of shadowing (arrowhead) is consistent with the area of microcalcifications on the mammogram. **D:** Ultrasound, 4/84. Note the large, relatively echo-free area in the upper left breast consistent with a large hematoma and seroma.

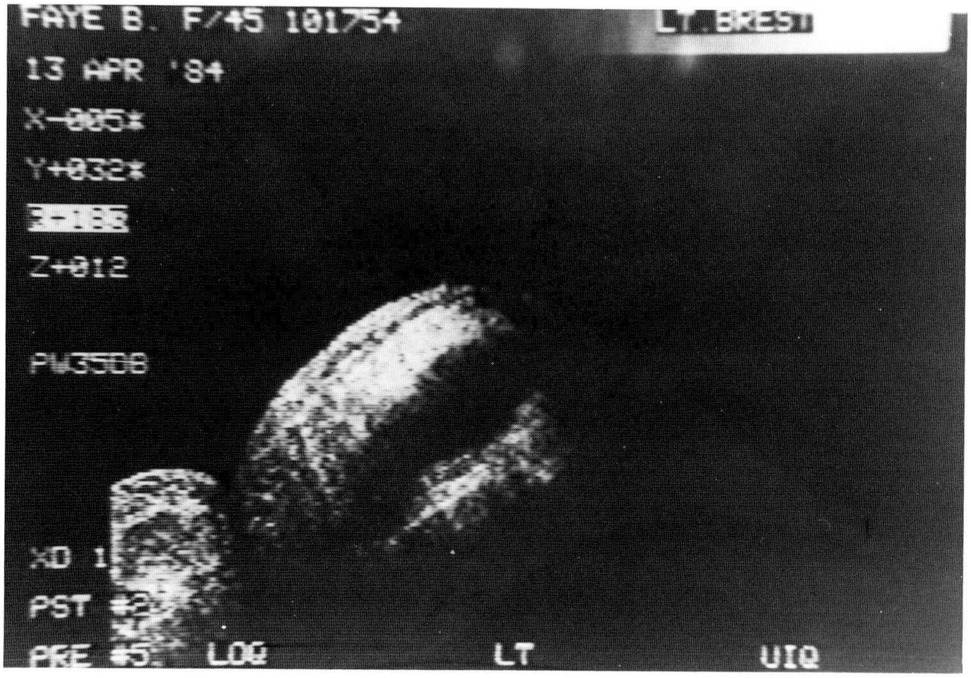

E

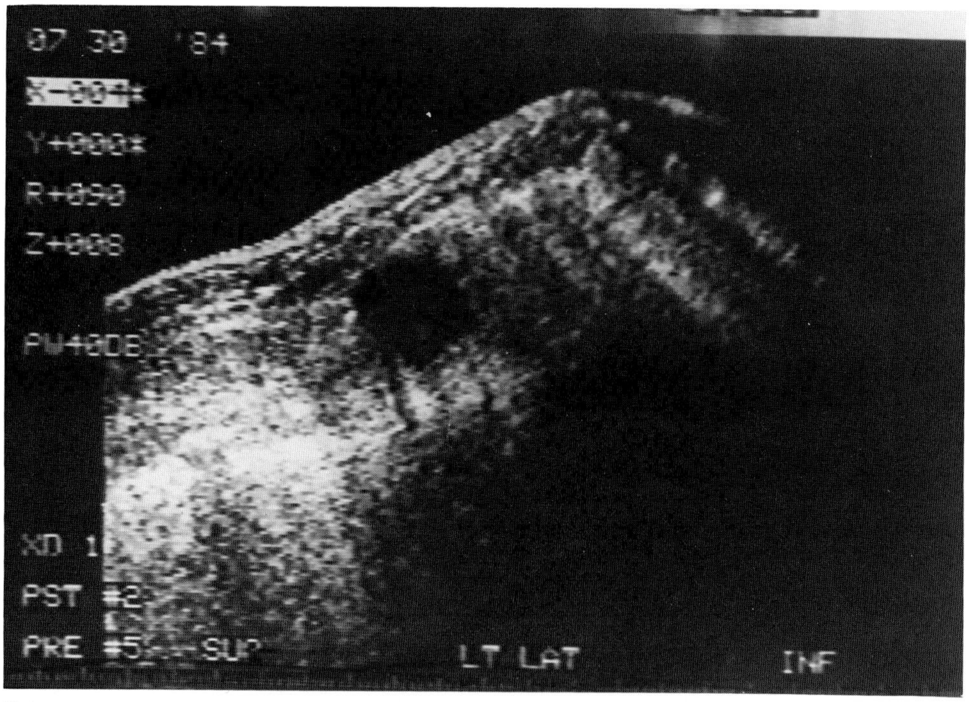

F

Fig. 24-5 E: Ultrasound, 4/84. Note the large, relatively echo-free area in the upper left breast consistent with a large hematoma and seroma. **F:** Ultrasound, 7/84, magnified. Note the decreasing size of the hematoma/seroma.

Case 6

L.P. is a 47-year-old woman who at the age of 5 had had radiation therapy to the left breast because of a breast lump. The amount of radiation is not known as the records are not available, but it is presumed to have been between 200 and 1000 rads, a not uncommon dose during the early 1940s for treatment of nodules and infections. In retrospect, at the age of 5 this lesion may have been either an infection or a very early prepubescent breast nodule.

On physical examination the left breast was about one-half the size of the right, and the nipple on the left was minimally developed. Thermograms demonstrated a slightly asymmetrical pattern with more vascularity on the right, but within normal limits. Diaphanography was normal. Mammograms and ultrasound demonstrated marked glandularity on the right and moderate glandularity on the left without a lesion.

Discussion

The follow-up of patients after lumpectomy and radiation therapy can be very difficult. In a patient with chronic radiation changes, as in case 2, the physical examination may be limited. The chronic changes can obscure small recurrences. In patients who develop radiation changes late, after the first year, it may be very difficult to differentiate these changes, as in case 1, from recurrent carcinoma. Case 3 points out the need for obtaining studies following biopsy and irradiation. Without previous studies it may be impossible to determine if the changes seen on imaging are due to recurrence or the irradiation. A formal biopsy in these patients can be fraught with difficulty, so that adequate needle biopsy is the procedure of choice when possible.

Case 4 points out the need for continued follow-up in these patients and the immense frustration that occurs when a patient refuses to be followed or to undergo life-saving therapy. Even though it is ultimately the patient's choice and life, it is nonetheless difficult to deal with a situation that goes against our medical training.

Case 5 demonstrates the need for close communication between the treating radiation therapist and the breast imager. Case 6 demonstrated one of the late effects of the indiscriminate use of radiation therapy to the breast in young patients. Hypodevelopment of the breast, or even lack of development, can follow radiation therapy in the prepubescent breast.

References

1. Fisher B, Bauer M, Margolse R, et al: Five-year results of a randomized clinical trial comparing total mastectomy and segmental mastectomy with or without radiation in the treatment of breast cancer. *N Engl J Med* 1985;312:665–673.
2. Moss WT, Brand WN, Battifora H: *Radiation Oncology: Rationale, Technique, Results*, ed 5. St. Louis, Mosby, 1979, pp 289–331.
3. Harris JR, Levene MB, Hellman S: Radiotherapy and breast carcinoma, in D'Orsi CJ, Wilson RE (eds): *Carcinoma of the Breast; Diagnosis and Treatment.* Boston, Little, Brown, 1983, pp 215–237.
4. Ohlsson B, Gundersen J, Nilsson DM: Diaphanography: A method for evaluation of the female breast. *World J Surg* 1980;4:701–707.
5. Gautherie M: Temperature and blood flow patterns in breast cancer during natural evolution and following radiotherapy. In Gautherie M, Albert E (eds): *Biomedical Thermology.* New York, Alan R. Liss, 1982, pp 21–64.
6. Bartrum RJ, Crow HC: Transillumination light scanning to diagnose breast cancer. *AJR* 1984;142:409–414.

7. DiMaggio C, Muzzio P, DiBello A, et al: Transillumination of the breast. *Radiol Med (Torino)* 1976;62:401–413.
8. Montgue ED, Ames FC, Schell SR, et al: Conservation surgery and irradiation as an alternative to mastectomy in the treatment of clinically favorable breast cancer. *Cancer* 1974;54:2668–2672.
9. Paulus DD, Libshitz HI: Breast, in Libshitz HJ (ed): *Diagnostic Roentgenology of Radiotherapy Change.* Baltimore, Williams & Wilkins, 1979, pp 55–68.
10. Dicker RH, Jellins J, Kossof G: The ultrasonic appearances of the breast following surgery and radiotherapy, in Jellins J, Kobayashi T (eds): London, Wiley, 1983.
11. Grant EG, Richardson JD, Ciglay OS, et al: Sonography of the breast: Findings following conservative surgery and irradiation for early carcinoma. *Radiology* 1983;147:535–539.
12. Libshitz HI, Southhard ME: Mammography following primary radiation therapy for carcinoma of the breast. *AJR* 1974;120:62–66.
13. Libshitz HI, Montgue ED, Paulus DD: Calcifications and the therapeutically irradiated breast. *AJR* 1972;128:1021–1025.
14. Libshitz HI, Montague ED, Paulus DD: Skin thickness in the therapeutically irradiated breast. *AJR* 1978;130:345–347.
15. Lipsztein R, Dalton JF, Bloomer WD: Sequelae of breast irradiation. *JAMA* 1985;253(24):3582–3584.

Index